Psychiatry:
Past Reflections–Future Visions

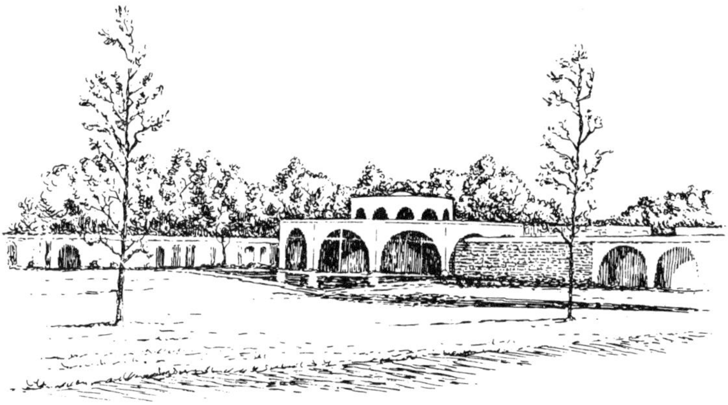

Taylor Manor Hospital

Psychiatry: Past Reflections–Future Visions

Proceedings of the Taylor Manor Hospital Psychiatric Symposium, held March 31-April 2, 1989, in Baltimore, Maryland

Editors

Bruce T. Taylor, M.D., F.A.P.A.
Associate Medical Director
Taylor Manor Hospital
Ellicott City, Maryland

and

Irving J. Taylor, M.D., L.F.A.P.A.
Medical Director
Taylor Manor Hospital
Ellicott City, Maryland

Elsevier
New York • Amsterdam • London

Elsevier Science Publishing Co., Inc.
655 Avenue of the Americas, New York, New York 10010

Sole distributors outside the United States and Canada:
Elsevier Science Publishers B.V.
P.O. Box 211, 1000 AE Amsterdam, The Netherlands

This book was printed on acid-free paper.

ISBN 0-444-01583-3

Current printing (last digit):
10 9 8 7 6 5 4 3 2 1

Manufactured in the United States of America

Contents

Foreword

While the documented treatment of the mentally ill has spanned centuries, the greatest advances in treatment have come in the last fifty years. Psychodynamic understandings have been augmented by biologic and social understandings of many of the illnesses. As we learn more about molecular events and systemic diseases, more disorders of behavior will be reclassified as disorders of biochemistry and the immune system.

This timely book addresses the practical applications of research and past experience to the present needs of our patients and social systems which affect us all. No matter how extensive these advances, holistic, interpersonal understanding and communication cannot be replaced by microscopic knowledge. Modern society faces many economic pressures which tend to drive funding of education, research and treatment. While these factors help to shape mental health policies, several authors address the ways in which concerned citizens and professionals can work together to create a brighter future based upon our past experiences.

Paul Fink, M.D., F.A.P.A., and Herbert Pardes, M.D., F.A.P.A., former Presidents of the American Psychiatry Association, address these issues from their unique perspectives. Research advances which have impacted or have the potential to make a significant impact on our practice and our society are discussed by Drs. Malcolm Lader, Solomon Snyder, Frank Ayd, Heinz Lehmann, Joel Elkes, Frederick Goodwin, Gerald Klerman and Sir Martin Roth, all former recipients of the Taylor Manor Hospital Psychiatric Award. These authors and the others in this volume have played a key role in the education and research which have helped to advance treatment of the emotionally ill. Their evaluation of the past and present provide a formative backdrop to evaluate the future needs and direction for modern psychiatry.

Taylor Manor Hospital has actively participated in developing and enhancing psychiatric treatments through the years. The symposium presented here was the culmination of a celebration of the 50th Anniversary of the Hospital's ownership and direction by the Taylor family. The achievements we have made could not have been possible without the efforts of our dedicated staff of skilled professionals working in concert with the patients and families who needed our assistance. It is ideas such as those presented here which enable us to maintain our development at a rapid pace while remembering that Psychiatry is both an art and a science at a very personal and human level.

Bruce T. Taylor, M.D., F.A.P.A.
Associate Medical Director
Taylor Manor Hospital

Preface

As these words are being written, the rate of change in mental health treatment is still accelerating, as if to keep pace with the unexpected and rapid changes in the governments in Eastern Europe. "Over-managed" case management has had the dramatic impact of Iraq invading Kuwait—with the resultant struggle for power and control—but not in a manner responsible or for the benefit of society.

Wondrous events and discoveries have occurred in the medical, including the psychiatric specialties field, and while these have been welcome, they have seemed to come at the expense of a loss of professional control and autonomy of the individual practitioner or hospital.

Most of these changes have benefitted the patients and their families, but some have caused anxiety and upheaval as well as less than definitive care due to the financial restrictions of the new health systems.

Regardless of everything, good treatment still boils down to the expertise and integrity, as well as the human kindness and empathy of the individual care giver. This book is dedicated to those professionals.

Irving J. Taylor, M.D., L.F.A.P.A.
Medical Director
Taylor Manor Hospital

Acknowledgment

The editors are extremely grateful for the able assistance of our support staff in preparing and proofing the text. We thank Kathleen Sappington, Joanne Byrnes and Virginia Levin for their tireless and competent efforts to help make this book a reality. We thank Rebecca Fleury for her skills in assisting with the computer.

Contributors

Frank J. Ayd, Jr., M.D., L.F.A.P.A., Emeritus Director of Professional Education and Research, Taylor Manor Hospital; Clinical Professor of Psychiatry, West Virginia Medical Center, Charleston.

Jay M. Baraban, M.D., Ph.D., Associate Professor of Neuroscience, Psychiatry and Behavioral Sciences, Johns Hopkins University School of Medicine.

Leon Eisenberg, M.D., F.A.P.A., Professor and Chair, Department of Social Medicine, Harvard Medical School.

Joel Elkes, M.D., L.F.A.P.A., Psychiatrist-in-Chief, Emeritus, Johns Hopkins Hospital: Professor of Psychiatry, Emeritus, University of McMaster, Ontario and Louisville, Kentucky: Director, Division of Attitudinal and Behavioral Medicine, University of Louisville.

Paul J. Fink, M.D., F.A.P.A., Medical Director, Philadelphia Psychiatric Center; Chairman, Department of Psychiatry, Albert Einstein Medical Center; Professor and Deputy Chairman, Department of Psychiatry, Temple University School of Medicine, Philadelphia.

Frederick K. Goodwin, M.D., F.A.P.A., Administrator of the Alcohol, Drug Abuse and Mental Health Administration.

Gerald L. Klerman, M.D., F.A.P.A., Professor of Psychiatry and Associate Chairman for Research, Department of Psychiatry, Cornell University Medical College.

Malcolm H. Lader, M.D., D.P.M., D.Sc.F.R.C. Psych., Professor of Clinical Psychopharmacology, Institute of Psychiatry, University of London.

Heinz E. Lehmann, M.D., L.F.A.P.A., Deputy Commissioner of Research, Office of the Department of Mental Health of New York State.

Paul R. McHugh, M.D., F.A.P.A., Director and Psychiatrist-in-Chief, Johns Hopkins University, Department of Psychiatry and Behavioral Sciences.

Stuart E. Nichols, Jr., M.D., Chief, Medical and Psychiatric Services, Methadone Maintenance Treatment Program.

Herbert Pardes, M.D., F.A.P.A., Vice President for Health Sciences; Dean of the Faculty of Medicine; Professor and Chairman, Department of Psychiatry, College of Physicians and Surgeons, Columbia University.

Domeena C. Renshaw, M.D., F.A.P.A., Professor of Psychiatry and Assistant Department Chairman, Department of Psychiatry, Loyola University of Chicago.

Martin Roth, M.D., Sc.D, F.R.C.P., F.R.C. Psych. (U.K.), Emeritus Professor of Psychiatry, University of Cambridge.

Solomon H. Snyder, M.D., F.A.P.A., Director, Department of Neuroscience, Johns Hopkins University School of Medicine.

Herman M. van Praag, M.D., Ph.D., Professor and Chairman, Department of Psychiatry, Albert Einstein College of Medicine.

Paul F. Worley, M.D., Assistant Professor of Neurology and Neuroscience, Johns Hopkins University School of Medicine.

chapter 1

Current And Future Trends In Psychiatric Education And Practice

Paul J. Fink, M.D., F.A.P.A.

The presidency of the APA provides an ideal platform from which to view the current and future trends in psychiatric education and practice. There are many concerns we face and many issues that seem to be overwhelming. I shall try to cover them in a way that will give a sense of how much we are doing, how much we have left to do, what are some of the positives, and what are some of the negatives.

To begin, practice is clearly driven by economics, and the economic climate in which we live is precarious and vulnerable. Psychiatry is the victim of enormous prejudice and stigma in many areas, including the economic sphere. No other medical specialty, no other series of medical illnesses suffers the amount of control of reimbursement as does psychiatry. We spend an enormous amount of money within the APA and within all the district branches just trying to keep even with the insurance business and trying to understand where we're going with HMOs, PPOs and other managed care systems. The reality of hospital work puts us in an unpleasant and difficult position. For instance, we have to admit as many patients as we can in order to balance the budget, and we have to do it in a way that doesn't shake our own ethical values too much. The longer you keep a patient the more money you make, unless you are dealing with capitated or HMO patients, in which case you not only don't want to admit them, you want to keep them as short a time as possible. In our hospital we do not tell the staff psychiatrists what the insurance of the patient is, and we in the front office then must struggle with the question of the economic balance between those whom we should and those whom we should not keep from the fiscal point of view. By the year 2000 almost all physicians will be employed. The movement is towards greater and greater control of medicine and toward giving doctors some semblance of control over their lives, over their finances, over their fringe benefits. They may find employment more commodious

Psychiatry: Past Reflections–Future Visions
B.T. Taylor and I.J. Taylor, Editors

than private practice. More and more doctors are moving out of solo practice into group practice as one way to solve the problem of total responsibility. As we move towards employment, we end with the question of for whom are we working--the patient or the company? For whom are we working--the patient or the hospital? For whom are we working--the patient or the insurance company, or the patient's employer who pays the insurance company for us to take care of the patient? These are questions that almost never affected physicians before this decade. I recall that I kept my first patient in the hospital for almost six months before anybody ever approached me. Now the average length of stay in most hospitals on the east coast is somewhere around 20-25 days; on the west coast even shorter. The average length of stay is watched with great care, particularly if the hospital gets paid by the case rather than the day. Everything is regulated, everything is reviewed, everybody is trying to get the doctor to do as little as possible to help the patient as much as possible. Pre-admission certification occurs on almost 95% of the patients who enter my hospital, concurrent review is constant, retrospective review is often, and we have a continuous erosion of confidence of the public in medicine and of physicians in themselves.

Psychiatry stands in a fairly good position compared to some of the other medical specialties, but we are still being battered by the prejudice in insurance. There's not an insurance policy sold in America in 1989 that is not prejudiced against the mentally ill. There is either a reduced lifetime benefit, a reduced series of total benefits, reduced number of days, reduced number of visits, reduced payment, a higher co-pay, etc., etc., etc. If someone has schizophrenia at the age of 20, it is anticipated that he will live until 60 and will have 40 years in which he will have a hospitalization every three years--the total bill of a lifetime will be close to $300,000 of which, if he has federal insurance that pays a lifetime of $75,000, he will have to pay $225,000 and if he has an average policy that is in the indemnity insurance which has a lifetime payment of $50,000, he will have to pay $250,000 out of pocket. Contrast that with ischemic heart disease--a man has the first heart attack at age 45, he's anticipated to live 10 years to 55--the total cost of his care over the next 10 years will be $110,000 including certain surgical procedures. Of the $110,000, if he has federal insurance, they will pay $97,000, and if he has indemnity insurance, they'll pay $95,000. Think about that. That makes heart disease so much better than mental illness in terms of its value in the community and the concern that people have for it. Those who say we have no science in our field are rationalizing a system of insurance coverage that is, in my opinion, unconscionable. One of the efforts being made through the courts is to redefine certain illnesses as physical and then get better insurance reimbursement for those illnesses. This grows out of the

National Alliance for the Mentally Ill's approach which is to define those illnesses about which they are concerned as brain diseases, a very dangerous thing for us in psychiatry because it dichotomizes our conditions and our diseases and our concerns in a way that will be very detrimental to the field. Three cases have been successfully tried and won along this line. In Arkansas, a lawyer-father of a manic-depressive daughter sued Blue Cross/Blue Shield of Arkansas and said this is a physical illness based upon the information we have about the genetics and so on. He won the case and they reimbursed him at 80%. We were joyous over it, we broke open champagne- it was a fabulous thing. Two months later, Blue Cross/Blue Shield of Arkansas in their wisdom decided to rewrite their policy so that they named every mental illness by name and said these are mental illnesses and we will only reimburse them at 50%.

The second case was in California in which the father of an autistic child sued and said this is clearly a physical illness--once again dichotomizing mental from physical. He, too, won. And in New York a case of anorexia was also tried and won on the same basis--not because she had a mental illness called anorexia nervosa, but because she had lost 40 pounds, she was malnourished, and she was about to die. The breakup of biopsychosocial into its components cannot help psychiatry in the future, and we're going to have to watch that tendency because our own ambivalence says we would like to get paid for those illnesses. If we have to do it one at a time, then we'll have to do it that way, but in the long run it will not benefit us to have this kind of piecemeal approach to better insurance coverage for the mentally ill as a class.

We continue to have in this country a non-system in the practice of psychiatry. We have a state hospital system, a community mental health system, a private psychiatric hospital system, a general hospital unit system, and private practice of psychiatrists in the community--five systems. Then we have a whole raft of agencies. These do not intersect in a meaningful way. Furthermore, those who have money get treated very differently from those who don't have money. Psychiatry has almost abandoned the public sector. I hope and long for the day when we return psychiatrists to a significant role in the care of the mentally ill poor, but it's very hard to do in a world where doctors who treat the poor are made to feel uncomfortable, where the bureaucracy is so overwhelming that it's much easier to go into private practice or to be in one of the other private systems. The *Psychiatric Times* ran a marvelous article by Randy Clark, M.D. in which he explained his continued loyalty and affiliation to the community mental health system, even though he had been battered and bruised. He is President of the American Association of Community Mental Health Center Psychiatrists and a very, very dedicated and bright man, but each time he tried to assert the authority of psychiatry in the public system he got hurt. Many of our colleagues have written to me over the year about their wish to take care of chronically mentally ill patients and how impossible it is in the fiscal climate in which they have to operate. In community mental health it means somebody else is going to do what doctors have traditionally done. In the insurance business it means let's manage the case to make sure we don't spend too much money. And if you just keep case management out there alone it sounds good, doesn't it? It sounds like a nice term, we're going to do good things. The only problem is that in both definitions it has nothing to do with people. We're also in a competitive marketplace under the gun from the Federal Trade Commission, making sure that we don't collude to take better care of people or making sure that the psychiatrists are seen as the enemy. In jurisdiction after jurisdiction in this country, I find as I travel that one of the biggest complaints has to do with the fact that you can't get a patient into a hospital. Often you even have to go to a court where the job of the public defender is to defend the patient against the psychiatrist. The psychiatrist becomes the enemy and in the adversary system you have to prove in front of the patient that the patient is crazy. My question to you is, which is crazy--the patient or the system? This is a bizarre way to handle what in every other situation ought to be a medical decision, a medical system.

We also are struggling in psychiatry with a tremendous problem about which professions do what for whom. I'm talking about organizational efforts to seek hospital privileges and prescription writing privileges by non-physicians, an area fraught with problems that we are going to be struggling with for the next few years. We've already spent an enormous amount of money in California on Capp v. Rank, a case in which the Psychology Association is attempting to get state authorization for full hospital privileges. We struggle with the political efforts of Pat DeLeon, the aide to Senator Inouye, to get prescribing privileges for psychologists in order to give them a greater breadth in their ability to care for and treat their patients. It is a complex and difficult problem. The battle over psychotherapy, however, is over. It is clear that all well-trained mental health professionals can do various forms of psychotherapy and do them well. There is no effort on the part of psychiatry to encroach upon psychological testing. But as neuroscience demonstrates the importance of organic treatments, the hospital becomes more and more a battleground. We need to define carefully what a psychiatrist is and then build the work of the psychiatrist, the professional psychiatrist, around that definition.

Another area of concern is education. Traditionally we've given a lot of our time to educating the next generation of psychiatrists; traditionally we've been proud to participate in programs for medical students and residents. There are an increasing number of young students going into psychiatry. It's seen as an important bastion for a different kind of process, while internal medicine last year had the fewest students ever because of the many kinds of stress in that field. I am not surprised that students are moving towards psychiatry because in psychiatry we have a built-in process of helping people grow. This is less evident in other medical specialties. There is something unique in psychiatry called individual supervision where students have an opportunity to sit down with a mentor and let feelings pour out. Individual supervision is a serendipitous miracle because it really creates an opportunity for people to grow in a way that, in fact, makes psychiatrists different from other physicians. We are different, and there's something very good about that difference. Can you imagine a young resident in internal medicine walking along making rounds and saying to his chief and the other five or ten people present, "It's absolutely going to tear me apart if this patient dies."? The most likely response in the medical education system is ridicule and humiliation. It is the reality, the tradition, but it's terrible. It is only in psychiatry that we've invented a method for getting people to look at themselves in the context of the therapeutic process. It is what makes psychiatry special and I don't want to lose that. Leon Eisenberg has said "Let's not trade the brainless psychiatry of yesterday for a mindless psychiatry of tomorrow." He is right. The mental part of our work is as valid and as important as the biological part of our work. We can't have a bizarre and arcane dichotomization in training, just as we can't have it in the categorization of illness as physical or mental.

Now the negative side of our training activity, unfortunately, is the fact that not all of our products, not all of our residents, not all of our training programs are good. We have determined that we will train people and we will test them by the Boards for minimal competency. We do not test, as they do in Britain, as they do in Australia, as they do in Canada--we do not test for *excellence*. I had the good fortune of going to Australia for several weeks and I learned a lot about the British and the derived-from-British systems. Let me tell you what a person has to do in order to become a full-fledged, certified psychiatrist in Australia. First of all, there is a five-year residency. In the fourth year, to qualify for the examination the candidate must submit five case histories: an acute psychiatric case, a patient with chronic psychiatric illness, a child case, a psychotherapy case (a minimum of 50 hours), and an organic case. This should give a sense of the biopsychosocial approach that they are taking; the five cases demonstrate breadth. Each case must be no less than 2,000 words, no more than 8,000 words, with the rules very well spelled out. Before you can even sit for the examination you have to demonstrate that you've done a little psychiatry, that you understand at least five segments of psychiatric interest, technique, and skill. Then you are allowed to sit for the examination--after three full years of training in a five-year program. Part 1 is written--it's all essay. The first day is three hours--four 45-minute questions. And the second day is three hours--ten 18-minute questions. In America, we are trained to take multiple-choice examinations. In Australia, if you pass this written part of the examination, you can take the orals. They are given in the fourth of five years. The first day you are assigned two patients. There's a one hour interview which you do alone; nobody watches you. Then there's a quarter of an hour so you can think. Then there's a half hour quiz with two examiners and an observer. On the second day you get one medical patient with an hour to see the patient, a half hour written quiz, and then a half hour oral quiz with two or three vignettes asking what would you do IF. Lastly, in the fifth year, you write a thesis or you write up five more cases that are joined together in a thematic way. Contrast that with the two skimpy hours of testing that we do in the American Board of Psychiatry and Neurology. I've been on the Residency Review Committee for six years. There are some fabulous programs like those in Baltimore. There are some terrible training programs where the people are needed to do clinical work and the training is an afterthought.

Another problem we face is that of undue familiarity, a euphemism for having sex with patients. It is a very, very difficult problem because of the trivialization of the concept of transference and countertransference. If one understands the danger that results from mishaps of transference and countertransference, one has a better chance of avoiding the ethical difficulties than if one is told in a way that essentially avoids any understanding of the mental functioning that goes on. There are about ten programs in this country that offer no training in psychotherapy. Outpatient work is considered tinkering with drugs. The education depends entirely upon a paradigm that makes sense, and it must be a broad, biopsychosocial paradigm. I have asked residents in my program to present cases to me as biopsychosocial ones. There is no case that doesn't have some kind of biological part because more and more we find that most of the psychoses and neuroses respond in some positive way to pharmacological intervention. I ask residents to talk about the psychodynamic nature of the case, to know what happened in the childhood, the early life experiences, the history, the intimate and intricate details that are necessary in order to be "psychiatric", and then I say to them--also tell me about the psychosocial context in which you find the patient. Not one of these paradigms alone really works thoroughly. As psychiatrists, we have to define ourselves as people who are knowledgeable of and capable of dealing with all three dimensions. When I went through residency, we weren't allowed to see the family--it contaminated the psychotherapy. Today family therapy is important. The science of psychotherapy really hasn't been tapped. I have called on the American Psychiatric Association, the National Institutes of Mental Health, and the American Psychoanalytic Association to develop national multi-centered studies on the efficacy of various forms of psychotherapy. If that isn't done in the next five to ten years we will lose the opportunity to have psychotherapy move from a skill to a science and thereby to a more legitimate part of the work of psychiatry. Efficacy studies that go beyond counting numbers are very important, and they're very difficult. It's much easier to do efficacy studies around pharmacology than it is to do efficacy studies around psychotherapy. Why don't we read our journals and do what they tell us? Why are the journals separate from the practice? Why are there so many journals--ever think of that? There are 75 journals published either monthly or quarterly in psychiatry, psychology, and social work, and we only read the journals that apply to us. We have a series of written documents which seem to have nothing to do with the reality of our practice and I think that's a major stumbling block, one of the psychosocial characteristics of the profession. I think that if you lock three psychiatrists in a room, when you let them out you'll have a new organization and a new journal.

This is partly a joke and partly not. One of the things I've tried to initiate is having the APA serve as an umbrella organization for the multiple other psychiatric organizations that exist in the United States. There are between 40 and 80 other psychiatric organizations, an enormous number. These include the American Academy of Child and Adolescent Psychiatry, the American Society for Adolescent Psychiatry, Biological Psychiatry, Geriatric Psychiatry, Drug Abuse Psychiatry, Alcohol Abuse Psychiatry--I could go on and on. Each of them has a valuable purpose, but I am concerned that in the move toward specialization, the fragmentation of our field will hurt us. We have a very strong Association. Eighty-five percent of all the psychiatrists in America and ninety-nine percent of all the residents in America belong to the APA. We are a very powerful lobbying group, even though our successes are only moderate. Congress is not that easy. We are powerful in our public affairs. We're working hard in economic affairs and we're paying a lot of attention to educational activities. I am hopeful that we will be able to reorganize over the next decade to serve as an umbrella to these 40 to 80 organizations to provide together in a single voice greater effectiveness in lobbying, in public affairs, in economic affairs, in government affairs, and in other activities, without spending enormous amounts of money over and over again through the separate organizations.

Finally, my major concern has to do with destigmatization--overcoming stigma. This is a two-edged sword. There are 40 million Americans who are afflicted with some kind of mental illness or substance abuse problem. Three million schizophrenics, 8 million depressives/manic-depressives, about 10 million alcoholics, 5 to 10 million drug abusers, 8 million panic and other anxiety disorders, and an infinite number of other types. As we destigmatize more people are going to want help, which puts us in an extraordinarily problematic position--in an era of cost cutting to work towards destigmatizing the field with the knowledge that somebody's going to come along and say we're going to have to cut the money--there's one pool of money and we're just going to have less per case. This is not a nation that is interested in taking care of those less fortunate. We are the only major democratic country in the world that does not have a national system of health insurance to take care of everybody. Thirty million Americans are without any kind of health insurance. Three million Americans are living on the street. That 3 million may grow to 6 million if the new law involving nursing homes is kept in effect; that is, the mentally ill cannot be kept in nursing homes unless there is a demonstrated treatment for them. And nursing home owners who are underpaid already are not going to provide a lot of care for the mentally ill; they're just going to exclude them. The end result is that we will have more people out on the street. Destigmatization, however, is beginning to take hold. We have had more good, positive programs about mentally ill patients this year than I can remember. "Peace of Mind," which featured Lionel Aldrich, a former football player, was a classic in which he told about living on the streets for ten years, hearing voices and hallucinating. "Strange Voices," produced by NBC, was a wonderful piece, sympathetic to the mentally ill. But for every one of those there are hundreds of occasions in which the papers blare out, "Ex-mental patient shoots so and so." I am waiting for the day when it says "Ex-orthopedic patient shoots so and so." It would be a lovely experience for me, but I am afraid it will never happen. We are stuck with the belief and mythology that seems absolutely inextricable from the mental functioning of America that all mentally ill patients are violent. In truth, only three percent of mentally ill patients are violent, yet on television, seventy-seven percent of mentally ill patients are depicted as violent. Ask why that is done and the answer is "it's good theater." Well, psychotics are good theater; violent psychotics are better theater. Writers have to have an excuse or a rationale for behavior on television, and if they have to write an entire scenario for a half hour with 23 minutes of air time or an hour show with 46 minutes, they had better use a lot of stereotypes. We have a lot of stereotypes in psychiatry--not only the patients, but also the psychiatrists. Sympathetic psychiatrists are few compared to non-sympathetic psychiatrists; psychiatrists who are bizarre, cruel or humorous are common. Glen Gabbard has written a wonderful book on psychiatrists in cinema--I recommend it to you--because he points out in a beautiful way 10 or 12 different scenarios of how psychiatrists and mentally ill patients are treated in the media. The media are much more powerful than organized psychiatry will ever be. Yet, progress is being made on the issue of destigmatization. We are seeing changes--partly because of the activities of the grassroots groups, the National Alliance for the Mentally Ill (NAMI), National Depression and Manic-Depression Association (NDMDA), National Mental Health Association, American Mental Health Fund, National Association for Research in Schizophrenia and Depression (NARSAD), and a variety of other groups throughout this country. There are now a half-million dues paying members in advocacy groups for the mentally ill. For the first time we have companions in the fight for destigmatization. By the year 2000, professional psychiatry and the care of the mentally ill patient will be moved much further along.

The role of psychiatry in the rest of medicine is the next frontier that we have to think about, one on which I am working. After my wife died I set up a program at Einstein called CAST--the Cancer Support Team. The leader of it is the head of consultation liaison psychiatry in my department. CAST has a staff of five social workers, and one sees every cancer patient who comes into the hospital. Last month they saw 180 different patients. That's triple the number of patients seen through the usual consult program. Every cancer patient gets a chance to work with somebody on his or her grief, pain, distress, and/or anxiety. In fact, we have an opportunity to look at cancer and to be involved in cancer from two directions, the cancer support team and neuropsychoimmunology. The role that stress plays in reorganizing our bodies and making us more vulnerable to viral conditions, to cancer conditions, to other conditions is currently being studied extensively. We are going to see that open up and blossom in the next ten years. We are going to play a signficant role in medicine, a role that we should play because of our knowledge and our willingness to move away from Descartes and to say that there is a mind and a body and a brain. The biopsychosocial paradigm is alive and well in American psychiatry.

chapter 2

Implications Of Research For Clinical Psychiatry

Herbert Pardes, M.D., F.A.P.A.

We are in a remarkable renaissance in psychiatric research. In science generally there are areas of extraordinary excitement today, including work in immunology, molecular genetics, and neurobiology. Some of these general basic sciences impinge upon the revolution in psychiatric research, but the revolution really is manifest through much of the breadth of psychiatric research. It is likely that clinical psychiatry will be profoundly affected in the next few decades by what is happening now in the scientific components of psychiatry.

I would like to offer a general survey of that excitement and the specific issues to which it is attached. I would also like to describe some of the broad themes which characterize psychiatric research and some of the exciting foci in problem areas of major concern in psychiatry. I should stress this is just a sampling of the many promising projects being done. Finally, I would like to talk about the professional, societal and governmental responses and reactions to this excitement.

That we are in a time of extraordinary excitement is an observation made by people out of psychiatry as well as in the field. Dr. Lewis Thomas stated in a review of the Lasker Awards that "The 1976-86 decade is already providing its own evidence that neurobiology is well under way as the most exciting of all fields in biological science." He went on to state that in the decades ahead we will see all of our early notions about the brain and about the mind that it operates or that operates it revolutionized.

Dr. Thomas's assessment is supported by the fact that in the last 8 or 9 years, in other words the eighties, there have been a number of Nobel Prizes, Lasker Awards and other major awards celebrating the advances in these sciences. It is interesting to look at the diverse nature of scientific investigation that has been commended. These

Psychiatry: Past Reflections–Future Visions
B.T. Taylor and I.J. Taylor, Editors

include elegant work by Hubel and Wiesel showing the developmental impact of sensory deprivation on the growing structure of the brain. It includes awards for new technology areas for the development of PET scanners and magnetic resonance imaging (MRI). It includes work on the elegant relationship between biology and behavior so nicely investigated by Dr. Eric Kandel. It includes genetic discoveries by people such as Drs. Baron and Egeland in manic depressive disease, work on biochemical and pharmacological systems such as the dopamine system in schizophrenia, and work on treatments such as that of Mogen Schou's work with lithium (Patty Duke). The fertile areas are extended further by some of the advances in epidemiology, which include more rigorous methodological approaches to the study of the psychotherapies as well as the pharmacotherapies resulting in documented proof of the effectiveness of psychotherapy in, for example, certain affective disorders.

BASIC THEMES

Individual findings are exciting but it is also important to see the overall fabric as psychiatry progresses.

One can see in the pattern of psychiatric research certain broad themes. For example:

1. There is a clear increase in basic data. This is true with regard to epidemiology's laying out the incidence and prevalence of psychiatric disorders, 15% of the United States population has a DSM-III diagnosable condition over a 1-month period; 19% in 6 months. Work in molecular genetics has also shown that there are 3-4,000 genes responsible for single gene diseases and that some 25% of the genes in the human genome have some impact on the brain and nervous system function. The data has shown an increasing number of transmitters, some fifty now (rather than the three known years ago) which play some role in brain function and have some potential impact on neurological and psychiatric disease. We have learned that there are 10^{11} nerve cells in the brain with an average of 10,000 connections per nerve cell which accounts for the enormously complicated system referred to as the mind and brain. These facts have helped us recognize what a marvelous system the human brain is and to account for the richness and the impressive capacity of the human mind. There is also an increasing recognition of what treatments may be helpful for what disorders in what amount. For example, it is now clear that some 60-70% of people with manic depressive disease respond to lithium.

There are estimates, too, that a third of the patients unresponsive to lithium respond to carbamazepine. In summary one sees increasing data, increasing quantification of illness, of the structures related to illness, and of data pertinent to treatment.

2. A further trend is that of disaggregation. Perhaps this is demonstrated most profoundly in the work that shows that one gene appears to be responsible for manic depressive disease, while some families with manic depressive disease show no gene to be operative. That means that there are at least two different types of manic depressive disease. But this is not too surprising. It is a follow-up to pre-existing trends. These include the differentiation of panic disorder from social phobia, from other anxiety disorders, and the distinction of atypical depressions from bipolar disease from unipolar disease. SAD is another example. Now more recently we find schizophrenia may include one subtype caused by a factor on chromosome 5, but this accounts for only a small component of the schizophrenias. So again research may introduce another focal point for disaggregation. We can see the same thing happening in Alzheimer's disease which may really be multiple disorders.

   A reasonable conclusion is that most major psychiatric disease diagnostic categories, which have heretofore been characterized as one disease, may really be groups of multiple disorders leading to a common outcome like mental retardation.

   This trend is not unique to psychiatric disease. Even in AIDS, there is the possibility of different forms of the disease being tied to different versions of the virus and to different target cells the viruses choose to invade. This disaggregation is important also because it offers some explanation of why some earlier research has left us with such confusing results. If one researches oranges and apples, the likelihood is one gets mixed results.

3. A third theme is the increasing access to key systems pertinent to the brain and to the psychiatric disorders. In many ways this is a function of the capacity from new technology. As Maya Pines has nicely articulated, the brain was shielded from investigation by the skull which protected it

and by the blood-brain barrier which discriminated what substances could flow in and out. We were restricted in looking at brain structure and function to skull x-rays and encephalograms and electroencephalograms until the modern era of brain imaging arrived. CAT scans and regional cerebral blood flow (rCBF) and SPECTS and MRIs and PETS have dramatically increased our access to systems of key interest. So does genetics.

4. A fourth trend is that of specificity. We have been looking at peripheral manifestations of diseases for so long; these methods of greater access bring us closer to basic causes and mechanisms of disease. For example, genetic causes and genetic factors offer us an insight into the very motor of the machine whereas earlier we were only able to access the manifestations of impairment by looking at the outside. Genes are able to turn off and turn on behaviors, functions, structures much as a fuse if turned can make lights go on or off. This kind of specificity has been relatively unknown in psychiatry. Thus, the marriage of molecular genetics and psychiatric disorders brings a degree of precision unknown to a field in which the human impact is vast. Often genetics has focused its attention on relatively infrequent disorders with far less impact on the human condition. But we have witnessed localization of genes in Alzheimer's, manic depressive disease, neurofibromatosis, and possibly panic disorder and schizophrenia.

   Further, technology allowing us to identify minute concentrations of transmitters in the brain and imaging technologies for visualizing receptors and receptor function promise further understanding of the brain and its relationship to behavior by virtue of access to these key physiological systems.

   The increased specificity is not restricted to genetic and imaging approaches. The progress in our diagnostic system has been largely responsible for the disaggregation and the insistence on observable criteria for disaggregating diseases. While it may have many shortcomings, the various versions of the diagnostic and statistical manual (DSM-III) have led to more and more agreement among scientists as to what phenomena they are studying. While we have to be careful about premature closure on diagnostic groupings, the advantages of enhanced reliability and better communication are monumental in terms of research as well as in clinical psychiatry, clinical advances, and their communicability to other people. Epidemiology using specific signs and symptoms which pertain to specific disorders has followed the diagnostic advances. This in turn has laid the groundwork for the American Psychiatric Association's effort to match treatment with specific illnesses. MAO inhibitors which had been discarded before as unhelpful in affective disorders seem to help in atypical depression. While carbamazepine helps some manic-depressives, it has recently been shown to be ineffective in panic disorder. Findings of negative therapeutic impact are as important in the process of refinement as are positive findings.

5. Another theme is our increasing awareness of the interactions of systems. It is remarkable that we are seeing laid out the linkage between biological and behavioral systems. The injection of a substance can create an anxiety episode. Kandel has led the way in showing how behavioral alterations can have an impact on brain function. Work on environmental enrichment suggests its effect on the vitality of brain structure. What these various advances tell us is that it is conceivable that when dealing with behavioral dysfunction, attention to the underlying biological systems may afford some therapeutic opportunity. Thus, the possibility exists that an understanding of the underlying physiological systems pertaining to learning and memory may offer potential answers for those suffering from Alzheimer's, other dementias and learning disabilities. The recognition of the impact of multiple transmitter and receptor systems on functions as diverse as eating, anxiety, pain regulation, etc., suggest that a better understanding of those systems will allow us to modify disturbances in the behavioral areas that involve those systems. Also the recognition of the plasticity of the nervous system encourages the thought that a dysfunctional brain may be susceptible of repair.

In another area of active current scientific investigation the interaction between behavior and immunology becomes important. In the *Archives of General Psychiatry*, January 1989, Keller, Bond, Schleifer, Cohen, and Stein reported an association between severity of depression, hospitalization, and immune system changes (absence of usual increased mitogen response and increased T4 lymphocytes). Also, depressed patients did not show the usual increases seen in controls with age. Some scientists, recognizing that psychiatric disturbances may compromise immune function, are examining the extent to which attention to psychiatric disease in a patient with AIDS who has both AIDS and a psychiatric disease might fortify the immune system and make the disease course less fulminating. Given the enormous variation in AIDS viruses and the differences in cells they attack, a behavioral handle might conceivably offer some therapeutic help, given the assumption that the clinical course of AIDS is not an all or none phenomenon.

6. Attacking areas of deficient capacity is also of interest. The increased amount of data and the increased specificity allows scientists to research those areas in which our therapies are most effective. We are increasingly able to quantify. This is shown, for example, in the recognition of the 30-40% of patients with manic depressive disorder unresponsive to lithium. Scientists' attention was drawn to treatments which may help the residual group, leading to the use of carbamazepine, which helps many unresponsive to lithium. Clozapine, too, has now been found to be helpful in patients who are unresponsive to typical neuroleptics. In like fashion, scientists have sought help for victims of substance abuse and found that certain antidepressant treatments may be helpful for a component of those patients. This does not mean that we should be disappointed at the fact that the treatments can't be effective in all patients with those disorders, but rather we should feel satisfaction from the fact that these treatments delineate at least one subgroup for which we can give help. For example, antidepressant drugs seem to be helpful in some patients suffering from cocaine abuse. Further, in schizophrenia, while the treatment generally is of modest effect, there is an increasing focus on the most untreatable problem; i.e., negative symptoms.

This focus on areas of deficiency includes the problem of high suicidal risk. Brent and colleagues have recently published a paper attempting to distinguish completed suicides from people who are at very high risk for suicide. He recommends specific criteria which may facilitate identifying the group which is in most danger.

The main point, however, is that by uncovering knowledge pertinent to areas where our treatment effectiveness is modest we constantly increase the field's ability to help.

These diverse research thrusts sum to an extraordinarily exciting and challenging intellectual era in psychiatric research. Data are being put on the table, new concepts are being tested, technologies are being applied, and marriages are being made between basic scientists and clinical scientists in a variety of ways.

MAJOR PSYCHIATRIC PROBLEMS

Having reviewed the broad themes, it is interesting to look at specific lines of attack on major psychiatric disorders. In schizophrenia, there has been a demonstration of altered numbers of dopamine receptors which has been disputed, but which is being actively investigated. In investigating this finding, another scientist has found a possible coupling between DA_1 and DA_2 receptors, and further that this coupling may be uniquely weak in S.R. Also, just reported is a follow-up on an earlier finding of a chromosome 5 location for a gene for schizophrenia. This had initially been introduced by Dr. Anne Bassett of Columbia University from a study of a small family in which two members had both a chromosomal aberration and also schizophrenia. Apparently Dr. Hugh Gurling in London has now followed up with large pedigrees and suggests that he has a linkage for chromosome 5. This has not been found in some other families to this point, and so it likely suggests, as with affective disorders, that schizophrenia is heterogeneous and that some schizophrenics will have chromosomal 5 abnormalities and some will not.

There are other approaches of interest in research on schizophrenia. A recent paper by Phil Holzman suggests that eye tracking dysfunction may be closely linked to schizophrenia. Holzman suggests that such dysfunction may be an expression of some autosomal dominant gene which manifests in eye tracking dysfunction or in schizophrenia or in both. There is other work on candidate genes for schizophrenia as well as on dopamine nerve cells placed in cell cultures and then studied for their response to various substances being injected into the media.

Scientists continue to look for alterations of ventricular size and brain content in schizophrenia. Recently an NIMH group, using MRI, reported replication of the increase in size in both the lateral and third ventricles in schizophrenia. They noted the difficulty finding the lesion responsible for this "ventriculomegaly." Still the fact that there are a number of studies showing some increase in ventricular volume suggests scientists are onto something which, with higher resolution MRI scanners and better image analysis systems, may become more specific.

Certainly, there has been a considerable amount of work showing that some of the abnormalities on CT scans (particularly lateral ventricular enlargement) are related to measures of function and clinical course such as cognitive impairment, diminished neuroleptic response, poor outcome, and a preponderance of negative symptoms over positive symptoms.

These research developments in schizophrenia also point up the richness of the lines of work necessary to understand psychiatric disease. Weinberger in an outstanding review in the *Archives of General Psychiatry* specifies the 3 inescapable clinical facts about schizophrenia:

1. The high probability of schizophrenia becoming clinically apparent in late adolescence or early adulthood.

2. The role of stress in onset and relapse.

3. The therapeutic efficacy of neuroleptic drugs.

He notes the likelihood that there is some fixed lesion in early life which then has to interact with maturational events that occur later in order that the disease be precipitated. He is stressing that there is some likely biological phenomenon early in life, but (1) the likelihood of stress that may be understood in behavioral or biological terms and (2) development and (3) maturation are also, in Weinberger's view, central to our best hypothesis about the pathogenesis of schizophrenia today.

Still there are studies of identical twins discordant for schizophrenia possibly showing brain changes in the schizophrenic patient and other early suggestions of differences between schizophrenic and non-schizophrenic brains on autopsy. There is also an early finding of possible abnormalities in schizophrenics in the relationship of D_1 and D_2 receptors.

ALZHEIMER'S DISEASE

Alzheimer's, which afflicts an estimated 1-2 million people and accounts for 50% of dementias over 65, is another major focus of research in psychiatry.

In Alzheimer's, excitement is related to the localization of a gene on chromosome 21 as responsible for Alzheimer's disease. Mohs, et al., had earlier suggested a common dominant autosomal gene. The notion of disaggregation holds here as well since while a sizable proportion of Alzheimer's patients are suffering from a genetic disorder others are not. In fact, there has been recent work from Yale University suggesting that a slow virus may be responsible for some Alzheimer's cases. What has become apparent is that the notion of one transmitter being defective and explaining Alzheimer's no longer seems likely. Certainly, acetylcholine is important, but it is not alone.

There is also new work on diagnostic assessment. Small and Greenberg point out that the agreement between clinical and histopathological diagnosis at autopsy formerly was low, but with development of vigorous diagnostic criteria, the degree of agreement approaches 90%. At Columbia, work using regional cerebral blood flow approaches has suggested a possibility for earlier diagnosis. The scientists have shown a characteristic perfusion deficit in the temporal parietal cortex. Not only is this important clinically, but it will facilitate research by identifying populations earlier. Research leading to earlier identification allows research otherwise not possible. Prohovnik in a recent paper has also suggested that it may be possible to discriminate Alzheimer's from other kinds of dementias through rCBF imaging. This means that if other forms are treatable, help is possible for at least some of the increasing number of patients with dementia.

AFFECTIVE DISORDERS

The advances in affective disorders have been profound. We are most effective amongst the various major psychiatric disorders in our treatment of affective disorders. Beyond the disaggregation of various genetic causes of bipolar disease, there is also the work demonstrating the utility of MAO inhibitors for atypical depression. There are many new treatments including Prozac, which is attractive in its specificity for the serotonin system. It is purely a blocker of serotonin uptake with no apparent effect on other transmitters and no acute effects on receptors. There is work to be done in refining how to give ECT. There is information showing the utility of psychotherapy. There is light treatment. There are also links between affective disorders and some of the substance abuse disorders. Noteworthy amongst these is the link between alcoholism and depression and also between drug abuse and depression.

More recently it has been shown that many people who have difficulty withdrawing from smoking, which is such a serious health risk, may have a history of depression in addition to the smoking addiction. There is new work showing that antidepressant treatment in conjunction with special treatment such as clonidine for reducing the craving may be effective in reducing smoking behavior.

OBSESSIVE COMPULSIVE DISORDERS

As a result of new epidemiological studies, obsessive compulsive disorders have been recognized as being far more widespread than were originally thought. Karno et al., in December, 1988, *Archives of General Psychiatry* say that lifetime prevalence rates for OCD diagnosed without DSM-III exclusions ranged from 1.9% to 3.3% and 1.2%-2.4% with such exclusion areas. As a result they are attracting renewed attention. In one set of studies Judy Rapaport and her colleagues point to the possibility of obsessive compulsive disorders being a function of selective basal ganglia dysfunction. She takes note of one study that showed decreased volume of the caudate nuclei bilaterally in obsessive compulsive patients while the venticular and the thalami did not differ from controls. Further, Baxter showed with PET scans increased metabolic rates bilaterally in the caudate nuclei and the lateral orbitofrontal cortex. Rapaport marshals other information to document this theory.

Of note, too, is the fact that chlomipramine has turned out to be a beneficial treatment for obsessive compulsive disorders. Clomipramine can be viewed as blocking the potentiation by serotonin of striatal neurons by driving down the number of serotonin receptors.

Rapaport is primarily interested in taking note of the fact that obsessive compulsive disease may involve much more in the way of biological mechanisms than we had thought. She still expresses reservations about her own theory, but she wants to put it forth in order to facilitate a discussion of these interesting new possibilities.

SUICIDE

The area of suicide is receiving increased attention with a variety of kinds of studies. The increase in suicides among teenagers in the United States over the last several decades has led to much more exacting epidemiological data on the numbers. The completeness of the data still represents a problem inasmuch as reporting of suicide is uneven. However, it has been found that some six thousand or so teenagers and young adults commit suicide in the United States each year, making it the second leading cause of death in that population. By virtue of the distressing and widespread nature of this phenomenon, there have been increasing efforts to understand what can be done to reduce those numbers; i.e., to prevent suicide.

There are suspicions that there may be a genetic factor involved in suicide. Adoption studies showed a 15-fold increase in suicide among biological relatives of index cases compared with biological relatives of controls.

From a different vantage point, the role of media information regarding suicide has drawn attention in the United States. Television movies depicting suicide and news accounts of suicides have in some studies been shown as factors in precipitating other suicides. There are controversial findings in the literature and the research is continuing, but it has led to caution on the part of the media as to how suicide is portrayed. If one romanticizes it and makes teenagers feel it is an ideal solution to their problems, the likelihood is great that one will have young people respond by imitating the behavior they have seen.

It has also been found that there are alterations in serotonin receptors which may be helpful in predicting suicide. This has not yet reached the level of clinical application, but increasing work in live patients and in post-mortem studies suggest that this may be a useful avenue for research.

In the United States there is also information regarding interventions and methods of prevention for suicide. It is generally felt that a suicide hotline attracts all kinds of callers and does not necessarily focus on those who would be likely risks for suicide. Also, suicide prevention programs are often aimed at wide general populations and as a result their potential impact is reduced. Let me elaborate that: If one has some 12 suicides per 100,000 population among youngsters and one has suicide prevention programs available to 100,000 youngsters from the general population, the greatest success would be precluding 12 suicides, but the two thousand teenage suicides in the country represent a vastly greater population. Researchers are evaluating these kinds of programs and determining whether and where they have impact and how to maximize their effect.

Researchers are also looking, under the leadership of people like David Shaffer, at the specific risk possibilities in different settings. Shaffer is focusing on young men and women in various settings to determine what factors make the risk.

Brent and his colleagues in Pittsburgh studied a group of twenty-seven adolescent suicide victims and compared them with a group of fifty-six who were at high risk for suicide (all of these controls were suicidal psychiatric inpatients--eighteen having seriously considered and thirty-eight having actually attempted suicide). These researchers were looking at how to get beyond some of the general factors known to be associated with suicide to those which distinguish patients who would be considered very risky from those who actually had completed suicide. They found several variables that significantly distinguised these two groups:

1. The group of completers had higher suicidal intent.

2. There was a high prevalence of bipolar disorder among completed suicide victims (22.2%) consistent with work done by other authors. They particularly pointed out that "early-onset bipolarity may be more malignant than the adult-onset variant, perhaps because of the tendency of younger bipolar patients to present in mixed states."

3. There was a high prevalence of non-affective comorbidity among the completers.

4. Only a third of the youth completers had had even one lifetime mental health contact. Only 1 of the 6 victims with bipolar disorder had been clinically identified as such. Thus, these patients who are completers seem to have gotten very little in the way of mental health attention.

5. They also found a heavy family loading for bipolar affective disorder and suicidal behavior.

6. They also showed, according to them for the first time, that the availability of firearms is much greater in the homes of completers than in the comparable group.

This study is interesting, it has limitations, but it is a further attempt to get more and more specific. We all know how formidable it is to predict violence either to others or to ourselves. This work, along with the work of Shaffer and Shafii moves in the direction of refining even more tightly these discriminations to help diagnosticians and to offer some badly needed guidance for treatment and prevention programs in an area where we have so far been dramatically ineffective.

CITIZEN AND GOVERNMENT RESPONSE

Given all this excitement in psychiatric research, it is important to take note of another phenomenon in the society which is important for the research effort. In the United States and in other countries there is a rising citizen involvement in advocating attention to mental illness. For years, the enormous stigma of mental illness had prevented the formation of advocacy groups, but this seems to be abating in the United States. This decreased stigma and increased citizen activity is related to the increasing knowledge of the medical and biological aspects of psychiatric disorders. Where formerly many people derided psychiatric care and patients with psychiatric illnesses as being weak, lazy, slothful, and having some character defect, that has changed dramatically. A number of organizations, the National Alliance of the Mentally Ill, the National Depressive and Manic Depressive Association, the National Consumers Association, and the Mental Health Association have been pressing harder and getting more people to join and become more effective in placing the issue of major mental illness higher on the public agenda.

At NIMH new programs are being launched on schizophrenia, depression, and also on a focus of neurobiology and genetics pertaining to psychiatric disorders. A new organization called The National Alliance for Research on Schizophrenia and Depression has developed. This is a private effort to complement the predominant government effort on research in mental illness. It awarded Lieber Awards of $250,000 in 1987, over $1 million in 1988, and projects $2-3 million in 1989. It will shortly announce $1.65 million in new awards. It will, with these, have awarded grants to almost 70 new and established scientists. This is all very heartening and in a sense it is circular. As citizens give more support to the research, the research is more productive, as the research is more productive, more citizens become encouraged, reveal themselves and enlarge this very rapidly rising constituency fighting for mental illness. We can help by making this our charity. It also is noteworthy that in the United States a number of well known figures who formerly tried to protect their public images are now associating themselves with mental illness and mental illness advocacy. Examples are Rosalynn Carter, Jennifer Jones, Patty Duke, Dick Cavett, Leonard Bernstein, and Senator Pete Domenici. This is further documentation of the destigmatizing trend in mental illness and the fact that mental illness as a problem in the United States will receive more and more attention. Although in the years from 1969-76 the NIMH budget for research went down from about $95 million to $90 million, the apparent figure for 1989 will be $294 million. So in the last 12-13 years there has been a 326% increase in government money for research in mental illness.

I make these points to say that intellectual excitement, genuine data advances, increased technology, and greater sophistication of the scientific enterprise are paralleled by community support, citizen activism and fiscal support. This all bodes well for research on psychiatric disorders and suggests a major effort in the next decade or so of advances in this field.

There are some specific concerns that we in the United States are trying to address and I suspect they may be problems for other areas of the world.

1) More and more young researchers are needed to come into the

field. The average age of the NIMH principal investigator is about 38. The field is really rather small, consisting of only a few hundred major investigators in the United States.

2) Substantial fiscal resources are needed to support the technology. The expansion of the psychiatric research group and attention to physical plant and to rapidly changing technology is critical.

3) All psychiatrists need education so that clinicians will foster research rather than feel threatened by it. I am sure that many clinicians find some of current research incomprehensible and alien. They may feel threatened. They may subtly or even overtly block the research. It is necessary when conducting research on a clinical unit to have the cooperation of clinicians.

   More important, however, is the fact that psychiatry is changing profoundly. The new answers and new knowledge we are getting is going to make our field enormously more effective. I can understand some of the concerns of those of us who trained 2-3 decades ago. At that time we had our psychotherapies, we had some convulsive therapies, and we had only the beginning of medications. The world has changed dramatically--for the good. Psychiatric disorders will be taken more seriously by society. Clinicians are going to have to work harder to get on top of some new approaches. But if they do, they are going to have many more patients coming for help and they are going to be much more effective in responding.

4) We require a policy that keeps the nature of our research efforts broad, since we don't know what disciplines will produce the answers to psychiatric illness. We need as much basic science and clinical science interaction as possible, so that both groups benefit from different questions that they ask and different perspectives in organizing scientific experiments. Increasingly, treatments are going to be combinations of psychotherapy and pharmacotherapy. New genetic information brings all kinds of psychiatric challenges and disturbing issues which require individual, group, and family therapy and counselling. What we have to do is become schooled in the new areas so that we can blend

our existing skills with new knowledge and skills and be even more responsive to the patient population.

I would say in closing that we are most impressed and encouraged by the possibilities of research in psychiatric disorders. The forties and fifties saw major advances in infectious disease treatment and were followed by a greater attention to cancer and heart disease in the sixties and seventies. It is our feeling that the eighties and the future (the nineties and the early 21st century) will bring major progress in the neuropsychiatric diseases and expand this remarkable revolution in the entire psychiatric field. Psychiatry truly is coming of age and it is our feeling that its regard among its medical colleagues and society in general will increase dramatically. In turn, with its increased capacity it will be able to render more and more useful care for the multitude of patients suffering from mental diseases.

chapter 3

Danger Zones In Depression Research

Herman M. van Praag, M.D., Ph.D.

PROGRESS IN PSYCHIATRY, A NON-LINEAR PROCESS

Psychiatry is in the process of being transformed into a science. A taxonomy of mental disorders has been developed as well as instruments to measure abnormal human behavior; systematic studies of biological, psychological and social determinants of abnormal behavior are being conducted; epidemiology, treatment outcome and long-term prognosis of psychiatric disorders are being studied. Progress, however, is generally a non-linear process and not every change in the name of progress turns out to be advantageous. I will discuss three trends in contemporary depression research I consider to be counterproductive. I qualified them as 1) codification of diagnostic confusion; 2) preoccupation with nosology and; 3) over-reliance on biology.

CODIFICATION OF DIAGNOSTIC CONFUSION

In 1958, the time when I started my residency training in psychiatry, diagnostic confusion reigned in the realm of depressive disorders. Diagnostic concepts were not operationalized, nomenclature was not standardized, and no taxonomy was generally accepted. What is the situation today, some 30 years later? Today we work under the patronage of the DSM-III classification of depression, a system in which diagnostic concepts *are* operationalized and nomenclature *is* both standardized and officially accepted in the U.S. and, *de facto*, in numerous countries all over the world. Did that system provide order where chaos reigned? The answer has to be in the negative and let me explain why I think this is so.

Syndromal Fogginess

The DSM-III holds the view of depression as syndromally heter-

Psychiatry: Past Reflections–Future Visions
B.T. Taylor and I.J. Taylor, Editors

ogeneous and recognizes two basic entities: major depression and dysthymic disorder. In delineating these entities it utilizes the "choice-principle." No fixed set of symptoms has to be present in order to qualify for either diagnosis, but y symptoms out of a series of y + x, no matter which ones. As a consequence, the same term covers a diversity of depressive syndromes. Moreover, the majority of symptoms listed under major depression are similar to those listed under dysthymic disorder; discriminating symptoms are few. The proposed dichotomy resembles two poorly focused slides, projected simultaneously and largely overlapping. Clarity is far to seek (Table 1 and 2).

This state of affairs is detrimental for research, in particular biological research, as well as for clinical practice. In biological psychiatry the search is for the biological underpinnings of specific syndromes or specific psychopathological dimensions and for specific biological interventions to eliminate them. These goals are ill-served by diagnostic ambiguities.

For the practitioner, the DSM system may seem handy but, in fact, it does not serve him well. Psychotropic drugs acquire ever greater biochemical specificity and thus probably a more narrowly focused therapeutic action. Working with unfocused diagnostic concepts, one could easily fail to discern specific therapeutic indications. It is true that many depressed patients do not fit rigidly defined diagnostic concepts, but it is better to recognize that and categorize them for the time being as "mixed states," or as "double depressions" or as "not yet classifiable with some degree of certainty" than to use labels that for all intents and purposes are meaningless and only provide pseudo-certainty.

When in the early sixties we introduced the concepts of vital and personal depression we rejected the "choice-principle" and defined these syndromes rigorously, and we categorized the patients in between the endpoints of the spectrum as mixed depressions (van Praag et al., 1965) (Table 3). Vital and personal depressions are the specified and operationalized equivalents of the syndromes described previously under the headings of endogenous and neurotic depression. The best fitting DSM-III diagnoses are major depression, melancholic type and dysthymic disorder, respectively.

Nosological Curtailments

The DSM-III aspires to be more than a syndromal depression classification and aims at delineation of disease entities, not only characterized by symptoms but by criteria such as intensity, duration and underlying personality structure. For example, dysthymic disorder is defined by symptoms as well as by mild intensity, chronicity and dis-

TABLE 1

SYMPTOMOLOGICAL CHARACTERISTICS OF DEPRESSION ACCORDING TO DSM III (1980)

MAJOR DEPRESSION	DYSTHYMIC DISORDER
Dysphoric mood or Anhedonia + 4/8 symptoms	Depressed mood or Anhedonia + 3/13 symptoms
SIMILAR SYMPTOMS	
Anhedonia	Anhedonia
Loss of energy; fatigue	Low energy level or chronic tiredness
Insomnia or hypersomnia	Insomnia or hypersomnia
Diminished ability to think or concentrate	Decreased attention, concentration or ability to think clearly
Suicidal ideation or suicide attempt	Recurrent thoughts of death and suicide
Feelings of worthlessness, self-reproach or excessive guilt	Feelings of inadequacy, loss of self-esteem or self-depreciation
Psychomotor agitation or retardation (not only subjectively)	Feels slowed down or restless
DIFFERENTIATING SYMPTOMS	
Poor or increased appetite	—
Weight loss or gain	—
—	Irritability or excessive anger
—	Tearfulness or crying
—	Decreased effectiveness at school, work, home and social withdrawal

ordered personality. The diagnosis major depression, melancholic type, is justified when certain symptoms are present and when the depression is severe and the premorbid personality basically normal. In other words, the DMS-III classification is firmly rooted in nosologic soil. That soil is traditionally polluted with wishful thinking; i.e., the hope that mental disorders will turn out to be classifiable as neat, separable packages each with its characteristic psychopathology, causation and course. I consider the nosological concept in depression classification as a *fata morgana.* Syndromal distinction is as far as one can go (van Praag and Leijnse, 1965). We demonstrated that factors like duration, intensity and personality structure do not relate specifically to a particular depressive syndrome but vary within one syndrome and hence should be assessed on an independent axis, that is, independent of syndromal diagnosis. I will illustrate this statement with three examples (van Praag, 1982, 1989).

1. The syndrome of vital depression (major depression, melancholic type) may occur in all degrees of severity, from mild to very severe. The same is true for personal depression

TABLE 2

SYMPTOMOLOGICAL CHARACTERISTICS OF DEPRESSION ACCORDING TO DSM III-R (1987)

MAJOR DEPRESSION	**DYSTHYMIC DISORDER**
5/9 symptoms at least one of them either 1) depressed mood or 2) anhedonia	Depressed mood + 2/6 symptoms
SIMILAR SYMPTOMS	
Insomnia or hypersomnia	Insomnia or hypersomnia
Fatigue or loss of energy	Low energy or fatigue
Feelings of worthlessness or excessive guilt	Low self-esteem
Diminished concentration or indecisiveness	Poor concentration or difficulty making decisions
Recurrent thoughts of death, or suicide plan or suicide attempt	Feelings of hopelessness
Decrease or increase of appetite; weight loss or gain	Poor appetite or overeating
DIFFERENTIATING SYMPTOMS	
Anhedonia	(All dysthymic symptoms feature in major depressive syndrome)
Psychomotor retardation or agitation	

TABLE 3

SYMPTOMATOLOGICAL CHARACTERIZATION OF VITAL AND PERSONAL DEPRESSION

VITAL DEPRESSION	PERSONAL DEPRESSION
1. DEPRESSED MOOD • Meaningless : i.e. no, for patient, under-standable connection between mood and precipitant (if any) • Often experienced "Leib-nah" rather than "Geist-nah"	DEPRESSED MOOD • Experiences congruence between mood and life experiences or personality make-up • Experienced as "Geist-nah"
2. MOTOR DISTURBANCES • Retardation • Agitation • Both	MOTOR DISTURBANCES • Agitation (usually not very pronounced)
3. SLOWING DOWN • Thought • Time experience	THOUGHT PROCESSING : UNDISTURBED
4. ANHEDONIA	EMOTIONAL RESPONSIVITY UNDISTURBED (Sometimes depersonalization)
5. SOMATIC DISTURBANCES • Fatigue, lack of energy • Decreased appetite • Early morning awakening • Disturbed sexual functions (impotence; decreased libido; disturbances menstrual cycle)	SOMATIC DISTURBANCES • Somatic anxiety equivalents (e.g. palpitations, atypical precordial pain) • Multiple sleep disturbances • Sexual functions not disturbed
6. DIURNAL FLUCTUATION	NO OR IRREGULAR FLUCTUATIONS
7. ANXIETY • Not manifest in retarded vital depression • Manifest in agitated vital depression, often linked to delusional thinking (e.g. poverty; guilt; hypochondriasis)	MANIFEST ANXIETY
8. NO SIGNS OF MANIFEST OUTWARD DIRECTED HOSTILITY	IRRITABILITY AND MANIFEST HOSTILITY
9. TAEDIUM VITAE	TAEDIUM VITAE
10. INABILITY TO CRY	CRYING SPELLS
11. GUILT FEELINGS; SELF-REPROACH	FEELINGS OF INADEQUACY; BLAMES OTHERS
12. ONCE GENERATED, THE COURSE IS INDEPENDENT OF PRECIPITANTS	PRESENCE OF SYMPTOMS CLOSELY RELATED TO PERPETUATION OF PRECIPITATING FACTORS

(dysthymic disorder). Severity is *not* a syndromal characteristic (Table 4).

2. The duration of vital (major) depression varies tremendously, from a few weeks to several years. The same, we showed, is true for personal (dysthymic) depression. It is erroneous to define dysthymia as a chronic depression (Table 5).

3. Personality disorders are ubiquitous in depressives, not only in dysthymic disorder. In vital depression (major depression, melancholic type) and mixed forms they are almost as prevalent as in personal (dysthymic) depression (Table 6). This observation has important implications. Therapeutic implications: major depression, melancholic type, in most cases, is as much a target for biological treatment as it is for psychotherapy. Research implications: biological variables found in major depression are not necessarily related to (features of) the depressive disorder, but they could be biological underpinnings of the co-existing personality disorder. For many years this was an entirely ignored consideration in affective disorder research.

TABLE 4

Syndromal Depression-Type and Severity of Depression

One psychiatrist made the syndromal diagnoses, another one determined the severity of the depression independently, i.e. not knowing the syndromal diagnosis made by the first psychiatrist. The factor severity was not linked to any one depression type.

	Number of patients with severe, moderate and mild depression			
	N	Severe	Moderate	Mild
Vital Depression	60	23	29	8
Personal Depression	55	20	24	11
Mixed Forms	62	18	30	14

TABLE 5

Duration of Present Dysthymic Episode and of Preceding Symptom-Free or Symptom-Reduced Interval

% of patients indicating that time interval (n = 100)

	Duration of the dysthymic episode	Duration of the preceeding symptom-free (-reduced) interval
< 1 week	-	6
1 month	6	38
1-3 months	19	35
3-6 months	22	19
6-12 months	29	2
12-24 months	14	-
< 24 months	10	-

By attaching nosological strings to syndromal depression concepts, one condemns many a depressed patient to be booked as Depressive Disorder not Otherwise Specified, that is, not to be diagnosed at all.

Etiological Prudery

The DSM-III aspires to be "atheoretical" and thus abstains from an etiological axis. This prudence is unnecessary. Potential etiological factors can be assessed with considerable precision: personality disorders with inventories or standardized interviews; recent life events with appropriate scales; hereditary factors via a detailed family history; physical factors through a thorough medical and neurological work-up. The issue of the etiological weight of these factors in a given case is a complicated one, but a consensus opinion can be reached most of the time, much the same as can be done regarding the presence and severity of particular psychopathological symptoms.

To make etiology a classificatory outcast is wrong. Etiology determines important therapeutic decisions, such as the initiation of systematic psychotherapy; and prognosis is difficult without taking

TABLE 6

Syndromal Depression Type and Personality Disorder

The data were collected with a structured interview. The interview was geared towards uncovering signs of character neurosis, i.e. signs the patient does not consider to be pathological, but part of his personality make-up but which negatively interfere with his interpersonal relations and his sense of well-being. The three factors were scored on a 10-point scale after the depression had subsided (van Praag, 1990).

	N	Basic feelings of discontent	Unhappiness with personal relations	Emotional instability
Vital depression	20	6.4	5.3	5.0
Personal depression	20	7.8	6.9	7.5
Mixed forms	20	6.1	4.9	7.2
Normal controls	20	1.0	0.7	1.1

etiological factors into account. An etiological analysis, or hypothesis if one wishes, is an indispensable part of psychiatric diagnosis. The DSM-III, as it stands now, imprints the trainees with the notion that such analysis is barely feasible and that it is preferable to make incomplete diagnoses. This is a harmful imprint, a veritable misprint.

Diagnostic Inequality

The DSM-III recognizes that the psychiatric condition of a given patient is often multi-syndromal in nature. To resolve this problem it does not recommend recording each of them but that all but one be disregarded. In other words, it resorts to a hierarchical principle whereby psychiatric disorders are rank-ordered according to severity and the more serious disorder takes precedence over the more minor one. Major depression, for example, cannot be diagnosed in the presence of schizophrenia, and generalized anxiety disorder has to be disregarded in the presence of a mood disorder. Compared to the DSM-III, the principle of multi-syndromal diagnoses gained some ground in the DSM-III-R, but the hierarchical system is by no means abandoned.

Psychiatry has little to gain from hierarchical diagnostic systems and much to lose. Loss of diagnostic information and loss of therapeutic opportunities, since little evidence exists that lower order syndromes will disappear if higher ranking syndromes have been combated successfully. Loss, finally, of validity of research, in particular biological research. How can one interpret biological findings, say in schizophrenia, if in one patient major depression co-exists and in the other it does not.

CONCLUSION

Today's depression classification is confusing, as it used to be some 30 years ago. All things considered, the present situation is worse. Then, psychiatrists were at least aware that diagnostic chaos reigned and many of them had no high opinion of diagnosis anyhow. Now, the chaos is codified and thus much more hidden. It is true, the codification is not sacrosanct and is periodically adjusted, so far, however, guided by experts, not by focused research. Modifications introduced today, then, will irrevocably be followed by modifications tomorrow, creating even more confusion both practically--not every clinician keeps up with the ever changing guidelines--and scientifically, because research conducted under the jurisdiction of the various DSM editions will be increasingly hard to compare.

There is nothing wrong in basing the first draft of an operationalized taxonomy on expert opinions. One should abstain, however, from proceeding on that route. Once having postulated a taxonomy, experts should be honorably discharged and replaced by researchers to study the merits of the system. In other words, I strongly feel that 1) an immediate moratorium should be laid on any further expert-opinion-based alterations in the classification of depression (or any other psychiatric disorder, for that matter) and, that 2) future changes should be based only on research, conducted in several centers simultaneously and specifically designed to resolve issues pertinent to the DSM (depression) classification.* In organizing, conducting and funding such a collaborative, goal-directed effort the National Institute of Mental Health could play a seminal role. A tall order, but the Diagnostic Manual deserves it.

---

*This paper was written before those of Spitzer and Williams (1988) and Zimmerman (1988). My recommendations are comparable with theirs, though definitely more stringent.

PREOCCUPATION WITH NOSOLOGY

Biological psychiatric research has been and still is very much under the spell of nosology. The search for biological markers and eventually causes of disease entities, such as depression, schizophrenia and panic disorder, is the major aim for most of these endeavors. Biological depression research is no exception. As an example, one needs only bring to mind the countless studies trying to prove that DST non-suppression is a marker of a disorder, in this case a particular depression type, despite abundant evidence suggesting this variable to be disorder-non-specific. The nosological focus has brought biological psychiatric research so far little return. Indeed, we discovered a lot of "biology" in psychiatric disorders. None of these variables, however, seems to possess any diagnostic specificity. Could the reason be that we have approached brain and behavior relationship in too restricted a fashion? This, I think, is indeed the case.

Nosological non-specificity of a given biological variable does not mean it is not specific at all. It could very well be that that variable relates not to a disorder as such but to a component of that disorder, to a particular (set of) psychological dysfunction(s). Psychological dysfunctions are seldomly nosologically specific but tend to occur in a variety of psychiatric disorders, clarifying why many biological variables in psychiatric disorders seem to defy nosological borders. The notion that biological dysfunctions might relate to psychological dysfunctions rather than to nosological entities is not a mere theoretical possibility but a viewpoint supported by facts, of which I will now discuss a few examples (van Praag et al. 1987; 1990a,b).

Dopamine and Depression

Some 20 years ago, we observed signs of diminished central DA metabolism in some depressed patients but not in others. In the former category, the postprobencid concentration of the major DA metabolite homovanillic acid (HVA) was lowered, an indication of decreased DA metabolism (van Praag and Korf, 1971). Guided by Parkinson's disease with its severe disturbances in motor functioning and profound DA depletion, we searched for correlations between lowered CSF HVA and motor retardation. In retarded depression post-probenecid CSF HVA was indeed twice as low as in non-retarded depression and in controls, and of the same order of magnitude as in Parkinson's disease (Fig 1).

The relationship between decreased DA metabolism in depression and motor retardation was substantiated by two therapeutic findings (van Praag and Lemus, 1986). l-DOPA, capable of boosting DA production in the CNS, ameliorated the motor condition of patients with retarded

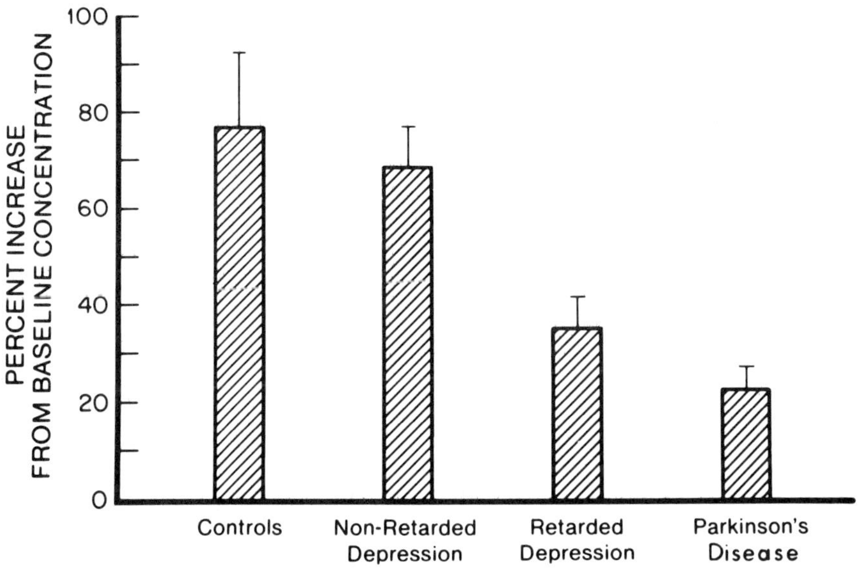

FIGURE 1. Post-probenecid concentration of HVA in CSF in controls (N=12), depression with (N=11) and without (N=13) motor retardation and in Parkinson's disease (N=14) (van Praag and Korf, 1971; Lakke et al., 1972).

depression, but was ineffective in elevating mood and decreasing anhedonia (Fig 2). It had no effect in non-retarded depressives. l-Tyrosine, which has a much weaker impact on DA synthesis than l-DOPA, had no measurable influence on motor retardation and neither on mood or anhedonia.

Based on these findings we hypothesized diminished DA metabolism to underly decreased motor activity and level of initiative, irrespective of nosological diagnosis (van Praag et al., 1975).

Serotonin and Depression

Decreased metabolism of serotonin (5-hydroxtyptamine, 5-HT) in the CNS, as reflected in lowered (post-probenecid) CSF 5-hydroxyindoleactic acid (5-HIAA), was initially considered to be indicative of a particular type of depression: the so-called 5-HT depression. In a series of precursor studies we showed this hypothesis to be untenable (van Praag and Lemus, 1986). Today it seems likely that the 5-HT disturbances are linked to particular psychological dysfunctions, most

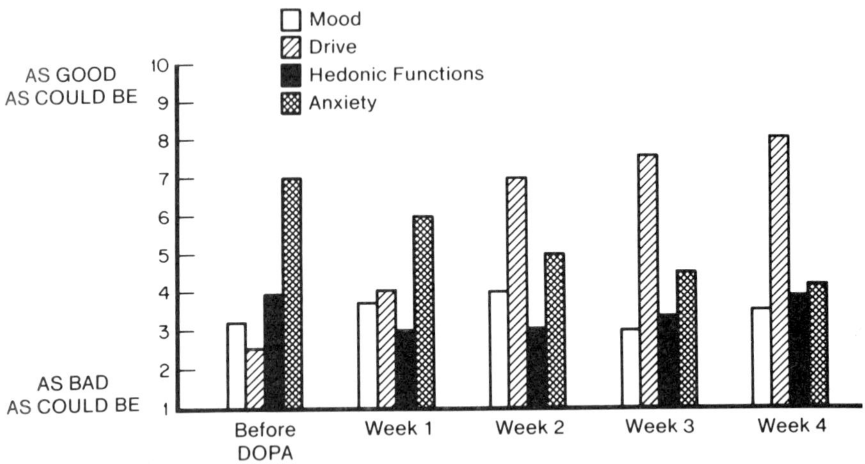

FIGURE 2. l-DOPA (average 260 mg/day) in combination with a peripheral decarboxylase inhibitor was administered for 4 weeks to 10 patients with major depression, melancholic type, pronounced motor retardation and low post-probenecid CSF HVA. Motor retardation and inertia ("drive") improved significantly. Mood and hedonic functioning were not significantly influenced. Post-probenecid CSF HVA was normalized. In melancholic patient with normal HVA response and without motor retardation DOPA was ineffectual and no better than placebo (van Praag and Lemus 1986).

notably to: *heightened anxiety* and *disregulated aggression*, dysfunctions which may occur in depression, but which may be absent as well and that are by no means specific for depression, thus explaining the capricious occurrence of 5-HT disturbances in depression as well as their nosological non-specificity.

The relation between lowered CSF 5-HIAA and *autoaggression* in depression was first reported by Asberg et al. (1976), but has now been confirmed by many investigators (Roy and Linnoila 1988; Cohen et al., 1988). Non-depressed suicide attempters, non-psychotic (Traskman et al. 1981) as well as psychotic (van Praag, 1983; Ninan et al., 1984) showed the same disturbance and so did individuals with uncontrolled outward directed aggression (Virkunnen et al., 1987; Roy et al., 1988).

Comparing depressed patients with low and with normal CSF 5-HIAA we found additional evidence for a relation: decreased 5-HT metabolism/disturbed aggression regulation. In the low 5-HIAA group, suicide rate was increased and so were signs of outward directed aggression (van Praag, 1988) (Table 7).

TABLE 7

Low 5-HIAA Depressives Compared to Normal 5-HIAA Depressives Present (van Praag and Lemus, 1986)

Finding	P
More suicide attempts	<0.01
Greater number of contacts with police	<0.05
Increased arguments with	
relatives	<0.05
spouses	<0.01
colleagues	<0.05
friends	<0.05
More hostility at interview	<0.05
Impaired employment history	
(arguments)	<0.05

The notion that 5-HT disturbances might be involved in states of increased anxiety is predicated on a number of observations. First, drugs that decrease 5-HT functioning have generally anxiolytic effects (Johnston and File, 1986; Gardner, 1988). Buspirone, a recognized anxiolytic, is an agonist of presynaptically (somatically) localized 5-HT1A receptors, thus reducing the impulse flow in 5-HT ergic neurons. 5-HT2 receptor antagonists like ritanserin have reportedly anxiolytic properties (Pangalila-Ratu Langi and Jansen, 1988) and so have 5-HT3 receptor antagonists (Jones et al., 1988). 5-HT uptake inhibitors, like fluvoxamine and fluoxetine, have been reported to exert therapeutic effects in panic disorder, often after an initial deterioration of the condition (Evans et al., 1986; Kahn et al., 1987). It has been hypothesized that the initial deterioration relates to increased synaptic availability of 5-HT and the amerlioration of symptoms to subsequent downregulation of post-synaptic 5-HT receptors (Kahn and van Praag, 1988).

A second set of data indicative of a relation between 5-HT and anxiety was arrived at with the MCPP challenge test. M-chlorophenylpiperazine is a 5-HT1 receptor agonist releasing prolactin and cortisol. Comparing patients with panic disorder, major depression and normal controls, we found the cortisol response in the former group significantly augmented (Kahn et al., 1988a) (Fig 3). Only in panic disorder did MCPP (0.25 mg orally) induce, moreover, anxiety

(Kahn et al., 1988b) (Fig 4). These findings are indicative of 5-HT receptor hypersensitivity in (some forms of) panic disorder.

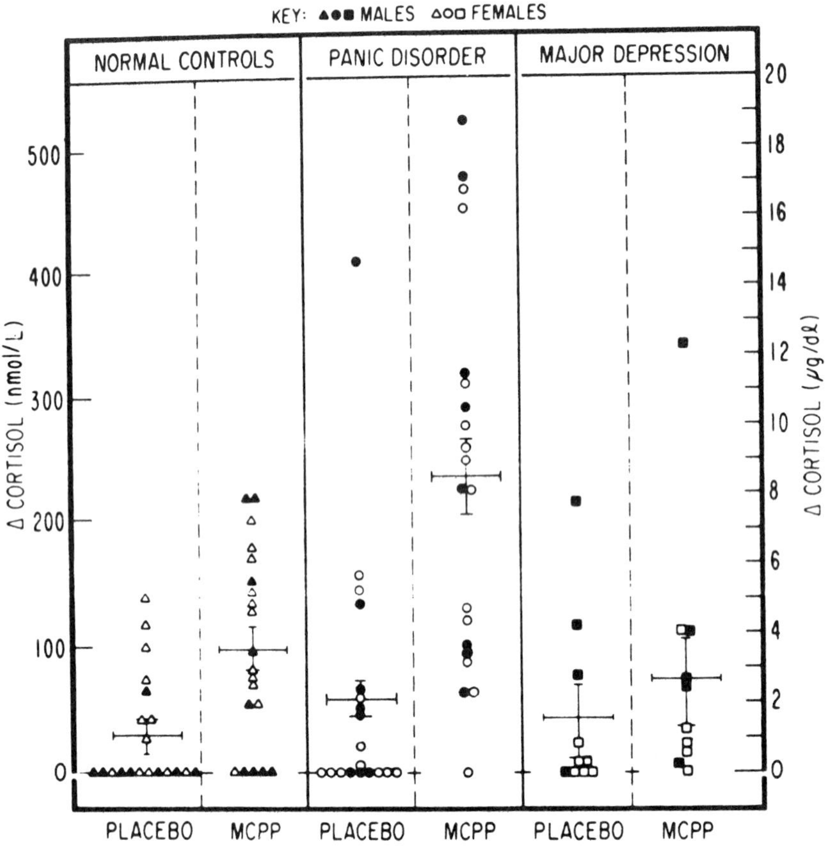

FIGURE 3. Individual delta cortisol response with group means and standard error of the mean (SEM), for normal controls (NC), patients with panic disorder (PD) and patients with major depression (MD) on placebo and 0.25 mg/kg MCPP p.o. Placebo-corrected delta cortisol response in PD vs NC $p<0.001$ and PD vs MD $p<0.005$; NC vs MD ns. Delta cortisol on MCPP vs on placebo in NC $p<0.005$ and in PD $p<.0001$, in MD $p<0.03$ (Kahn et al., 1988a).

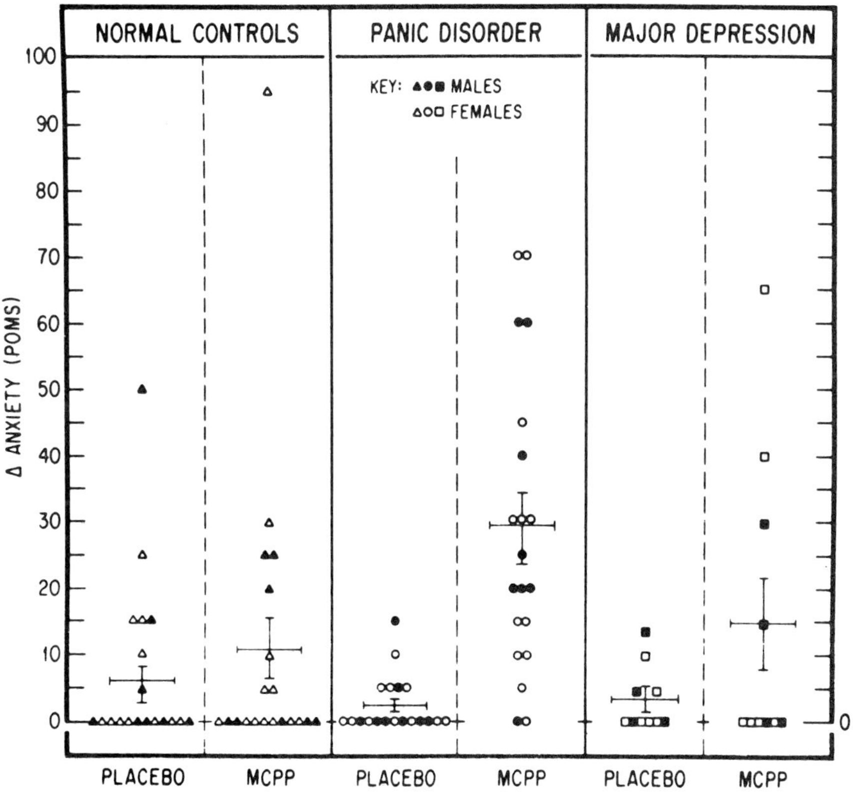

FIGURE 4. Individual delta anxiety response on Profile of Mood States with group means and standard error of the mean (SEM) for normal controls (NC), patients with panic disorder (PD) and patients with major depression (MD) on placebo and 0.25 mg/kg MCPP p.o. Placebo corrected delta anxiety response in PD vs NC $p<0.05$, PD vs MD ns, NC vs MD ns. Delta anxiety on MCPP vs on placebo in PD $p<0.001$; in NC and MD ns (Kahn et al., 1988b).

Finally in depression a negative correlation has been found between anxiety ratings and CSF HIAA (Banki, 1977; Ryden et al., 1982).

These data justify the hypothesis that low CSF HIAA, rather than being indicative of a particular depression type, is related to particular psychopathological dimensions; i.e., disturbed aggression regulation and heightened anxiety, irrespective of diagnoses (van Praag et al., 1987).

Noradrenaline and Depression

In animals, evidence exists that noradrenergic (NA ergic) mechanisms as well as DA ergic circuits are involved in brain reward systems. DA neurons constitute a "go-system" directing animals to areas in the environment associated with reward, while NA ergic systems are supposed to be involved in the coding of naturally occurring, rewarding experiences (Crow, 1973, 1977; Stein, 1978; Crow and Deakin, 1985; Ashton, 1987). They play a role in what I have called "emotional memory," that is in the consolidation and retrieval of the emotional arousal induced by certain behaviors. Simply put: NA neurons may enable the animal to couple the experience of reward or anticipated reward to a particular activity.

We found tentative evidence that the same might be true in humans (van Praag et al., 1989). I mention here only one piece of evidence. In our tyrosine studies in depression we found the precursor to be overall ineffective but not inert. It seemed to improve anhedonia, as well as to increase anxiety (Fig 5). Tyrosine is the precursor of

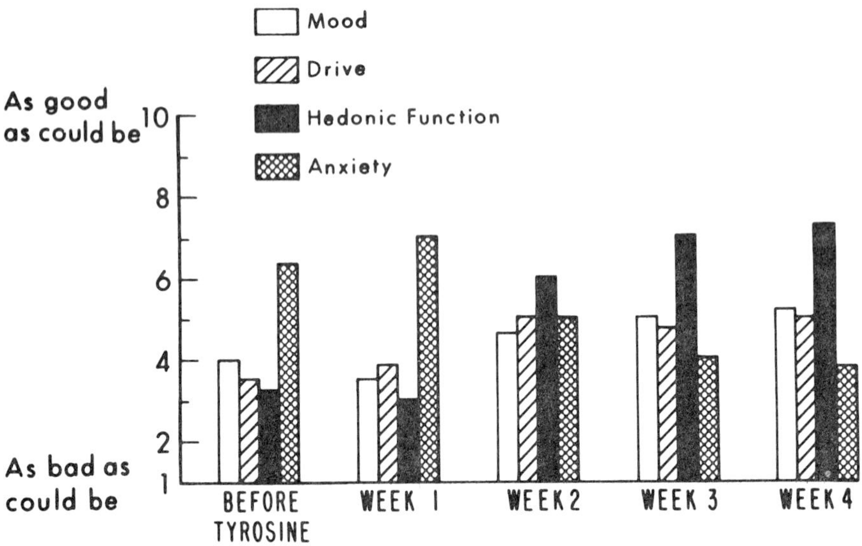

FIGURE 5. In 10 patients with major depression, melancholic type, l-tyrosine (100 mg/kg/day for 4 weeks) did not change the overall Hamilton score. Discrete components of the syndrome, however, did change significantly. Hedonic functioning improved while anxiety levels increased. Placebo did not change these psychopathological dimensions (van Praag et al., 1990a).

both DA and NA. After oral administration to humans, the CSF concentration of 3-methoxy-4-hydroxyphenylglycol (MHPG), the major NA metabolite, in the CNS was raised considerably, the HVA concentration only slightly. The reverse occurs after oral DOPA administration. We concluded that tyrosine's effect on NA synthesis is pronounced and seemingly greater than on DA synthesis (van Praag and Lemus, 1986).

The data relating NA ergic dysfunctioning to anhedonia are so far tentative at best, but the hypothesis is sufficiently intriguing to be further explored.

CONCLUSION

Our monoamine (MA) studies suggest a dimensional involvement of these transmitter systems in depression, DA ergic systems being related to drive, 5-HT systems to the affects of anxiety and aggression and NA ergic systems to hedonic functioning (Fig 6). Dimensional analysis of biological data is thus a fruitful approach and seems to be a necessary complement to the nosological approach.

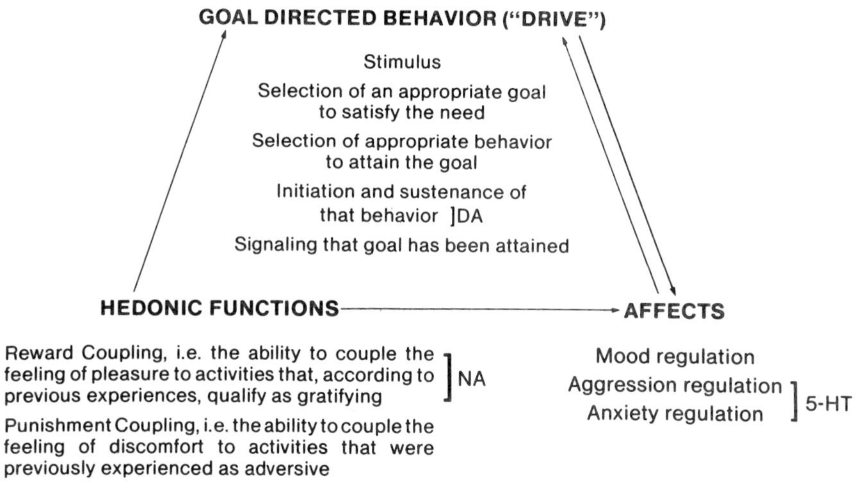

FIGURE 6. Depiction of the major domains of psychological dysfunctioning in major depression, melancholic type and the hypothesized MA-ergic dysfunctions underlying these psychological dysfunctions (van Praag et al., 1990b).

OVERESTIMATION OF BIOLOGICAL DETERMINANTS OF DEPRESSION

The impact of psychological factors in depression

Biology is dominating research into the origins of depression. We learn that most depressions are "biological," that depression is a "brain disease" and that they usually can be treated adequately with medication alone. This is what the French call "terrible simplification." Let's have a look at the syndrome that is being particularly referred to if the subject of "biological depression" comes up. Major depression, or more stringent even: major depression, melancholic type, the syndrome we have called vital depression.

1. Does that syndrome usually occur in the absence of psychological stressors?

   Not at all: in 73% of a cohort of 100 patients, stressful events had occurred in the six months prior to the depression (psychosocial 59%; physical 14%) (Table 8).

TABLE 8

Precipitants in the Three Months Preceding the Depression in the Two Major Syndromal Depression Types

	Number of patients indicating precipitants	
	Major depression melancholic type (Vital depression) (n=100)	Dysthymic disorder (Personal Depression) (n=100)
No Precipitants:	27	33
Precipitants:	73	67
Psychosocial:	59	56
Biological:	14	11

2. Do the patients themselves think the depressions to be detached from psychological events?

   Not at all: 63% of that same cohort experienced a causal connection.

3. Do "important others" consider depression and psychological events as independent?

   Not at all: in that same cohort, 83% of those referrents suggested a causal relationship.

4. Is the personality make-up generally undisturbed in this type of depression?

   Not at all: the score for "character neurosis" in vital depression (major depression, melancholic type) proved to be very significantly higher than that in a control group (Table 6).

5. Are antidepressants helpful in this type of depression?

   Without question: an abundance of evidence demonstrates that a majority of patients improve on antidepressants.

6. Another question is: do they improve sufficiently; do they generally return to the premorbid level? Is the recovery complete? The answer is: in a majority of patients, this is not the case.

   To a cohort of 61 patients, who all were considered to be good responders to antidepressant medication, we addressed the question whether they felt again the way they used to be before the first depressive episode. They recorded this judgement on a ten point scale, in which 10 represented being again the usual self; the score 1, feeling miserable and the score 5, feeling so-so. All patients had improved more than 50% on the Hamilton Depression Scale. The well-being scale was scored at 6m, 9m and 12m after the start of antidepressants, while the patients were still on antidepressants, but not involved in systematic psychotherapy.

   The great majority of patients (85%) remained definitely

improved as manifested by a 50% or more reduction of Hamilton score, compared to the pre-treatment score. However, between 50-60% of the cohort indicated not to be fully recovered on antidepressants. Their "well-being score" fluctuated between 6 and 8 (Average 6.9) (Fig 7).

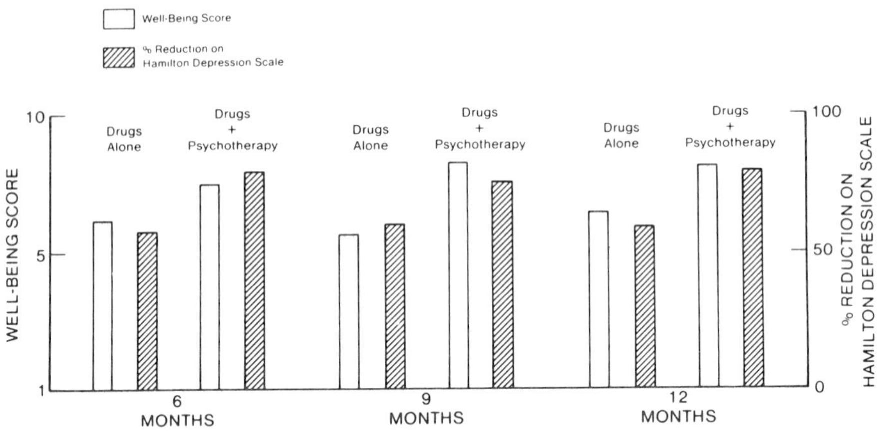

FIGURE 7. Hamilton scores and well-being scores in two cohorts of patients with vital depression (major depression, melancholic type). One (n=61) was treated with various antidepressants but no systematic psychotherapy. The second (n=39) was treated with various antidepressants and systematic psychotherapy of different kinds, depending upon individual diagnosis. Assessments were made 6, 9 and 12 months after the beginning of treatment.

7. Is it possible to improve those treatment results by adding focused psychotherapy and psychosocial interventions?

Definitely. In a second cohort of 39 patients, antidepressants were combined with different kinds of psychotherapy (made to measure, so to say) from the time significant improvement had ensued. Improvement scores were systematically higher in the second than in the first cohort (average 52% and 71% respectively) and so were the well-being scores, fluctuating from the sixth month on between 6 and 9 (average 8.2) (Fig 7).

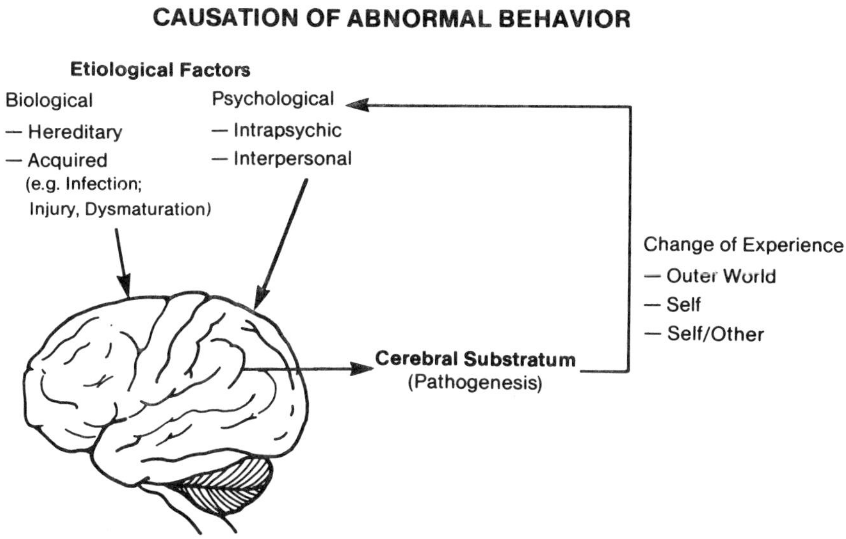

FIGURE 8. In the causation of mental disorders, two components have to be distinguished: 1) the disturbances in the functioning of the brain that underly the behavioral pathology (*pathogenesis*) and 2) the factors responsible for these cerebral dysfunctions, the so-called *etiological* factors. The latter can be psychological or biological in nature. The (pathological) state of the brain does influence the way the self, the other and the environment is experienced. These experiential changes in their turn may contribute to the cerebral pathology (van Praag and Leijnse, 1964, 1965).

CONCLUSION

Let me then, finally, kick in an open door, or better, a door that should be open, but is not: in depression psychological factors do count. Even in the "biological prototype" i.e., major depression, melancholic type. When patients are being told that they are suffering from a chemical imbalance in the brain they are being put off with acommonplace. All behavior is biologically determined, dependent on a functioning brain, and *ipso facto* abnormal brain functioning is a necessary precondition for abnormal behavior. The relevant question is: to what extent do psychological factors contribute to the dysfunctions in the brain underlying depressive behavior (van Praag and Leijnse, 1964) (Fig 8). In a majority of cases, the answer seems to be: they do and to a significant extent. When patients are being told that the depression can be fixed with medication, they are being put off with a half truth. Drugs help, but without appropriate psychotherapy the job done is sloppy. As far as depression is concerned, a glass filled to the middle is half empty, not half full.

For too long, biological psychiatry has ignored psychological factors as a major jammer of the brain. Ignoring the mind as a substance *sui generis* is ignoring an essential ingredient of the human condition as well as an essential generator of the functioning brain. Hence, mind/brain relationships have to become an essential part of biological psychiatry.

Dr. Fink (1988) recently pleaded strongly for reintroduction of psychosocial considerations in psychiatry. He, however, sees "the psychosocial as the human element in disease and health," and that viewpoint I do not share. Psychosocial factors should be taken seriously in a scientific sense and be as much a subject of systematic scrutiny as biological factors. Going on to characterize, or better, to condemn, non-material factors as being the soft belly of medicine is doing serious injustice to their probably substantial pathogenic weight. The human element is indeed a serious matter in medicine. It is the emotional tone in which medical matters--research and health care--should be conducted. It pertains to a particular mind set and is not to be confused with scientific exploration of psychological and environmental determinants of physical and mental disorders.

I submitted in this treatise some of my professional concerns. Be convinced that I do not want to posture as an alarmist. As a psychiatrist, I am profoundly proud of the scientific achievements of our profession over the past three decades. I submit my concerns precisely for the reason that they seem to me roadblocks on the way ahead.

SUMMARY

The progress of psychiatry over the past few years is impressive. That process, however, is non-linear and I think that the three developments in depression research discussed in this paper are counter productive. First, the depression classification as institutionalized by the DSM-III is an unfocused and confusing one. The regular revisions, moreover, largely based on the opinions of experts rather than on the research by experts, add to the confusion. Second, the preoccupation of biological psychiatry with nosology is seen as a growth-inhibiting factor. The functional/dimensional approach searching for correlations between biological and psychological dysfunctions, an approach we have been advocating for many years, seems to have great potential and deserves to be included in mainstream biological psychiatry. Finally, the "biologization" of depression research went too far.

The conception of depression as a brain disease is a "terrible simplification," even for the syndrome considered to be the most "biological" of all: major depression, melancholic type. Psychological determinants of the brain dysfunctions underlying depressive disorders deserves as much scientific scrutiny as their biological counterparts. The mind should not be the soft belly of (biological) psychiatry.

REFERENCES

Ashton H (1987): Brain or systems disorders and psychotropic drugs. Oxford:Oxford University Press.

Asberg M, Traskman L, Thoren P (1976): 5-HIAA in the cerebrospinal fluid: a biochemical suicide predictor? Arch Gen Psychiatry 33:1193-1197

Banki CM (1977): Correlation of anxiety and related symptoms with cerebrospinal fluid 5-hydroxyindoleacetic acid in depressed women. J Neural Trans 41:135-143

Cohen LS, Winchel RM, Stanley M (1988): Biological markers of suicide risk and adolescent suicide. Clin Neuropharmacol 11:423-435

Crow TJ (1973): Catecholamine-containing neurones and electrical self-stimulation: 2. A theoretical interpretation and some psychiatric implications. Psychol Med 3:66-73.

Crow TJ (1977): A general catecholamine hypothesis. Neurosci Res Prog Bull 15:195-205

Crow TJ, Deakin JFW (1985): Neurohormonal transmission, behavior and mental disorder. In Shepherd M. (ed.), Handbook of Psychiatry Part 5. Cambridge: Cambridge University Press.

Evans L, Kenardy J, Schneider P, Hoey H (1986): Effect of a selective serotonin uptake inhibitor in agoraphobia with panic attacks. Acta Psychiatr Scand 73:49-53

Fink PJ (1988): Response to the Presidential Address. Is "biopsychosocial" the psychiatric shibboleth? Am J Psychiatry 195:1061-1067

Gardner CR (1988): Potential use of drugs modulating 5HT activity in the treatment of anxiety. Gen Pharmacol 19:347-356

Johnston AL, File SE (1986): 5-HT and anxiety: Promises and pitfalls. Pharmacol Biochem & Behavior 24:1467-1470

Jones BJ, Costall B, Domeney AM, Kelly ME, Naylor RJ, Oakley NR, Tyers MB (1988): The potential anxiolytic activity of GR38032F, a 5-HT_3-receptor antagonist. Br J Pharmacol 93:985-993

Kahn RS, van Praag HM (1988): A serotonin hypothesis of panic disorder. Human Psychopharm 3:285-288

Kahn RS, Wetzler S, van Praag HM, Asnis GM (1988a): Neuroendocrine evidence for 5-HT receptor hypersensitivity in patients with panic disorder. Psychopharmacol 96:360-364

Kahn R, Wetzler S, van Praag HM, Asnis GM, Strauman T (1988b): Behavioral indications for serotonin receptor hypersensitivity in panic disorder. Psychiatry Res 25:101-104

Kahn RS, Westenberg HGM, Verhoeven WMA, Gispen-de Wied CC, Kamerbeek WDJ (1987): Effect of a serotonin precursor and uptake inhibitor in anxiety disorders: a double-blind comparison of 5-hydroxytryptophan, clomipramine and placebo. Int Clin Psychopharm 2:33-45

Lakke JPWF, Korf J, van Praag HM, Schut T (1972): Predictive values of the probenecid test for the effect of l-DOPA therapy in Parkinson's disease. Nature 236:208-209

Ninan PT, van Kammen DP, Scheinin M, Linnoila M, Bunney WE, Goodwin FK (1984): CSF 5-hydroxyindoleacetic acid levels in suicidal schizophrenic patients. Am J Psychiatry 141:566-569

Pangalila-Ratu Langi EA, Jansen AAI (1988): Ritanserin in the treatment of generalized anxiety disorders: A placebo-controlled trial. Human Psychopharmacol 3:207-212

Roy A, Linnoila M (1988): Suicidal behavior, impulsiveness and serotonin. Acta Psychiatr Scand 78:529-535

Roy A, Adinoff B, Linnoila M (1988): Acting out hostility in normal volunteers: Negative correlation with levels of 5HIAA in cerebrospinal fluid. Psychiatry Res 24:187-194

Rydin E, Schalling D, Asberg M (1982): Rorschach ratings in depressed and suicidal patients with low CSF 5-HIAA. Psychiatry Res 7:229-243

Spitzer RL, Williams JBW (1988): Having a dream. Arch Gen Psychiatry 45:871-874

Stein L (1978): Reward transmitters: catecholamine and opioid peptides. In Lipton MA, DiMascio A, Killam KF (eds.), Psychopharmacology: A Generation of Progress. New York:Raven Press, pp, 569-581

Traskman L, Asberg M, Bertillson L, Sjostrand L (1981): Monoamine metabolites in CSF and suicidal behavior. Arch Gen Psychiatry 38:631-636

van Praag HM (1982): A transatlantic view of the diagnosis of depression according to the DSM-III. I. Controversies and misunderstandings in depression diagnosis. Compr Psychiatr 23:315-329

van Praag HM (1983): CSF 5-HIAA and suicide in non-depressed schizophrenics. Lancet ii:977-978

van Praag HM (1988): Serotonergic mechanisms and suicidal behavior. Psychiatr and Psychobiol 3:335-346

van Praag HM (1989): Diagnosing depression. Looking backward into the future. Psychiat Developm 4:375-394

van Praag HM, Leijnse B (1964): Die bedeutung der psychopharmakologie fur die klinische psychiatrie. Systematik als notwendiger ausgangspunkt. Nervenarzt 34:530-537

van Praag HM, Leijnse B (1965): Neubewertung des Syndroms. Skizze einer funktionellen Pathologie. Psychiatr Neurol Neurochir 68:50-66

van Praag HM, Korf J (1971): Retarded depression and the dopamine metabolism. Psychopharmacologia 19:199-203

van Praag HM, Lemus C (1986): Monoamine precursors in the treatment of psychiatric disorders. In: Wurtman RJ and Wurtman JJ (eds.), Nutrition and the brain. Raven Press, New York. Vol. 7, pp. 89-138

van Praag HM, Uleman AM, Spitz JC (1965): The vital syndrome interview. A structured standard interview for the recognition and registration of the vital depression symptom complex. Psychiatr Neurol Neurochir 68:329-346 van Praag HM, Korf J, Lakke JPWF, Schut T (1975): Dopamine metabolism in depression, psychoses and Parkinson's disease: the problem of the specificity of biological variables in behavioral disorders. Psychol Med 5:138-146

van Praag HM, Asnis GM, Brown SL, Korn M (1990a): Monoamines and abnormal behavior. A multidimensional perspective. Brit J Psychiat (In press)

van Praag HM, Asnis GM, Brown SL, Korn M, Harkavy Friedman JM, Wetzler S (1990b): Beyond serotonin. A multi-aminergic perspective on abnormal behavior. In: Brown SL, van Praag HM (eds.), Serotonin in psychiatric disorders. Brunner/Mazel, New York. (In press)

van Praag HM, Kahn RS, Asnis GM, Wetzler S, Brown SL, Bleich A, Korn ML (1987): Denosologization of biological psychiatry or the specificity of 5-HT disturbances in psychiatric disorders. J Affect Dis 13:1-8

Virkkunen M, Nuutila A, Goodwin FK, Linnoila M (1987): Cerebrospinal fluid monoamine metabolite levels in male arsonists. Arch Gen Psychiatry 44:241-247

Zimmerman M (1988): Why are we rushing to publish DSM-IV? Arch Gen Psychiatry 45:1135-1138

This chapter is reprinted by permission of Professor J. Mendlewicz, Brussels, Belgium. The article containing the same information and entitled "Moving ahead yet falling behind. A critical appraisal of some trends in contemporary depression research" was printed in the Journal of Neuropsychobiology.

chapter 4

Second Messenger Systems And Psychoactive Drug Action: Focus On The Phosphoinositide System And Lithium

Solomon H. Snyder, M.D., F.A.P.A.
Jay M. Baraban, M.D., Ph.D.
Paul F. Worley, M.D.

Most of the major drugs used in psychiatry were introduced some 3 decades ago. In intervening years much progress has been made in understanding their mode of action in eliciting both therapeutic and side effects. Essentially all of the known actions of psychotropic drugs involve a handful of neurotransmitter systems. Specific sites of action vary among the different drugs: influences are exerted on metabolic enzymes, storage processes in synaptic vesicles, release mechanisms, and neurotransmitter receptors. Thus, reserpine depletes biogenic amines from the brain by impairing their storage in synaptic vesicles. Monoamine oxidase inhibitors block a key metabolic enzyme. Amphetamines enhance the release of catecholamines, and nearly all tricyclic antidepressants inhibit the reuptake inactivation of biogenic amines.

During the past 15 years, the ability to measure drug and neurotransmitter receptors by simple binding techniques (first developed for studies of opiate receptors) has helped clarify actions of numerous drugs (1). Blockade of the D_2 subtype of dopamine receptors may account for the therapeutic action of a wide range of antipsychotic agents (2,3). The same drugs appear to exert their sedative effects by blocking α_1 adrenoceptors (4). The tendency of drugs in this group to elicit extrapyramidal side effects varies inversely with their muscarinic cholinergic antagonist potency (5). Psychedelic drugs appear to act primarily by mimicking serotonin at one class of serotonin receptors, the 5-HT_2 subtype (6-8).

Recently, increased attention has been devoted to amino acid neurotransmitters as sites of psychotropic drug action. Benzodiazepines have long been known to act by facilitating synaptic effects of γ-aminobutyric acid (GABA) (9). This action involves subtle interactions

Psychiatry: Past Reflections–Future Visions
B.T. Taylor and I.J. Taylor, Editors

between subunits of the GABA receptor that have been characterized in detail by molecular cloning studies (10). GABA and benzodiazepines bind to different sites and possibly different subunits of the receptor protein. The binding of benzodiazepines increases the ability of GABA to interact with its recognition site. Barbiturates, meprobamate, and alcohol all appear to act through the GABA receptor protein complex but at different sites than the benzodiazepines or GABA itself. In contrast to these sedating and anticonvulsant drugs, agents that block GABA receptors cause excitation and convulsions. This is true for bicuculline which blocks the GABA recognition site. The convulsant picrotoxin blocks GABA transmission but not at the GABA recognition site. Instead, picrotoxin acts at a site related to the chloride ion channel portion of the GABA receptor protein. GABA exerts its inhibitory, hyperpolarizing synaptic effects by opening chloride ion channels in synaptic membranes. Interestingly, the chloride ion channel is part of the same receptor protein complex as the GABA recognition site. Molecular cloning studies have shown that the nicotinic acetylcholine receptor and its associated cation channel are also part of the same protein complex (11) as the inhibitory glycine receptor and its chloride ion channel (12).

These GABA, glycine, and acetylcholine receptors represent a group of neurotransmitter receptors that directly influence ion channels. Many other neurotransmitters, perhaps the majority of the biogenic amines and neuropeptides, act through biochemical second messenger systems that enzymatically amplify the signal generated by the neurotransmitter-receptor binding events. Following a chain of molecular events, neurotransmitters that act through these second messengers may ultimately open or close ion channels in the plasma membrane or influence neuronal excitability through other intracellular metabolic events. During the past 15 years, neurotransmitter receptors have been extensively characterized at a molecular level and the drug actions mediated by these receptors have been thoroughly explored. Recent progress in understanding second messenger systems has clarified our understanding of neurotransmitter actions and focused attention on these systems as sites of psychotropic drug action.

This review will emphasize the phosphoinositide system, a major second messenger system in the brain, which has been extensively elucidated only in the last few years and which may be involved in the therapeutic actions of lithium. To introduce several general features of second messenger systems, we will also outline briefly the organization of the cAMP system and focus on the role of GTP binding proteins that form the interface between transmitter receptors and both the phosphoinositide and cAMP systems.

cAMP AND GTP BINDING PROTEINS

Second messenger systems are triggered by neurotransmittei receptor stimulation (see figure 1). The transmitter-receptor complex then interacts with a GTP binding protein, usually designated as a G-protein. Interaction of the G-protein with the receptor increases its affinity for GTP. For the cAMP system, activation of the G-protein in this manner enables it to dissociate from the receptor and stimulate the enzyme adenylate cyclase, enhancing synthesis of cAMP from ATP. In turn, cAMP activates a phosphorylating enzyme called cAMP-dependent protein kinase or simply protein kinase A. This kinase then phosphorylates a wide range of substrate proteins that regulate diverse cellular function.

Some transmitters, such as catecholamines acting at β-adrenoceptors, stimulate adenylate cyclase, while others, such as enkephalin acting at opiate receptors, inhibit the enzyme. Distinct G-proteins mediate these two effects, G_s for stimulation and G_i for inhibition of adenylate cyclase (13). These differential effects involve the subunits of G-proteins. G-proteins consist of three subunits, designated alpha, beta, and gamma (14). Adenylate cyclase is directly activated by the alpha subunit of G_s. When alpha is bound to beta and gamma subunits, the G-protein is inactive. When the transmitter-receptor complex binds to the G-protein, GTP is enabled to interact potently with the G-protein, triggering dissociation of the beta and gamma subunits from the G_s protein. The resultant free alpha subunit then activates adenylate cyclase. At this point the alpha subunit, which also possesses intrinsic GTPase activity, cleaves GTP to GDP, whereupon the beta and gamma subunits reassociate with the alpha subunit, terminating activation of adenylate cyclase.

The way in which G_i inhibits adenylate cyclase has not been established definitively. However, one prominent model suggests that the initial events parallel activation of G_s and that the beta and gamma subunits dissociate from the alpha subunit when neurotransmitter receptor activation takes place. However, since the concentration of G_i is substantially greater than G_s, the beta and gamma subunits released from G_i are free to complex with the alpha subunit of G_s, preventing it from stimulating adenylate cyclase. Thus, transmitters that inhibit adenylate cyclase may do so indirectly, by preventing the activation of the enzyme by G_s. Another model suggests that the alpha subunit of G_i directly inhibits adenylate cyclase (14).

Besides regulating adenylate cyclase activity, G-proteins can directly influence ion channels. In the heart, acetylcholine through muscarinic receptors slows pacemeker cell firing by opening potassium channels. Patch-clamp recordings of individual potassium channels in the heart indicate that a unique G-protein, designated G_k, opens potassium

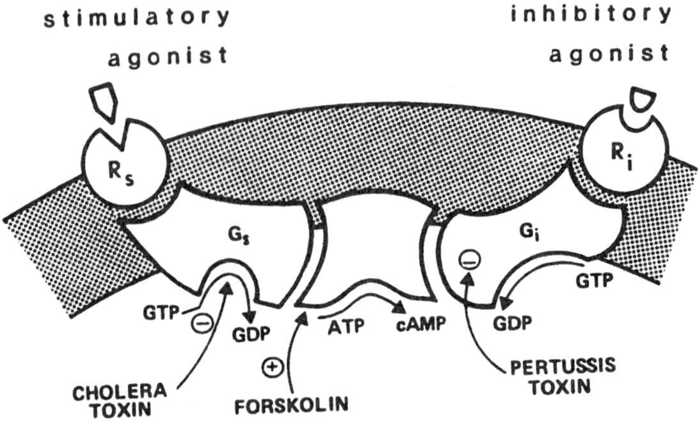

[a]A stimulatory agonist is recognized by a receptor (R_s), and together they activate the stimulatory GTP-binding regulatory unit for adenylate cyclase (G_s). Activation of G_s is associated with its binding of GTP, which displaces GDP. A parallel system is shown as inhibiting adenylate cyclase by activating the inhibitory regulatory unit for adenylate cyclase (G_i). Cholera toxin blocks the GTPase activity of G_s, causing its persistent activation. Pertussis toxin blocks the inhibitory action of G_i. At low concentrations, forskolin enhances the stimulatory interaction of G_s and adenylate cyclase; at higher concentrations, forskolin directly activates adenylate cyclase.

FIGURE 1. Bidirectional Regulation of Adenylate Cyclase[a]

channels without any other intervening metabolic steps (15, 16). Similarly, G-proteins may directly affect calcium channels in certain cell types in the dorsal root ganglion (17, 18). The alpha subunit of the G-protein is thought to interact with the ion channels and the beta and gamma subunits are thought to serve only to inactivate alpha subunits. However, some recent studies suggested that beta subunits can themselves have direct messenger functions at potassium channels (19) or at the prostaglandin precursor, forming enzyme phospholipase A_2 (20).

Besides the three G-proteins already mentioned (G_s, G_i, and G_k), molecular cloning techniques have revealed at least four others and many more may exist (21). One reason researchers formerly doubted the feasibility of drugs targeted at second messenger systems is that only a few principal second messenger systems have been identified, in contrast to the hundred or more distinct neurotransmitters and receptors. If only two or three second messenger systems mediate the bulk of neurotransmitter actions, drugs acting through second messengers might exert diffuse, global effects that would not be therapeutically useful. However, the considerable heterogeneity of the G-proteins and other aspects of second messengers suggest that selective drugs can be developed.

Improved understanding of the different G-proteins may indicate how they affect different brain functions discretely. The three best studied G-proteins in the brain are G_s, G_i, and G_o, a protein whose function is not yet known. Although G_s has been best characterized, it is least abundant, present at only half the levels of G_i and one-tenth the levels of G_o (22). Discrete localizations throughout the brain of G-proteins and other components of second messenger systems, to be discussed below, have considerably clarified these functions.

Although no therapeutic drugs have yet emerged in the cAMP system, some agents provide useful research probes. Forskolin is an al-

FIGURE 2. The Multiple Actions of Individual Neurotransmitters on Second Messenger Systems[a]

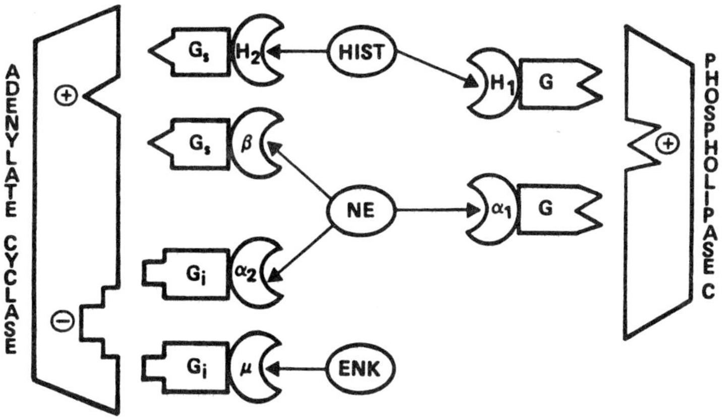

[a]These actions are carried out by their receptor subtypes, which are coupled with specific G-proteins. Histamine (HIST) stimulates adenylate cyclase by acting at H_2 receptors coupled to its stimulatory G-protein (G_s). Histamine also stimulates phospholipase C of the phosphoinositide second messenger system by acting at H_1 receptors linked to a distinct G-protein. Similarly, norepinephrine (NE) can stimulate (β receptor) or inhibit (α_2 receptor) adenylate cyclase or stimulate (α_1 receptor) phospholipase C. Conversely, each G-protein pool is coupled to several receptor subtypes: G_s is coupled to H_2 and β receptors, and the inhibitory G-protein for adenylate cyclase (G_i) is coupled to α_2 receptors and μ-opiate receptors (one of the enkephalin [ENK] receptor subtypes). An as yet unidentified G-protein (G) couples H_1 receptors and α_1 receptors to phospholipase C.

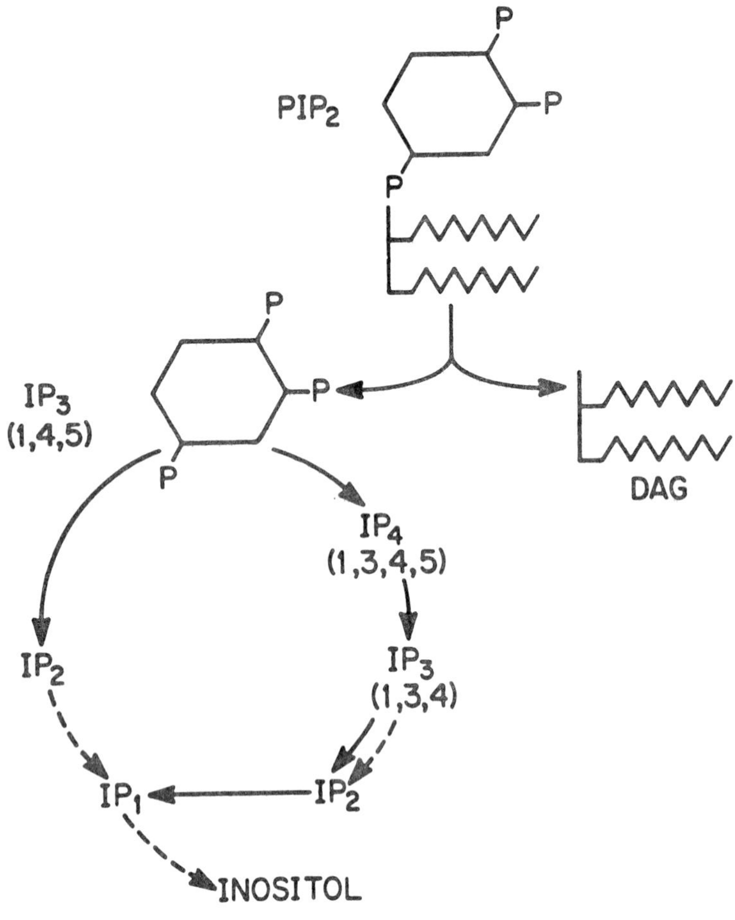

[a]Phosphatidylinositol-bis-phosphate (PIP_2) is hydrolyzed by phospholipase C, generating diacylglycerol (DAG) and inositol 1,4,5-trisphosphate (IP_3[1,4,5]). IP_3(1,4,5) is acted on by either a kinase or a phosphatase, generating 1,3,4,5-tetrakisphosphate (IP_4[1,3,4,5]) or inositol 1,4-bis-phosphate (IP_2[1,4]), respectively. IP_4 (1,3,4,5) is hydrolyzed to IP_3(1,3,4) and then to IP_2. Specific phosphatases hydrolyze the various IP_2 isomers to inositol. Several inositol phosphatases are inhibited by lithium. These are shown as dotted arrows. In some steps both lithium-sensitive and lithium-insensitive enzymes are involved (27) so both solid and dotted arrows are shown.

FIGURE 3. Inositol Phosphate Metabolism[a]

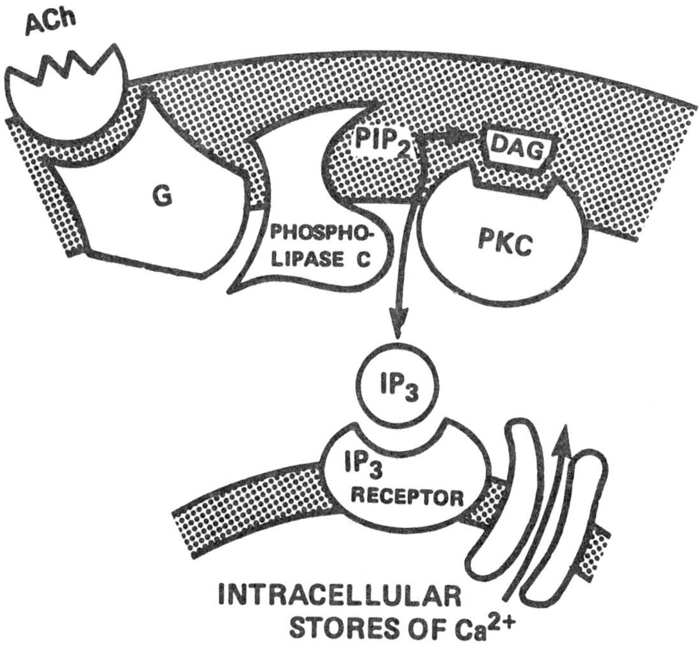

[a]A transmitter such as acetylcholine (ACh) binds to its receptor, which in turn activates a G-protein (G). Activated G-protein stimulates phospholipase C, which hydrolyzes phosphatidylinositol-bisphosphate (PIP_2), generating inositol trisphosphate (IP_3) and diacylglycerol (DAG). IP_3 interacts with a specific receptor and causes the release of nonmitochondrial intracellular stores of calcium. DAG activates protein kinase C (PKC), which phosphorylates a broad range of substrates. Like DAG, phorbol esters activate PKC.

FIGURE 4. Receptor-Mediated Phosphoinositide Turnover[a]

kaloid extracted from an Indian herb, *Coleus forskohlii*, which has been used for centuries to treat heart disease, insomnia, and convulsions. Forskolin potently activates adenylate cyclase (23), so that biological functions influenced by forskolin are candidates for being mediated by cAMP. Cholera toxin irreversibly activates adenylate cyclase by selectively modifying G_s enzymatically. By contrast, pertussis toxin selectively modifies G_i and G_o but not G_s (14).

THE PHOSPHOINOSITIDE SYSTEM

In contrast to the more than three decades of research on the cAMP system, the phosphoinositide cycle has been widely appreciated as a major second messenger system only in the past 5 years (24-26). The two systems display several similarities. They both work through G-proteins as well as phosphorylating enzymes. Both display considerable heterogeneity in their individual molecular components, so that subtle regulation in discrete parts of the brain are achievable.

A variety of receptors can trigger the phosphoinositide cycle. It is difficult to tabulate those neurotransmitters which act through adenylate cyclase versus those which act through phosphoinositides because most neurotransmitters act through both. The discrimination comes in the receptor subtypes involved. For instance, norepinephrine acting at β-adrenoceptors stimulates adenylate cyclase, but norepinephrine inhibits the enzyme through α_2 adrenoceptors and stimulates the phosphoinositide cycle through α_1 receptors (see figure 2).

Receptor stimulation activates a phospholipase C enzyme selective for phosphatidylinositol and phosphorylated derivatives of this lipid. Phosphatidylinositol, which contains one phosphate group, is a major component of cell membranes. The phospholipid that appears to play a more prominent role as a second messenger contains an additional two phosphate groups and is termed phosphatidylinositol-bis-phosphate (PIP_2) (see figures 3 and 4). Phospholipase C triggers the breakdown of PIP_2 to the sugar phosphate inositol trisphosphate (IP_3), which contains the three phosphate groups of PIP_2. The other product of phospholipase activity is diacylglycerol (DAG). This action of phospholipase C requires a G-protein whose identity has not yet been established definitively.

Both IP_3 and DAG influence cellular function in major ways. IP_3 binds to a unique receptor on the endoplasmic reticulum within the cell to trigger the release of calcium, which in turn can regulate cell function in many different ways. Thus, the IP_3 receptor is thought to be a crucial final common pathway for the phosphoinositide cycle. The IP_3 receptor represents a novel extension of the "receptor" concept because it is an intracellular recognition site in a second messenger system rather than a binding site for a neurotransmitter localized to the external surface of the plasma membrane. We (28,29) and others (30) have been able to label IP_3 receptors through the binding of radiolabeled IP_3. We have purified the IP_3 receptor protein to homogeneity (31). The IP_3 receptor is a large protein comprising four identical subunits each of a molecular weight of about 260,000 daltons so that the full protein has a molecular weight greater than 1,000,000 daltons. When it occurs in intact membranes, binding of IP_3 to its receptors is potently inhibited by calcium in the submicromolar concentrations that normally occur within cells (see figure 5). This suggests a feedback mechanism whereby calcium released by IP_3 acts back on the IP_3 receptor to block further calcium release. The ability of calcium to inhibit IP_3 binding is mediated by a protein that is distinct from the IP_3 receptor, designated

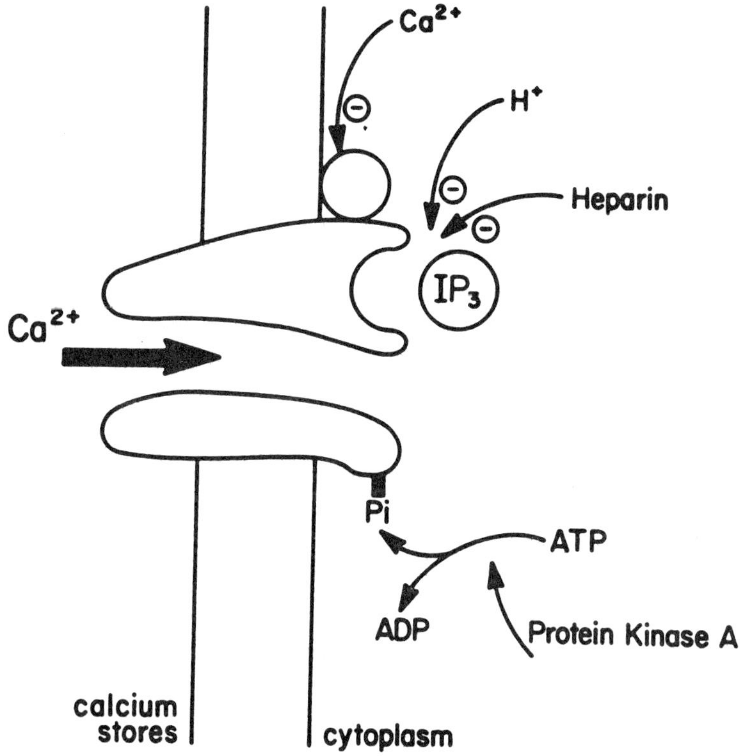

[a]Inositol trisphosphate (IP_3) binds to a high-affinity binding site on the cytoplasmic face of the IP_3 receptor, which is shown as a membrane-spanning protein containing a channel for passage of calcium out of intracellular stores. Binding of IP_3 to the receptor is inhibited by heparin in a competitive fashion and enhanced at slightly alkaline pH. Inhibition of IP_3 binding by calcium appears to be mediated by a distinct membrane-associated protein. Activation of the cAMP-dependent protein kinase leads to phosphorylation of the receptor protein.

FIGURE 5. Schematic Model of IP_3 Receptor Regulation[a]

"calmedin" (32). We suspect that calmedin may be an important intracellular protein regulating numerous actions of calcium, perhaps in ways similar to the well-characterized calcium binding protein calmodulin.

The IP_3 receptor is selectively phosphorylated by cAMP-dependent protein kinase decreasing the potency of IP_3 in releasing calcium (33). This suggests a specific mechanism for "cross talk" between the cAMP and the phosphoinositide second messenger systems. In other words, cAMP formed in response to neurotransmitter action would modulate the actions of transmitters that act through the phosphoinositide system by phosphorylating the IP_3 receptor and altering its function.

IP_3 formed by hydrolysis of PIP_2 can be phosphorylated further to inositol 1,3,4,5-tetrakisphosphate (IP_4) (34,35). The exact function of IP_4 is not as well characterized as that of IP_3. IP_4 may facilitate the entry of calcium into the cell through the plasma membrane possibly directly into a pool of calcium that is susceptible to release by IP_3. Alternatively, IP_4 may trigger a movement of calcium within the cell into IP_3-releasable pools (36). Recently, inositol 1,3,4,5,6-pentakisphosphate (IP_5) has been demonstrated in rat brains and shown to have pharmacological actions, suggesting a neurotransmitter role (37).

DAG represents the second "limb" of the phosphoinositide system. Elegant studies by Nishizuka (38) have clarified the biological role of DAG, which involves the activation of protein kinase C. Protein kinase C is a phosphorylating enzyme that is dependent on calcium and phospholipids for its activity and is distinct from protein kinase A, the cAMP-dependent protein kinase. Protein kinase C within the cytoplasm moves to the cell membrane when calcium is elevated within the cell, in part by IP_3-induced release of calcium, or with a rise in DAG, a lipophilic chemical that remains in the cell membrane after its formation from membrane phosphoinositides. DAG activates protein kinase C by enhancing its sensitivity to activation by calcium ions.

Among the numerous proteins that can be phosphorylated by protein kinase C are proteins involved in signal transduction. These substrates include receptors for a wide variety of signaling molecules such as those for acetylcholine, insulin, and epidermal growth factor, transmitter-synthesizing enzymes such as tyrosine hydroxylase, and certain G-proteins such as G_i (38-40).

Protein kinase C exerts prominent feedback effects on several aspects of the phosphoinositide system. It inhibits the ability of transmitters to produce IP_3 (41,42). In addition, protein kinase C phosphorylates the IP_3 phosphatase enzyme which degrades IP_3 and, thus, increases its enzyme activity (43,44). Protein kinase C even phosphorylates itself, enhancing its sensitivity to calcium, thus producing a feed-forward regulation of its own activity (45).

A direct role for protein kinase C in neurotransmitter actions has been established in various excitable tissues. In our own laboratory, we first showed protein kinase C to regulate cholinergic mechanisms in smooth muscle (46). In the hippocampus, protein kinase C activation blocks a calcium-activated potassium channel, which leads to increased neuronal excitability (47). Protein kinase C also blocks the prominent inhibitory actions of several neurotransmitters, such as serotonin and adenosine (48). The effects of protein kinase C on calcium-activated potassium channels (49) and on adenosine inhibition are also produced by acetylcholine acting through muscarinic receptors. Thus, these effects of acetylcholine presumably involve the phosphoinositide system and protein kinase C.

HETEROGENEOUS LOCALIZATION OF SECOND MESSENGER SYSTEMS IN THE BRAIN

Since the major second messenger systems interact with many of the same neurotransmitters, one would tend to assume that the two systems are ubiquitously distributed throughout the brain. However, although a given second messenger might be present in virtually every cell in the brain, its levels may be orders of magnitude greater in some than in others. Moreover, the existence of multiple subtypes for the various proteins involved in each second messenger system provides other opportunities for regional variations. Molecular cloning techniques have revealed marked biochemical heterogeneity of key components of the phosphoinositide system: seven distinct protein kinase C enzyme subtypes and five phospholipase C have been identified (50,51). Differences in their localization, and potential differences in their regulation, may provide yet another means for selective drug action on the phosphoinositide system. Direct investigations have supported the existence of regional specificity and have identified substantial differences in the localizations of components in both the cAMP and phosphoinositide systems.

We localized adenylate cyclase throughout the brain by using ^{3}H-forskolin, which binds to the enzyme selectively (52). Forskolin binding was localized by autoradiography, a technique in which the radioactive agent bound to thin frozen sections of the brain is visualized. In this technique sections are exposed to photographic emulsion so that development of silver grains occurs wherever the radioactive probe is bound to receptors. We observed striking differences among brain regions. Densities of adenylate cyclase in the caudate and olfactory tubercle were much greater than they were in most other brain areas. In these areas, the adenylate cyclase was contained in the cell bodies of neurons that descend to terminate in the substantia nigra, since lesions of the caudate abolished forskolin binding in the substantia nigra. These cells are recipients of the largest dopamine neuronal input in the brain. Since D_1 dopamine receptors, which are linked to adenylate cyclase activity, are also concentrated in these areas, the high levels of adenylate cyclase in the caudate olfactory tubercle are probably linked to dopamine receptors.

Several different elements of the phosphoinositide system have been localized in the brain. Our first studies visualized protein kinase C throughout the brain by autoradiography using a tritiated phorbol ester. Phorbol esters are chemicals extracted from croton oil that trigger inflammation and promote tumor development in extremely low concentrations (53). Phorbol esters bind to and activate protein kinase C in similarly low concentrations (54-56). We found striking differences in the densities of protein kinase C throughout the brain (52,57). In addition, the anatomical pattern observed for protein kinase C differs greatly from the localization of adenylate cyclase.

Recent studies revealed differences in the localizations of subtypes of protein kinase C (50). Four of the seven subtypes of protein kinase C have been physically separated and measured in different areas of the brain. mRNAs for three types of protein kinase C have also been visualized by *in situ* hybridization showing differential distribution of the different subtypes among neuronal populations.

At least four distinct forms of phospholipase C have been separated and molecularly cloned (51, 58, 59). We have visualized and localized mRNA for these four enzyme subtypes by *in situ* hybridization, which has revealed strikingly distinct localizations that correlate with specific neurotransmitter receptors (60). For instance, mRNA for the enzyme form designated type A (60) or form I (51) is selectively concentrated in the choroid plexus and the serotonin-containing raphe nuclei, implying a link to serotonin 5-HT-lc receptors (60). This same enzyme subtype is localized to Purkinje cells of the cerebellum, where it presumably mediates the major glutaminergic synaptic input to Purkinje cells from the granule cells (61).

We do not fully understand the functional implications of high levels of adenylate cyclase and phosphoinositide system markers in particular neuronal populations. Nevertheless, by reflecting on the maps of localizations of the two second messenger systems, it might be possible to conceptualize characteristics of brain function that are attributable to one or the other system. For example, since protein kinase C has been implicated in certain forms of synaptic plasticity (i.e., long-term changes in synaptic responses), neurons containing high levels of this pathway may be more versatile in regulating their excitability. Conceivably, insights into the response characteristics of brain systems will be possible by focusing on their repertoire of second messengers.

Within the phosphoinositide system, protein kinase C represents one limb that may be quite distinct from the inositol phosphate component. Therefore, although the activity of phospholipase C on PIP_2 generates both DAG and IP_3, DAG may be formed to a much greater extent from phosphatidylinositol or other phospholipids such as phosphatidylcholine, which occur in very high levels in the brain, than from PIP_2, whose levels are much lower. IP_3, on the other hand, can be derived only from PIP_2. To obtain insight into possible differences in the disposition of the IP_3 and DAG limbs of the phosphoinositide cycle, we localized IP_3 receptors by autoradiography (29, 62).

In general, IP_3 receptors show a similar distribution to that of protein kinase C. For instance, both protein kinase C and IP_3 receptors occur in neurons projecting from the caudate to the substantia nigra and in Purkinje cells of the cerebellum. However, there are some marked regional variations in relative abundance. In the cerebellum, concentrations of protein kinase C and IP3 receptors are similar. However, in the cerebral cortex and corpus striatum, protein kinase C densities are about 10 times those of IP_3 receptors. Even more dramatic, the substantia gelatinosa of the spinal cord, where sensory afferent fibers terminate, displays an extremely dense band of protein kinase C but is devoid of IP_3 receptors. Similarly, the external plexiform layer of the olfactory bulb, which contains synaptic interactions of incoming olfactory neurons, possesses very high densities of protein kinase C without detectable IP_3 receptors. Accordingly, in these latter two regions it is likely that DAG is formed from phosphatidylinositol with no substantial formation of IP_3 and few IP_3 receptors.

Using antibodies raised against the purified IP_3 receptor protein, we have successfully visualized IP_3 receptors by immunohistochemistry (C. Ross, personal communication). Localization at the light microscopic level reveals essentially the same distributions of IP_3 receptors as were observed by autoradiography with ^3H-IP_3. At the electron microscopic level, IP_3 receptors can be localized intracellularly to a discrete part of the endoplasmic reticulum, confirming earlier studies that this intracellular compartment contains IP_3-sensitive stores of calcium.

LITHIUM: POTENTIAL ACTIONS THROUGH INOSITOL PHOSPHATASES AND G-PROTEINS

Clarifying the therapeutic actions of lithium in psychiatry has proved far more difficult than for many other psychotropic drugs. There are several reasons. Most drugs occur in homologous series of chemical structures that vary in their therapeutic potencies. If a molecular action shows a similar variation, one can feel more confident with a relationship between the biochemical and therapeutic effects. For example, the close correlation between blockade of dopamine D_2 receptors and therapeutic potency in a large series of neuroleptics established a convincing link between dopamine receptor blockade and antipsychotic activity (2, 3). In the case of lithium no such series exists.

Lithium is also intrinsically difficult to understand, since it often relieves both manic and depressive symptoms as well as prevents recurrence of both poles of manic-depressive illness. One can readily conceptualize how a drug such as a neuroleptic can influence receptors for a given neurotransmitter to diminish manic symptoms. Similarly, facilitating the actions of certain biogenic amines may explain antidepressant drug effects. In theory, one might postulate that lithium exerts separate and distinct actions on different neurotransmitter systems to relieve mania or depression. However, abundant clinical evidence suggests that the effects of lithium on the two poles of the illness involve similar mechanisms, since they seem to go hand in hand in individual patients and across patient groups. Indeed, the action of lithium is usually regarded as a "normalizing" effect, preventing excessive excursion away from a euthymic mood level (63).

Actions on a second messenger system might well explain the normalizing effects of lithium on mood. One neurotransmitter system might be hyperactive in mania and another one hyperactive in depression. Through a second messenger system, lithium could block movements of either neurotransmitter system into a hyperactive state. Since second messenger systems are intimately involved in mediating neuronal responsiveness to monoamine and cholinergic systems hypothesized to be involved in affective disorders (64), actions of lithium on the phosphoinositide system and on G-proteins discussed later in this paper may be relevant.

One aspect of the phosphoinositide metabolism not reviewed until now has been the mechanism whereby the phosphate groups are sequentially removed from inositol phosphates (see figure 3). IP_3 (1,4,5) is inactivated by a phosphatase that removes the phosphate in position 5. IP_4 is also metabolized by a phosphatase that removes the 5 phosphate. This gives rise to an isomer of IP_3, IP_3 (1,3,4), which is different from the active IP_3 (1,4,5). The IP_3 (1,3,4) has no known biological activity and is thought merely to be a breakdown product. It is metabolized further to isomers of IP_2 that are distinct from that formed from the breakdown of IP_3 (1,4,5). All of the various IP_2 isomers are metabolized to corresponding isomers of IP_1, and these in turn are degraded to free inositol. Inositol is then attached to phosphatidic acid to form phosphatidylinositol. Phosphatidylinositol is then sequentially phosphorylated to PIP_2.

A team of investigators at Washington University beginning in 1971 showed that lithium administration to rats depletes brain levels of inositol due to an increase in IP_1 levels, which in turn derives from a selective inhibition of the IP_1 phosphatase (65,66). With the emergence of the phosphoinositide cycle as a second messenger system, Berridge et al. (67) suggested that lithium's psychoactive effects involve depletion of inositol to slow down the phosphoinositide cycle by preventing the formation of PIP_2 and thereafter IP_3. The extent of "shortfall" of inositol mediators would be proportional to the overall activity of the cycle. One would predict a dampening of synaptic activity associated with the phosphoinositide cycle, particularly for those synaptic systems which are overactive. This formulation would fit nicely with the types of effects needed to explain the normalizing action of lithium.

Studies measuring the biochemical turnover of phosphoinositides and levels of inositol phosphates as a function of lithium treatment have provided evidence that lithium clearly affects inositol phosphate metabolism (68-75). To assess the physiological significance of these observations, we felt it would be important to investigate a synaptic system in the brain directly to determine whether therapeutic concentrations of lithium would influence synaptic activity in the predicted direction.

We took advantage of the system whereby acetylcholine, through muscarinic cholinergic receptors, activates phosphoinositide turnover in slices of the hippocampus (48). In this system, cholinergic agonists that act through the phosphoinositide cycle block synaptic inhibition caused by adenosine. This effect involves protein kinase C because it is mimicked faithfully by phorbol esters.

In this model system, we elicited cholinergic stimulation by applying the cholinergic agonist carbachol and demonstrated that therapeutic concentrations of lithium impair the ability of carbachol to block adenosine (76). The effect of lithium was apparent at 0.5 mM and near maximal at 1 mM of lithium, corresponding to therapeutic concentrations. We observed ionic selectivity, since rubidium had no effect. If lithium were to act by affecting phosphoinositide turnover, this effect should occur before protein kinase C activation. We would predict that lithium should not block the effects of phorbol esters. Indeed, at a time when carbachol effects were abolished by lithium, phorbol esters still reversed the effect of adenosine.

In an earlier study we showed that therapeutic concentrations of lithium influenced neurotransmitter-induced smooth muscle contraction elicited by histamine or cholinergic receptors by acting through the phosphoinositide cycle in smooth muscle (77). This result may also reflect a diminished activation of protein kinase C.

The changes in synaptic transmission we observed with lithium certainly take place through the phosphoinositide system. However, we do not have any direct evidence that inhibition of inositol phosphatases is the mechanism involved. An alternative way in which one could influence the phosphoinositide or other second messenger systems would be through G-proteins. If lithium were to diminish the coupling between G-proteins and receptors, it would also dampen excessive excursion of synaptic transmission involving any transmitter that acts through G-proteins. Avissar et al. (78) have obtained evidence for this type of action. They measured the interactions between receptors and G-proteins in two ways. In one system they measured the ability of carbachol or the β-adrenergic agonist isoproterenol to influence ^{3}H-GTP binding to brain membranes. In another, they monitored the influence of GTP on the competition by muscarinic agonists for radioligand binding to muscarinic cholinergic receptors. In this system, GTP acting through a G-protein decreased the potency of agonists in competing for receptor binding. Using both systems, lithium decreased apparent interactions of neurotransmitter receptors with G-proteins. Similar results were evident in intact rats administered lithium for 12-21 days to produce therapeutic blood levels of 0.6-1.0 mM. These results suggest that lithium interferes with the activity of G-proteins, perhaps by competing with magnesium ions, which are essential for the binding of GTP to G-proteins. Recent studies indicate that lithium's effect on G-proteins may influence phospholipase C activity (79,80).

These animal studies raise the possibility that effects of lithium on second messenger systems, such as the phosphoinositide system, may contribute to the therapeutic effects of lithium. This suggestion can be tested directly. One could design a series of organic chemical drug-like structures that potently inhibit IP_1 phosphatase or phospholipase C. Such agents may have the therapeutic benefits of lithium but without the substantial toxicity that comes from lithium's ionic competition with sodium.

In summary, molecular characterization of second messenger systems has advanced greatly in the last few years. Like the great multiplicity of neurotransmitters and their receptors, second messenger systems, especially the phosphoinositide system, display marked heterogeneity with multiple subtypes of regulatory proteins. It is likely that new psychoactive agents will emerge from the tailoring of molecules for proteins that are key components of these second messenger systems. Studies of the actions of lithium already suggest promising directions.

ACKNOWLEDGEMENT

This chapter is adapted from an article in the *American Journal of Psychiatry*, 146:10, October 1989.

REFERENCES

1. Snyder SH: Drugs and neurotransmitter receptors in the brain. Science 1984; 224:22-31

2. Seeman P, Lee T, Chau-Wong M, et al: Antipsychotic drug doses and neuroleptic/dopamine receptors. Nature 1976; 262:717-719
3. Creese I, Burt DR, Snyder SH: Dopamine receptor binding predicts clinical and pharmacological potencies of antischizophrenic drugs. Science 1976; 192:481-483
4. Peroutka SJ, U'Prichard D, Greenberg DA, et al: Neuroleptic drug interactions with norepinephrine alpha receptor binding sites in rat brain. Neuropharmacology 1977; 16:549-556
5. Snyder SH, Greenberg D, Yamamura HI: Antischizophrenic drugs and brain cholinergic receptors. Arch Gen Psychiatry 1974; 31:58-61
6. Glennon RA, Titeler M, McKenney JD: Evidence for 5-HT_2 receptor involvement in the mechanism of action of hallucinogenic agents. Life Sci 1984; 35:2205-2211
7. Titeler M, Lyon RA, Glennon RA: Radioligand binding evidence implicates the brain 5-HT_2 receptor as a site of action for LSD and phenylisopropylamine hallucinogens. Psychopharmacology (Berlin) 1988; 94:213-216
8. Rasmussen K, Aghajanian GK: Effect of hallucinogens on spontaneous and sensory-evoked locus coeruleus unit activity in the rat: reversal by selective 5-HT_2 antagonists. Brain Res 1986; 385:395-400
9. Tallman JF, Gallager DW: The GABAergic system: a locus of benzodiazepine action. Annu Rev Neurosci 1985; 8:21-44
10. Schofield PR, Darlison MG, Fujita N, et al: Sequence and functional expression of the $GABA_A$ receptor shows a ligand-gated receptor super-family. Nature 1987; 328:221-227
11. Noda M, Takahashi H, Tanabe T, et al: Structural homology of Torpedo californica acetylcholine receptor subunits. Nature 1983; 302:528-532
12. Grenningloh G, Rienitz A, Schmitt B, et al: The strychnine-binding subunit of the glycine receptor shows homology with nicotinic acetylcholine receptors. Nature 1987; 328:215-220
13. Schramm M, Selinger Z: Message transmission: receptor controlled adenylate cyclase system. Science 1984; 225:1350-1356
14. Gilman AG: G proteins: transducers of receptor-generated signals. Annu Rev Biochem 1987; 56:615-649
15. Pfaffinger PJ, Martin JM, Hunter DD, et al: GTP-binding proteins couple cardiac muscarinic receptors to a K channel. Nature 1985; 317:536-538
16. Breitwieser GE, Szabo G: Uncoupling of cardiac muscarinic and B-adrenergic receptors from ion channels by a guanine nucleotide analogue. Nature 1985; 317:538-540
17. Holz GG, Rane SG, Dunlap K: GTP-binding proteins mediate transmitter inhibition of voltage-dependent calcium channels. Nature 1986; 319: 670-672

18. Dolphin AC: Nucleotide binding proteins in signal transduction and disease. Trends in Neurosciences 1987; 10:53-57
19. Logothetis DE, Kurachi Y, Galper J, et al: The beta gamma subunits of GTP-binding proteins activate the muscarinic K^+ channel in heart. Nature 1987; 325:321-326
20. Axelrod J, Burch RM, Jelsema CL: Receptor-mediated activation of phospholipase A_2 via GTP-binding proteins: arachidonic acid and its metabolites as second messengers. Trends in Neurosciences 1988; 11: 117-123
21. Itoh H, Kozasa T, Nagata S, et al: Molecular cloning and sequence determination of cDNAs for alpha subunits of the guanine nucleotide-binding proteins G_s, G_i, G_o from rat brain. Proc Natl Acad Sci USA 1986; 83:3776-3780
22. Neer EJ, Lok JM, Wolf LG: Purification and properties of the inhibitory guanine nucleotide regulatory unit of brain adenylate cyclase. J Biol Chem 1984; 259:14222-14229
23. Seamon KB, Padgett W, Daly JW: Forskolin: unique diterpene activator of adenylate cyclase in membranes and in intact cells. Proc Natl Acad Sci USA 1981; 78:3363-3367
24. Berridge MJ: Inositol trisphosphate and diacylglycerol as second messengers. Biochem J 1984; 220:345-360
25. Berridge MJ, Irvine RF: Inositol Trisphosphate, a novel second messenger in cellular signal transduction. Nature 1984; 312:315-321
26. Hokin LE: Receptors and phosphoinositide-generated second messengers. Annu Rev Biochem 1985; 54:205-235
27. Majerus PW, Connolly TM, Bansal VS, et al: Inositol phosphates: synthesis and degradation. J Biol Chem 1988; 263:3051-3054
28. Worley PF, Baraban JM, Supattapone S, et al: Characterization of inositol trisphosphate receptor binding in brain: regulation by pH and calcium. J Biol Chem 1987; 262:12132-12136
29. Worley PF, Baraban JM, Colvin JS, et al: Inositol trisphosphate receptor: biochemical and autoradiographic demonstration in brain and variable stoichiometry with protein kinase C. Nature 1987; 325:159-161
30. Spat A, Bradford PG, McKinney JS, et al: A saturable receptor for ^{32}P-inositol-1,4,5-trisphosphate in hepatocytes and neutrophils. Nature 1986; 319:514-516
31. Supattapone S, Worley PF, Baraban JM, et al: Solubilization, purification, and characterization of an inositol trisphosphate receptor. J Biol Cnem 1988; 263:1530-1534
32. Danoff SK, Supattapone S, Snyder SH: Characterization of a membrane protein from brain mediating the inhibition of inositol 1,4,5-trisphosphate receptor binding by calcium. Biochem J 1988; 254:701-705

33. Supattapone S, Danoff SK, Theibert A, et al: Cyclic AMP-dependent phosphorylation of a brain inositol trisphosphate receptor decreases its release of calcium. Proc Natl Acad Sci USA 1988; 85:8747-8750
34. Batty I, Nahorski SR, Irvine R: Rapid formation of inositol 1,3,4,5-tetrakisphosphate following muscarinic receptor stimulation of rat cerebral cortex slices. Biochem J 1985; 232:211-215
35. Irvine RF, Letcher AJ, Heslop JP, et al: The inositol tris/tetrakisphosphate pathway--demonstration of Ins (1,4,5) P_3 3-kinase activity in animal tissues. Nature 1986; 320:631-634
36. Hill TD, Dean NM, Boynton AL: Inositol 1,3,4,5-tetrakisphosphate induces Ca^{2+} sequestration in rat liver cells. Science 1988; 242:1176-1178
37. Vallejo M, Jackson T, Lightman S, et al: Occurrence and extracellular actions of inositol pentakis--and hexakisphosphate in mammalian brain. Nature 1987; 330:656-658
38. Nishizuka Y: Studies and perspectives of protein kinase C. Science 1986; 233:305-312
39. Jakobs KH, Bauer S, Watanabe Y: Modulation of adenylate cyclase of human platelets by phorbol ester, impairment of the hormone-sensitive inhibitory pathway. Eur J Biochem 1985; 151:425-430
40. Katada T, Gilman AG, Watanabe Y, et al: Protein kinase C phosphorylates the inhibitory guanine-nucleotide-binding regulatory component and apparently suppresses its function in hormonal inhibition of adenylate cyclase. Eur J Biochem 1985; 151:431-437
41. Labarca R, Janowsky A, Patel J, et al: Phorbol esters inhibit agonist-induced [^{3}H]inositol-1-phosphate accumulation in rat hippocampal slices. Biochem Biophys Res Commun 1984; 123:703-709
42. Watson SP, Lapetina EG: 1,2-Diacylglycerol and phorbol esters inhibit agonist-induced formation of inositol phosphates in human platelets: possible implications for negative feedback regulation of inositol phospholipid hydrolysis. Proc Natl Acad Sci USA 1985; 82:2623-2626
43. Connolly TM, Lawing WJ Jr, Majerus PW: Protein kinase C phosphorylates human platelet inositol trisphosphate 5'-phosphomonoesterase, increasing the phosphatase activity. Cell 1986; 46:951-958
44. Molina Y, Vedia LM, Lapetina E: Phorbol 12,13-dibutyrate and 1-oleyl-2-acetyldiacyglycerol stimulate inositol trisphosphate dephosphorylation in human platelets. J Biol Chem 1986; 261:10493-10495
45. Huang KP, Chan KFJ, Singh TJ, et al: Autophosphorylation of rat brain Ca^{2+}-activated and phospholipid-dependent protein kinase. J Biol Chem 1986; 261:12134-12140
46. Baraban JM, Gould RJ, Peroutka SJ, et al: Phorbol ester effects on neurotransmission: interaction with neurotransmitters and calcium in

smooth muscle. Proc Natl Acad Sci USA 1985; 82:604-607
47. Baraban JM, Snyder SH, Alger BE: Protein kinase C regulates ionic conductances in hippocampal pyramidal neurons: electrophysiological effects of phorbol esters. Proc Natl Acad Sci USA 1985; 82:2538-2542
48. Worley PF, Baraban JM, McCarren M, et al: Cholinergic phosphatidyl-inositol modulation of inhibitory G protein-linked, neurotransmitter actions: electrophysiological studies in rat hippocampus. Proc Natl Acad Sci USA 1987; 84:3467-3471
49. Cole AE, Nicoll RA: The pharmacology of cholinergic excitatory responses in Hippocampal pyramidal cells. Brain Res 1984; 305:283-290
50. Nishizuka Y: The molecular heterogeneity of protein kinase C and its implications for cellular regulation. Nature 1988; 334:661-665
51. Bennett CF, Balcauk JM, Varrichio A, et al: Molecular cloning and complete sequence of form-I phosphoinositide-specific phospholipase C. Nature 1988; 334:268-270
52. Worley PF, Baraban JM, DeSouza EB, et al: Mapping second messenger systems in the brain: differential localization of adenylate cyclase and protein kinase C. Proc Natl Acad Sci USA 1986; 83:4053-4057
53. Blumberg PM, Jaken S, Konig B, et al: Mechanism of action of the phorbol ester tumor promoters: specific receptors for lipophilic ligands. Biochem Parmacol 1984; 33:933-940
54. Kikkawa U, Takai Y, Tanaka Y, et al: Protein kinase C as a possible receptor of tumor-promoting phorbol esters. J Biol Chem 1983; 258: 11442-11445
55. Leach KL, James ML, Blumberg PM: Characterization of a specific phorbol ester aporeceptor in mouse brain cytosol. Proc Natl Acad Sci USA 1983; 80:4208-4212
56. Niedel JE, Kuhn LJ, Vanderbank GR: Phorbol diester receptor co-purifies with protein kinase C. Proc Natl Acad Sci USA 1983; 80: 36-40
57. Worley PF, Baraban JM, Snyder SH: Heterogeneous localization of protein kinase C in rat Brain: Autoradiographic analysis of phorbol ester receptor binding. J Neurosci 1986; 6:199-207
58. Suh, P, Ryu SH, Moon KH, et al: Cloning and sequence of multiple forms of phospholipase C. Cell 1988; 54:161-169
59. Suh P, Ryu SH, Moon KH, et al: Inositol phospholipid-specific phospholipase C: complete cDNA and protein sequences and sequence homology to tyrosine kinase-related oncogene products. Proc Natl Acad Sci USA 1988; 85:5419-5423
60. Ross CA, MacCumber MW, Glatt CE, et al: Brain phospholipase C isozymes: differential mRNA localizations by *in situ* hybridization. Proc Natl Acad Sci USA 1989; 86:2923-2927
61. Blackstone CD, Supattapone S, Snyder SH: Phosphoinositide-linked glutamate receptors mediate cerebellar parallel fiber-Purkinje cell

synaptic transmission. Proc Natl Acad Sci USA 1989; 86:4316-4320
62. Worley PF, Baraban JB, Snyder SH: IP_3 receptor autoradiography in rat brain. J Neurosci 1989; 9:339-346
63. Klein DF, Gittelman R, Quitkin F, et al: Diagnosis and Drug Treatment of Psychiatric Disorders: Adults and Children, 2nd ed. Baltimore, Williams & Wilkins, 1980, pp 810-818
64. Janowsky DS, Risch SC: Role of acetylcholine mechanisms in the affective disorders, in Psychopharmacology: The Third Generation of Progress. Edited by Meltzer HY. New York, Raven Press, 1987
65. Allison JH, Stewart MA: Reduced brain inositol in lithium treated rats. Nature 1971; 233:267-268
66. Hallcher LM, Sherman WR: The effect of lithium ion and other agents on the activity of myo-inositol-1-phosphatase from bovine brain. J Biol Chem 1980; 255:10896-10901
67. Berridge MJ, Downes CP, Hanley MR: Lithium amplifies agonist-dependent phosphatidylinositol responses in brain and salivary glands. Biochem J 1982; 206:587-595
68. Whitworth P, Kendall DA: Lithium selectively inhibits muscarinic receptor-stimulated inositol tetrakisphosphate accumulation in mouse cerebral cortex slices. J Neurochem 1988; 51:258-265
69. Sherman WR, Munsell LY, Gish BG, et al: Effects of systemically administered lithium on phosphoinositide metabolism in rat brain, kidney and testes. J Neurochem 1985; 44:798-807
70. Batty I, Nahorski SR: Differential effects of lithium on muscarinic receptor stimulation of inositol phosphates in rat cerebral cortex slices. J Neurochem 1985; 45:1514-1521
71. Batty I, Nahorski SR: Lithium inhibits muscarinic receptor stimulated inositol tetrakisphosphate accumulation in rat cerebral cortex. Biochem J 1987; 274:767-780
72. Kendall DA, Nahorski SR: Acute and chronic lithium treatments influence agonist and depolarization stimulated inositol phospholipid hydrolysis in rat cerebral cortex. J Pharmacol Exp Ther 1987; 241: 1023-1027
73. Drummond AH: Lithium and inositol lipid-linked signalling mechanism. Trends in Pharmacological Sciences 1987; 8:129-133
74. Downes CP, Stone MA: Lithium-induced reduction in intracellular inositol supply in cholinergically stimulated parotid gland. Biochem J 1986; 234:199-204
75. Casebolt TL, Jope RS: Chronic lithium treatment reduces norepinephrine-stimulated inositol phospholipid hydrolysis in rat cortex. Eur J Pharmacol 1987; 140:245-246
76. Worley PF, Heller WA, Snyder SH, et al: Lithium blocks a phosphoinositide-mediated cholinergic response in hippocampal slices. Science 1988; 239:1428-1429

77. Menkes HA, Baraban JM, Freed AN, et al: Lithium dampens neurotransmitter response in smooth muscle: relevance to action in affective illness. Proc Natl Acad Sci USA 1986; 83:5727-5730
78. Avissar S, Schreiber G, Danon A, et al: Lithium inhibits adrenergic and cholinergic increases in GTP binding in rat cortex. Nature 1988; 331:440-442
79. Volonte C: Lithium stimulates the binding of GTP to the membranes of PC-12 cells cultured with nerve growth factor. Neurosci Lett 1988; 87:127-132
80. Volonte C, Racker E: Lithium stimulation of membrane-bound phospholipase C from PC 12 cells exposed to nerve growth hormone. J Neurochem 1988; 51:1163-1168

This article was printed in the American Journal of Psychiatry, 146:10, October 1989, pages 1251-1260, copyright 1989, The American Psychiatric Association. Reprinted by permission.

chapter 5

Psychobiology, Communication And The Future Of Medicine

Joel Elkes, M.D., L.F.A.P.A.

INTRODUCTION: ADOLF MEYER AND PSYCHOBIOLOGY

I am honored to participate in this memorable symposium. It brings to mind 1967 when, on a windy day, we stood on a beautiful knoll near Ellicott City to lay the foundation stone of a new hospital center at Taylor Manor and to join in another landmark symposium (1) at which many of us met at the invitation of the Taylor family to review old beginnings and, jointly, to look ahead. Now the Doctors Taylor and their families have brought us together again to celebrate with them another festive occasion. Our warm good wishes go out to the Taylor family for a long life of this remarkable and innovative institution. As for us, I can honestly say that we are all here to learn.

Seventy-six years ago an historic event which we commemorated recently took place here in Baltimore. The Phipps Clinic was dedicated on April 16, 1913. It was a ceremony in the grand manner, attended by Osler, McDougall, Eugen Bleuler, Cushing and Ernest Jones, among others. Speaking briefly on the purposes of a psychiatric clinic, Adolf Meyer said:

> "For the first time in English speaking countries, a university and large general hospital serving a medical school received, as not merely affiliated but as an intrinsic part of its facilities, a well equipped clinic to take care of its patients with mental disorders.... At last science begins to take up with new and forceful methods the great problems of mental life... This work does not stop in

Published 1990 by Elsevier Science Publishing Co., Inc.
Psychiatry: Past Reflections–Future Visions
B.T. Taylor and I.J. Taylor, Editors

> the sanctum of the investigator. Just as bacteriology studies the water supply, air and food of communities, schools, and homes, so we psychopathologists have to study more effectively the atmosphere of the community, and must devise safeguards [in the environment]... from which patients come and to which patients come and to which they must return (2)."

There was a comprehensiveness about Adolf Meyer's vision of Psychiatry. Brain, body, thought and behavior were to him a biological continuum; and symbolic life, an aspect of general biology. He connected, like few before him and long before the life sciences were ready for such a connection, Psychiatry to the Life Sciences and the Life Sciences to Psychiatry, probing the relation of Claude Bernard's Inner Environment, (and later Cannon's homeostasis) to the forces and influences playing upon an ordinary person's life from birth to maturity into old age. He emphasized early bonding in human development and learning and saw the family as the most important school of man. He recognized the web of social support as a healer of great power. Long before the present emphasis on life events, he focussed, by way of the autobiographical essay, on life events. Long before cybernetics, autoregulation, social field theory and the analog computer, he sensed and thought and wrote about the importance of systems in human affairs. He travelled light and he travelled far, crossing boundaries from his neuroanatomical laboratories (which literally comprised brains from lizards to elephants) to the clinic and to mental hygiene in school and community, and back again; and he did so with great élan and vitality. In a word, he saw *connections* between the disparate fields which related medicine to psychiatry and psychiatry to medicine. Soma and Symbol, the society within the skin and the society without, were to him aspects of a vast realm of communication which he termed "Psychobiology." All his life he struggled valiantly with the awesome comprehensiveness of the term. His Salmon Lectures on the subject were delivered in 1932 but not published until seven years after his death in 1957 (3). Long before modern neurochemistry, molecular biology, and concepts that we take totally for granted today, Adolf Meyer had a view of psychiatry which remains astonishingly modern. Communication was to him at the heart of psychobiology; communication reaching beyond psychiatry into the body of medicine at large. It is this theme of somatic and symbolic communication in relation to psychiatry and medicine which I would like to address. For psychiatry is about communication: intercellular communication by way of special signal molecules in brain and body; communication and coding in neural and immunological nets; communication between brain and organ systems and between brain and the world, including the duplicate world we encode in our symbols. I would like to examine some of the attributes of the languages--molecular and symbolic--which make up the matrix of modern psychiatry; to point to certain features which these languages may have in common; to examine the implications of this new knowledge for our day-to-day practice and training in psychiatry and in related areas of medicine; and to indicate the steadily lessening contradiction between brain chemistry, its exquisite susceptibility to the environment, and the so called psychosocial approaches. The observations I wish to put before you are by now well known; I have examined some of these issues on previous occasions (4,5,6,7,8). I hope I may be forgiven for certain repetitions.

MOLECULAR COMMUNICATION, SYMBOLIC COMMUNICATION, AND THE PRESERVATION OF THE SYMBOLIC SELF

A Society Within the Skin

The society of cells residing within the human skin forms an entity which throughout evolution has continued to function with remarkable smoothness, efficiency, and resilience. This entity, the human body, is built up of interacting units of varying size and complexity--from mitochondria, microsomes and membranes to cell ensembles, tissues, organs and organ systems. These units interact and communicate; the whole is informed of the parts and the part is informed of the needs of the whole. In a word, the biological machine is a self organizing system. In the exchange of matter and energy, precise information is the key. Information, in turn, is linked to time and timing. From the picoseconds of a charge transfer reaction to the opening of ion channels, to the recurrent contraction of the heart, to the ebb and flow of the tides of biological rhythms, information arriving at the right place at the right time appears to be the cardinal rule of biological order. Somehow, cell ensembles have developed plans and schemata for cooperation--a sort of inner altruism. Homeostasis and constancy are achieved in the face of the opposite, continuous change and exchange. The primary goal of this remarkable arrangement would appear to be the maintenance of the intactness of that society. Normally we take this arrangement totally for granted. Only when we are ill are we shaken out of our insensibility, to become aware of the ever-renewing miracle within us.

Communication within the skin is effected by the exchange of electrochemical signals between cells coded for function through specific genetic instructions. These are very precise. The advance in our understanding of intercellular communication has been very rapid and has recently been the subject of comprehensive and far reaching reviews (9,10,11). Cells govern themselves by signals from membrane to interior (the first and second messenger system) or from membrane to membrane. The agents are relatively small molecules, some of them remarkably simple in structure, which allosterically interact with receptors of specific configuration. The interaction conveys precise instructions which initiate and terminate specific processes, be they ion fluxes across a membrane or the transport or induction of an enzyme in a specific plan of protein synthesis. The action is usually optimal for the conditions which pertain at the time.

While cell to cell communication pertains in plants and simple marine organisms, and in ourselves operates in regulating and limiting growth, we are endowed with three broad systems which decisively influence intercellular and intracellular message transmittal. One is a fixed system which, like a giant plant emanating from a central trunk and core, pervades the farthest reaches of the body through its finest tendrils and arborizations. I speak, of course, of the nervous system and its broad divisions of voluntary and autonomic control. The second system is composed of clusters of specialized fixed cells contained in glandular tissue which release signalling molecules into the blood stream, molecules that reach their target receptors by that route. This system is the endocrine system. The third is made up of colonies of cells which are partly fixed and partly mobile, which carry out a surveillance function for the body and scan for molecular information which is "foreign" to the body. This system, the immune system, comprises thymus, spleen, lymph nodes, bone marrow and lymphoid tissue scattered in mucosa and elsewhere. The weight of the brain is about three pounds, the weight of the immune system, about two, and the weight of the endocrine system, less than a pound. Yet, it is these systems which guard our identity and preserve our biological and symbolic self. There is not a cell in the society within the skin which is not irrigated by blood, bathed by lymph, and exposed to continuous fluxes of the autonomic nervous system. The final common path of these convergent communication systems is the exquisite micro apparatus of the cell membrane. The numbers operating in these processes are stupendous. There are twelve to fourteen billion neurons, each capable of making some two hundred connections; millions of lymphocytes, and some hundred million billion antibodies are produced per second (12). All this tremendous variation is derived from a relatively small genetic pool. The three communication systems are internally connected. The nervous system, by way of the hypothalamic pituitary axis, guides the endocrine system; and the endocrine system, in turn, transduces information from the nervous to the immune system. More direct pathways between the nervous and the immune systems both ways have been recently identified (13). Integrity, coordination and decision making--the right information at the right time--are all of a piece. The linking of the society within the skin to the society without involves a miraculous piece of chemical engineering.

The Brain: Molecular Communication, Symbolic Forms and the Sense of Self

The human brain emerges as the most remarkable biological machine to appear in the evolution of this planet. In the briefest moment of human history it has radically transformed our ecology and established the dominance of our able and dangerous species on earth. The exosomatic extensions which have become the instruments and agents of our culture are products of the brain; it is to these that our body-mind must now adapt.

The organ in question is relatively young and carries within it the regional chemical footprints of its own evolution. It is a system of systems, an ensemble of biased homeostats which has grown exponentially in cellular mass and cytoarchitectural elaboration in the last few minutes (a mere two million years or so) of the evolutionary calendar of life on this planet. Despite its complexity, its component subsystems, cables and connections, and the teeming interneuronal molecular traffic, certain functional, regionally organized groupings can be clearly distinguished.

The so-called amphibian brain which is connected to the hypothalamus pituitary apparatus subserves decisions concerning individual survival--hunger, thirst, elimination, sexuality, territoriality and the like. The plans here are genetically "wired," the sensory apparatus is extraordinarily elaborate and precise; the responses released by very specific cues are swift, stereotyped and effective. Like any neural net it can learn. There is more latitude in the programs of the Limbic System (14) which are concerned with species survival. The behavior patterns related to sexuality, pair bonding, tropisms of attraction and repulsion--pleasure and displeasure, love and hate--appear to be coded by cell ensembles which, as has been shown by Nauta (15), have deep and pervasive connections into the brain stem, the spinal cord, and upward into the thalamus and the neocortical mantle. However, the explosive growth of the neocortex is man's most characteristic acquisition; a process re-enacted ontogenetically in remarkably sped up fashion in intrauterine and early postnatal life. This, as has been said many times, makes for both plasticity and vulnerability of the immature brain.

With cortical development came an ability to code, store, and model perception and forms of behavior in symbols and, through myriads of inner schemata and maps, to create a duplicate inner representation which made it possible to be aware, to think, and to plan. Kenneth Craik, in his "Nature of Explanation" (16), discussed the role of modeling long before the age of the computer. A primary model of the world within the skin is the construction of the Body Image, or to use a better term--Body Schema (17). We suspect that visceral representation is laid down relatively early and stored silently, only to intrude when disturbed in illness or brought into awareness through biofeedback and visceral training (18). The world without is scanned through distance receptors and modeled through thought and language. This continuous modeling engages distinct, hierarchically organized cell groups in successive convergences, transformations and condensations of information (19). Such concepts owe a great deal to the study of the process of perception and learning in primitive organisms. The simpler the brain, the more stereotyped the responses, the clearer the chemical coding. The larger the brain, the higher the redundancy, the more discriminate the selection, the more massive the selective inhibition and "banking" of the inappropriate and the irrelevant. It is this massive capacity to selectively delay, inhibit and ignore which makes decisive and discriminate performance possible. The human brain, indeed any brain, in a series of successive transforms, condenses more and more information into less and less. I have suggested elsewhere (20) that these transforms employ shifting and highly discriminate inhibitory mechanisms in laminar, cellular hierarchies in the elimination of redundant information; that they are matched for fit against stored programs, and tested in a sort of internal rehearsal for adaptive value to the organism until a decision and commitment is either imagined or enacted. The final product, the emerging whole--be it a percept or a motor act, or idea--represents a condensed symbolic model of a succession of operations which always, always comprise informational traces, shared properties of the antecedent phases in a temporally coded pattern.

There is thus in the brain continuous communication, a sharing of properties, a matching, weighing and feature extraction through the use of electrochemical languages in these processes. To put it another way, there proceeds in the brain a continuous evolution by natural selection of symbolic forms which employ communicating cell populations, or groups, or ensembles (21). This evolution of informed cell assemblies is, of course, non-genetic; and in man can be transferred from generation to generation in sight and sound. Languages--silent or articulate--are the tools of evolution. We are what we are because of the continuous evolution proceeding in our head. If you will, the brain may be regarded as a fashioner of wholes.

We will note too some aspects in these successive transformations. The process operates both in series and parallel modes, asking and answering the questions one at a time, and asking the questions all at once. It operates in very rapid automatic stages: a search; a scanning for fit against coded or genetically or cognate acquired schemata; a recognition and affective labeling in terms of adaptive value of the schema to the organism; inhibition of other inappropriate response repertories; re-entry to test for validity; commitment to bring a particular cell ensemble to a particular course and action; and action through speech or another motor act. We will note two features of this sequence: First, the key role of informed inhibition in structuring a response. What is not happening--banked, as it were--is as important as what emerges. Second, the inexorable nature of commitment--a stage which, once reached, is difficult to reverse.

This process of inner communication and evolution and non-genetic transmittal of information has populated our world with the exosomatic products of our culture. From brain, to libraries, to computers, communication remains our principal attribute. In this respect the brain underwent an interesting evolutionary twist. For quite early, it distinguished and parcelled out two modes of operation in information transfer, putting the sequential or digital-linear and the parallel-analagous mode into two separate hemispheres, interacting by way of the corpus callosum. Something else probably happened as well. Just as species-specific behaviors appear to have been stored and encoded in the amphibian and limbic system, so culturally valuable schemata--rituals, ceremonies, myths, racial memories if you will--may have found their repository in the right hemisphere, leaving the left hemisphere to plan and enact--by way of sequential speech--the ever present Now. While we know a good deal of the dominant hemisphere and its role in the genesis and maintenance of consciousness, we know far too little of the non-dominant hemisphere. Far from silent, it speaks to us distinctly in our trade. Dreaming and daydreaming may be related to its activity. Symbolic form constants emerge impressively, from James Frazer (22) to Jung (23) to Campbell (24), and lately, Stanislav Grof (25). These symbolic forms, in their incessant transformations, are accessed not through words but through means of communication which are both preverbal and postverbal--metalanguages of the inner self. Dreaming, daydreaming, music and dance, painting and poetry, deep meditation and religious experience, practiced individually and in a group, are our avenues to them; and, strangely significant, experiencing them gives us a feeling of loss restored, a sense of completeness, wholeness, connectedness, communication and knowing. We must ask why this should be so. What is it about art that restores? Restores to what? What is it about the best of religious practice that communicates and makes whole like nothing else? What is the "a-part-ness" that is healed? We must suspect that ancient psychobiological processes, pervading the whole structure of the body-mind, from Soma to Symbol, are at play in the experience and expression of these states; and conclude, then, that their study is very much the business of modern Psychobiology.

IMMUNITY: MOLECULAR COMMUNICATION AND THE PRESERVATION OF THE BIOLOGICAL SELF

The explosive growth of modern immunology, stimulated by advances of molecular genetics and the pressing exigencies of AIDS, coincides with a mounting recognition of the connection between the nervous system, the endocrine system and the immune system, and the influence of psychological and behavioral factors on immune function. The pioneering work establishing these connections has now been documented (26,27,28,29). It records a story with profound implications for the behavioral scientist. As findings accumulate, the vast array of specialized cells comprising the immune system (we will recall the numbers mentioned earlier) emerges as an exquisitely balanced, self-monitoring information network, communicating by chemical signals. It monitors the invading "without" against the "familiar" within. This network employs strategies reminiscent of the processing of information by the nervous system, and even more than the nervous system impresses by its stupendous biological reserve, manifested as "degeneracy" and redundancy (21). Somewhat like the construction of the body image and visceral schemata, self recognition and other recognitions proceed continuously; the molecular intactness of the biological self is preserved through a miraculous, continuous process of inner communication. I may perhaps be forgiven if, in an informal discussion some years ago, I referred to the immune system as a "liquid brain," an all-pervasive embodiment of mind.

It is beyond my scope here to detail the different functions assigned to different kinds of cells. There are some excellent reviews for the general reader (28,29). Nossal uses six key words to capture the task confronting the system. They are *Encounter*, *Recognition*, *Activation*, *Deployment*, *Discrimination* and *Regulation*. "The invading antigen must *encounter* cells capable of responding....molecular mechanisms of *recognition* must exist... the system must possess the capability of responding to any conceivable antigen, including "new" substances synthesized by man.... Having recognized the antigen, lymphocytes must be *activated* to respond either by producing antibodies or by acting in the inflammatory response... They have furthermore to cooperate in an elaborate *deployment* strategy, amplifying and distributing defense functions... The evolutionary process has ensured that the system can *discriminate* between self and non-self, thereby avoiding autoimmune damage.... The mechanisms establishing such tolerance are part of a wider series of control loops that constitute immune *regulation* in which the intensity of the immune response is corrected for a particular antigenic load" (30).

More and more it looks like a coordinated *network* (12,26). The network has an afferent pathway comprising a specific recognizing and a non-specific parallel set. Indeed, the immune system has been called a sensory organ, scanning for molecular fit (31). One can also envision an efferent "imaging" component and an effector loop which is held in check by a process of internal inhibition. This is selectively modulated to lead to clonal selection and proliferation of the appropriate lymphocytes. Scanning, recognition, selection, modulation and selective inhibition, leading by way of a sort of internal rehearsal to *commitment*, steps which remind one of communication in the nervous system. Induction of antibody production is irreversible once it has occurred and is remembered for the future.

Moreover, a two way connection between the nervous, endocrine and immune systems is now established (32). Selective damage or stimulation of brain areas, particularly hypothalamus, affects immune function (33). The suborgans of the immune apparatus (thymus, spleen, lymph nodes, bone marrow, mucosal parenchyma) receive rich autonomic innervation from both the parasympathetic and sympathetic systems (34,35); communication goes both ways. There is also *afferent* communication *back* from the immune system to the nervous system, particularly the thymus (32). Most significantly, too, as shown in the now classical studies, the immune system responds to environment and can be conditioned (36). Alteration in immune function is seen, e.g., examination of stress (37), and related to style of coping (38). There is evidence suggesting impaired immune function in depression (39,40). The complex field of the relation of personality type, coping style and emotion to the onset or remission of cancer is full of promising leads and inconsistencies (41,42,43,44) which should be resolved in the next decade. The same applies to the old/new field of possible immune dysfunction in the genesis of schizophrenia (45,46). On a slightly different note, one cannot leave this field without referring to the enormous benefit experimental neuroscience has derived from the advent of the fluorescent antibody techniques, making, literally, regional neurochemistry shine in the dark.

FAMILIES OF NEUROREGULATORY COMPOUNDS AND "INFORMATIONAL SUBSTANCES"

"The body of a worm and the face of a man

> alike have to be taken as chemical responses. The alchemist dreamed of old that it might be so. The dream however supposed a magic chemistry. There they were wrong. The chemistry is plain everyday chemistry. But it is complex. Further, the chemical brew has been stirring unceasingly throughout some millions of years in the service of a final cause. The brew is a selected brew (47)."

The chemistry of which Sherrington spoke began not in the brain but in the gut and in the heart. It began with acetycholine, histamine, and later norepinephrine and serotonin. It is hard, in an age which takes ligand techniques and the *in vivo* PET scanning of metabolic pathways in the brain totally for granted to grasp how improbable a coherent chemistry of the brain seemed forty years ago. I, for one, was warned by my elders; they told me that the brain was a "sticky mess" which would prove one's professional undoing. Yet I still recall vividly the excitement with which I read the classical paper of Feldberg and Vogt (48) questioning the universal transmitter role of acetycholine in the brain, and I remember listening to Marthe Vogt as she presented her evidence for the distribution of norepinephrine in the very areas of the brain where (on electrophysiological evidence) Bradley and I suspected the existence of a biogenic amine (50). Those were heady days, labor notwithstanding. It took two PhD students two years each to map the distribution of an enzyme system in the brain.

Between 1953 and 1957 (50,51), on the basis of electrophysiological and neurochemical evidence I suggested that "Perhaps rather than thinking in unitary terms, it might be advisable to think in terms of the possible selection by chemical evolution of small *families* of already closely related compounds which by mutual interplay would govern the phenomena of excitation and inhibition in the central nervous system." I spoke of the operation of chemical fields in nodal regions of the brain which would depend on the rate of liberation, diffusion and destruction of locally produced neurohumoral agents. I stressed the uneven distribution of cells with different chemical endowment in various areas of the brain--some cells condensed in nodes, others colonized in particular layers, some scattered randomly. I proposed that the agents in question might either be identical with or, more likely, were derived from neuroeffector substances familiar to us in peripheral neural nets. I stressed the importance of interaction and interdependence between molecules governing and modulating the gating, storage and flow in self-exciting neural loops. As I put it, "The number of those substances was probably quite small but the influence upon the integrative action of higher nervous activity could be profound; the basic states of consciousness might well be determined by variation of local concentration of these agents" (52).

The substances we knew at the time were acetycholine, norepinephrine, serotonin and GABA. We all know what has happened since. We are no longer talking of small families, but hierarchies perfected by evolution; generations of families of compounds, from GABA, glycine, and cyclic AMP to prohormones, peptides and opiate-like substances. The brain is emerging as a huge organ of internal secretion; and to synaptic transmission there is now being added the very important concept of *para*synaptic communication--local hormone-like effects of messenger substances, reaching brain cells through the extracelluler fluid bathing the cell surface.

In a seminal paper, F.O. Schmitt, a towering figure in modern neuroscience, has proposed as a working hypothesis the concept of Informational Substances as molecular regulators of brain function (53). His list of classical neurotransmitters numbers about ten, comprising members of the small families to which I referred earlier. The lists of neuropeptides and neurohormones, as we know, comprise some forty members; it has grown considerably since. The extraordinary import of this paper is twofold. First, it traces the evolutionary origin of the neurotransmitters, suggesting that they may have evolved from being intracellular messengers to a role in rapid intercellular communication through synaptic discharges. Secondly, it argues for a twofold mode of communication: a precise, familiar mode of neuron-to-neuron synaptic transmission (We will recall that each neuron carries about 200 junctional sites.); and a more direct information transmission "in parallel" or alongside (not instead of, or in competition with) neuronal circuitry. This may take place through the release and diffusion of informational substances through extracellular fluid and their attachment to ligands on the cell surface, coding for a particular behavioral repertoire (as in sex hormones, releasing appropriate behavior) or for components of a mosaic which makes up the repertoire. It is this combination of serial, synaptic, and parallel parasynaptic communication which makes for extraordinary flexibility in the repertoires of a particular neural net. Scanning, analysis, recognition and discharge would seem to depend on recognizers for a particular configuration being in place. There appears to be "cross-talk" between recognizing sites as well. Once again, one is reminded of the immune system.

The awed sense of wonder grows as some of the very same informational substances familiar to us in the nervous system turn up on the surfaces of lymphocytes. Lymphocytes have receptors for acetycholine, epinephrine, norepinephrine, histamine, dopamine, testosterone, insulin and a number of other hormones. The list is growing steadily (54).

In these electrochemical conversations between different sites, another very important principle emerges. Somehow the informational substances act in concert; their effect depends on the presence of each other. As in spoken language, not only do molecules signal, they communicate and interact; the net meaning depends on *context*. What a particular substance will do at a particular time, at a particular site, will depend on 'who' and 'what' else is, or has been, there at that time. This brings to mind early observation on the interaction between acetycholine and norepinephrine at peripheral receptor sites (55). One grapples for an analogy which could comprise both space and time. The image of a molecular combination code--a sort of evanescent combination lock--spread throughout the body provides a rough approximation of the idea.

MOLECULAR LANGUAGES IN THE TRANSCRIPTION OF BODY-MIND EVENTS

The pervasive presence of neuroregulatory and informational substances throughout the body makes it possible to think of the transcription of symbolic events in molecular terms. The classical studies of Kandel in a simple organism, aplysia (56), have furnished us with one molecular model of a memory trace. This model emphasizes the role of calcium as a critical regulator of transmitter release. However, the molecular transcription of psychosocial cues is evident in other areas (57,58). Social factors, especially in early life, influence drug responsiveness and affect enzyme induction, with deep influence on an organism's social reactivity. Handling, stroking, and touch may affect growth hormones, liver enzymes and development (59). More significantly, hormones, and some peptides--informational substances in their own right--deeply affect learning (60). It has even been argued that information molecules themselves may exhibit a "plasticity" (i.e., variation in number and distribution) in the acquisition of new behavior (61). We will note, too, some regional chemical features relevant to the establishment of a visceral memory trace. The system of subserving attention and vigilance is dopaminergic, with special reference to the locus coeruleus. The cell ensembles subserving pleasure and avoidance (the so called reward and punishment system), engaged in a preliminary scanning and grouping of patterns in terms of their appetitive or aversive connotation, and subsequent encoding and recall, are found in discrete nodal areas of the limbic system, the amygdala, and the hippocampus--areas which are rich in peptides and other informational substances mentioned above (62,63). The hypothalamic pituitary axis is replete with prohormonal and finished chemical messengers which, by way of local routes and the bloodstream, can potentially reach every cell in the brain and body, particularly during stress (65). If, as one suspects, these critical nodal cell ensembles were to participate in the laying down of an affectively labeled memory trace, it is conceivable that, by mechanisms still unknown, informed and specifically responsive neural nets may be established as representational maps of a particular configuration of psychological events. We will remember that informational substances, particularly peptides and substance P substances, abound in the autonomic nerve endings of viscera, and that even the heart has its hormones (64).

In an important series of papers, Rossi (66,67) has argued that learning, any learning, is conditioned by the chemical state of the organism--particularly the brain--in which it occurs. The model, which is derived from the study of addiction, is that of *State Dependent Learning*. Behaviors learned under the influence of drugs are exquisitely susceptible to these same drugs or related social cues (68). Similarly, it is argued that behaviors and/or memories, or visceromotor responses acquired during a particular state of neurohormonal arousal (a particular hormonal "mix") are susceptible to cognate cues. Such memories, in Rossi's experience, are evoked in low arousal states by the use of an Eriksonian approach of gentle hypnosis and guided imagery. The somatic specificity of such responses is certainly impressive and suggests widespread cell communication and extensive representation and discrimination in the memory trace. Whether this is due to a widespread dissemination of molecular recognizers (62), or to a peculiar and specific chemical wiring, or to some form of molecularly conditioned, trancellular "resonance," or, to my mind, quite likely electromagnetic and/or electrochemical fields (69) is unknown. One is, however, certainly reminded of tissue hypersensitivity.

DISEASE AS A DISORDER OF MOLECULAR AND SYMBOLIC COMMUNICATION

The evidence briefly reviewed above brings us to the point with which we began. The society within the skin emerges as a miraculously coordinated communication system in which the whole is informed of the part, and the part is informed of the whole. Constancy of body function is maintained throughout adult life through an extraordinary array of signal exchange. Evolution in man manifests mainly in symbolic life. The core and content of our life is symbolic; and--be it in soma or symbol--we consciously sample only the tiniest fraction of the ancient symbolic structures with which we are endowed and which inform our day-to-day being.

The messaging system of the body-mind is truly stupendous. The chemical languages, honed by many millions of years of biological evolution--far transcending our species--are extraordinarily precise. Compared with the precision of these messages, our language, developed as a tool of social evolution, is paltry, clumsy, and imprecise in the extreme. Thc parable of the Tower of Babel still holds. Just listen to the verbal clutter invading our living room every night.

Within our skin and skull, then, there exists a vast laboratory of symbolic forms in ongoing transformations which we only dimly perceive unless things go very wrong or very right. When things go wrong we "know it in our body." When things go right we are inwardly aware how good things can be. In the first we say we are uneasy, concerned, anxious, angry, furious or depressed; in the other we experience the joy of simply being. We are signalled when communication is out of phase. Anxiety is a warning and signifies that a problem is unsolved and demands solution. Depression is an act of adaptive coping by not coping; pain (including mental pain) signals severing of organismic integrity; an invasion or an incipient (or actual) parting of the part from the whole. As Bakan put it, "Disease is estrangement (70); and healing, as the word implies, is a restoration of communication--a coming together, a return to wholeness. When communication is good, we amble along. When it falters, we are warned to attend to it; when it is impaired or lost, we get sick." Curious that in our profession we know so much about anxiety, pain, and depression, and much, much less about joy. We know more about the biology of despondency than the biology of expectation and hope. A Science of Sorrows is still waiting for a Science of Joys.

In a very significant paper, still in press, Herbert Weiner (9) has argued that disease may in fact be a manifestation of disturbed intercellular and organ communication. He regards an altered relationship between messenger, mediator, and receptor as crucial; and postulates several levels of organization at which this might occur. A cognate model has been very ably argued by Cunningham (71). Rubenstein too has examined the suggestive evidence, speaking of diseases related to defects in intercellular communication (10).

The examples of this model in somatic diseases, though still sparce, are suggestive. There is Graves disease caused by a circulating autoantibody binding preferentially to the receptor for thyrotropin and interrupting the normal feedback loop to TRH; Myasthenia gravis, where the ACh receptor is blocked by an autoantibody, impairing neuromuscular transmission and ultimately destroying the receptor; a deficiency of low density lipoprotein LAL receptor which leads to dangerous elevation of cholesterol in familia hypercholesteremia, and reduction of the number of insulin receptors in diabetes in relation to stressful life events (10).

But surely the richest field in support of this thesis is our own field of biological psychiatry. For here, through the evolution of modern psychopharmacology and the refined methodologies of receptor identification *in vivo* and purification *in vitro*, the elegant ligand techniques (72,73), metabolic loading techniques, and brain imagery have given us a plethora of new findings and generation upon generation of working hypotheses.

For evidence, I refer you to the section on Biological Psychiatry in *Psychopharmacology: The Third Generation of Progress*, edited by Dr. Herbert Meltzer and published last year in association with our own American College of Neuropsychopharmacology on its 25th Anniversary (74). The volume numbers 1,840 double columned pages--a one volume encyclopedia. The section on Biological Psychiatry covers 541 pages by distinguished invited authors and comprises forty-one articles with up-to-date statements on the biology of the affective disorders, schizophrenia, psychiatric disorders of childhood, dementia, and anxiety, among others. Norepinephrine, dopamine, serotonin, acetycholine, opioid peptides, corticotropin, somatostatin and thyroid hormone appear involved in affective disorders; dopamine, GABA, the prostaglandins and peptides, and prolactin and growth hormone in schizophrenia; norepinephrine in attention disorders in children, cholinergic, serotonergic, and neuropeptides in Alzheimers Disease. The locus coeruleus, with the implied dysregulation of the norepinephrine system and the GABA, benzodiazapine receptor complex appears to be involved in anxiety and panic. Again and again the same players come up. We will hear in much more detail in this program from some of the builders of these seminal hypotheses.

Some years ago, at the 3rd International Neurochemical Symposium in Strasbourg in 1960 (20), I considered possible chemical factors which, in schizophrenia, might interfere with the information processing in the brain. I spoke of "a fundamental organizing process which during wakefulness in the normal, and at tremendous speed, registers, codes, matches, and correlates new against stored information, and in a succession of such transactions computes the probabilities which are of optimum service to the adaptive needs of the organism." I furthermore suggested that "these transformations proceed simultaneously as different yet closely interrelated neural levels; that they employ shifting reciprocal and highly discriminate inhibitory mechanisms in a successive elimination of redundant information." In the same paper I speculated on the chemical topology (involving the norepinephrine/dopamine/serotonin system) possibly underlying a *mis*processing of information, emphasizing interplay and interaction, possibly involving the Globus Pallidus and Caudate Nucleus.

We did not really have the help of the computer modeling of information processing at the time, and the chemicals in question were a mere handful. Today one is deeply encouraged by what has happened. For the various disorders we know as mental diseases may indeed turn out to be manifestations of dysregulation of molecular communication in the regionally organized, chemically mediated organ of information which we carry in our skull.

RESTORING COMMUNICATION: MOLECULAR LANGUAGES, VERBAL LANGUAGES AND THE METALANGUAGES OF THE INNER SELF

It would seem then, that the core element of our work is to restore communication, to re-pair, to re-connect the parted parts into a smoothly functioning whole. At the level of intercellular and inter-organ commerce the organism evidently employs precise molecular languages. These have been selected by evolution to exercise these functions. The symbolic "releasers" of innate and specific behaviors are chemically coded. The verbal languages used in day-to-day human commerce are much, much younger and much less precise. They are also the backbone of modern psychotherapy. Younger still is the astonishing array of the languages of science which, over the shortest span of evolution, have given us the products of our culture; and beyond these, as a sort of common ground of our humanity, there are the ancient symbolic metalanguages treasured by our race from culture to culture. These have special reflective attributes; for used in appropriate settings--be it individual, be it in a group--they have the power to evoke certain unmistakable experiences of wholeness, identity, selfhood and meaning. In some strange non-verbal way, these metalanguages appear to restore and re-connect. Art, religion and spirituality are the terms reserved for this realm. One is tempted to inquire into their mode of operation. Here one moves away from the realm of traditional science: Asking "how" is more appropriate than posing an immodest "why."

I submit that at a molecular level of communication we are way ahead. The astonishing explosion of knowledge, of which this symposium is a celebration, has carried the *in vivo* regional chemical topology of the brain from anatomical and histochemical to the molecular level. It has given us insights into regional metabolic shifts in relation to thought and intention and in mental disorder. Now receptor configuration is amenable to precise analysis; a taxonomy, a sort of periodic table (75) of informational substances is afoot. Add to it the miracles of modern genetic engineering, the isolation of genes fashioning receptors, and the crafting, literally harvesting, of transmitters and receptors in vitro and you have the advent of a rational chemotherapy of mental disorders which none of us thirty years ago would have dreamt in our philosophy.

However, as we enter the area of verbal communication and the languages of psychotherapy, things become at once more human and more complex. For languages, while depicting and reflecting experience, also shape experience. The rules governing their structure are ancient rules; quite probably, the brain is coded for them at birth (76). These rules--rules of astonishing logic and economy--go, as argued by Whorf (77), into the structure of even quite primitive languages; they order the fact symbols to each other and to the world they represent, and they make for the smooth use of language as an instrument of social adaptation and communication. Again, as in molecular languages, we come up against the key concept of *context*. Conventional logic imposes a linear, sequential, discursive quality upon them which seriously limits their informational power. For while carrying certain meanings in one context, words may carry a totally different meaning in another; and even standing alone they may--as anyone who has traced the origin of a word in a dictionary can see--carry an accretion of different meanings in a strange calculus of their own. Words are thus not mere labels, cards stacked for reference in one of Brocas areas. They are states, sets, depending on relation and context. They carry multiple meaning. The "unspeakable" metalanguages of the inner self are as different from the "speakable" as the structure of a dream is from deliberate, planned action. In such symbolic forms totality is apprehended simultaneously at different levels; mutually occlusive elements coexist; time is of no consequence; and serial ordering in time--that backbone of causal reasoning--gives way to simultaneously perceived relationships. I have elsewhere examined these issues in relation to the languages of physics (5). In this context, listen to William James (78):

> "What must be admitted is that the definite images of traditional psychology form but the smallest part of our minds as they actually live. The traditional psychology talks like one who should say a river consists of nothing but pailsful, spoonfuls, quartpotsful, barrelsful and other moulded forms of water. Even were the pails and pots all actually standing in the stream, still between them the free water would continue to flow. It is just this free water of consciousness that psychologists resolutely overlook. Every definite image in the mind is steeped and dyed in the free water that flows round it. With it goes the sense of its relations, near and remote,

> the dying echo whence it came to us, and
> the dawning sense whither it is to lead."

Traditional and Non-Traditional Psychotherapies

Jerome Frank, in his classic *Persuasion and Healing* (79) and a thoughtful series of papers (80,81), and Drs. McHugh and Slavney, in their monograph on "Perspectives on Psychiatry," (82) have examined the qualities and limitations of language in psychotherapy. Dr. Frank has argued for a comparison of psychotherapy to both rhetoric and hermeneutics. Rhetoric may be defined as the use of words to form attitudes and induce actions. Clearly this is an active mode. Hermeneutics is interpretive--the original word pertains to the interpretation of a religious text to discover intended meaning. In rhetoric, there is the common ground of emotional arousal followed by a cognitive process of argument. In hermeneutics, the patient is read like a text. Patient and therapist jointly engage in a quest to improve communication within. Contradictory aspects of functioning, forgotten memories, and subpersonalities are engaged in conversation. A web of *meaning* is derived, one which represents the best schema to account for past and present difficulties and offers an alternative interpretation of the future. This meaning is not absolute; on the contrary, it is relative and individual. Yet with meaning comes a sense of connectedness, and with this connectedness and communication, a reduction of despair and a raising of morale, competence, and a return of Hope. The biology of these positive states is relatively unknown. I suggest that they present a central theme for a psychobiology of the future.

It is deeply significant that in this quest for a sense of wholeness, for meaning, modern psychotherapy no longer depends solely on the verbal transaction. To the analytical interpretive and the deeply significant developments in cognitive therapy (83), there have now been added the Group approaches (84), where, as in a lens, interpersonal forces of great power are focused on an individual (especially when led by a professional who is also a peer [85]) and interpreted, as in psychosynthesis, with special reference to establishing communication between subpersonalities. The Gestalt "Body" and Movement techniques mobilize somatic memories "frozen" into a "body armor" (86); the powerful techniques of guided imagery in low states of arousal mobilize the imagination and illuminate true needs and choices (87); approaches which deliberately call on the devotional and sacred elements in a person's life are experienced as healing (88). We will readily admit that some of these approaches are a long, long way from the sciences which inform traditional medicine; yet, since they are reported to work, they should be included in our future agenda of research. Significantly, they provide bridges to the other ancient modes of self communication invented to allay the travails of the spirit. The arts and religion are old partners in the practice of healing. Like few branches of modern medicine, they have provided avenues into meaning which emerge as cornerstones of modern psychotherapy. We must ask why they have persisted; what has been their biological function for so long? I have never understood the so called contradiction between the practice of science and an acceptance of religion. I suspect it is contrived by persons who do not understand either science or religion. If the need for belief has so long an evolutionary history, religion--not doctrine, but the need to believe--is surely the business of psychobiology.

Arts, and the Spiritual Element

It would require a separate paper to review the place of the Arts in therapy. Their time-honored role in psychiatry is well established; professional associations and journals attest to their effectiveness. What is regrettable is that they have remained at the periphery of medicine. Music, for example, is establishing for itself a firm place in therapeutics (90). Analgesic, anxiolytic, and hormonal effects of music have been noted (92,93), as have the effects of music and imagery on adrenal corticosteroids and circadian rhythms. Moreover, certain temporal musical patterns have grammatical patterns akin to languages (91) and appear to be related to certain common emotional states, the so called sentic cycle (94).

Similarly, the languages of the visual and plastic arts are related to therapy and have been used for at least a century. They offer a fascinating field of inquiry lying in the borderlands of sickness and creativity (95).

A spiritual element can be central to a patient's life. As healers, we should inquire after this dimension in our patients. A recently introduced Spiritual Inventory for the Medically Ill Patient takes stock of this important dimension in the medically ill (96). It inquires how one's patients see and interpret the meaning of their illness: Do they see it as a challenge? An enemy? A punishment? Weakness? Relief? It asks how they see their values, their belief and faith; the function of love in their lives; the place of forgiveness, and the place of prayer; the capacity for private meditation or worship in a group. As we said earlier, if restoration of meaning is central to successful psychotherapy, these aspects of inner life would appear central to meaning. I suggest that we look beyond the traditional therapies into the restorative and healing powers of these old/new approaches, and that we do so in a systematic way by established tools of biomedical research. Private institutions have an extraordinary opportunity in this regard. Nor can we do it alone. New professions, new mixes of professions are needed. Of necessity, they will emerge in time.

TOWARDS A SCIENTIFIC HUMANISM: THE CATALYTIC FUNCTION OF PSYCHIATRY IN A MEDICINE OF THE FUTURE

Psychiatry as a Statement of Human Biology

I hope that by now we have noted some attributes of our field which are a source of both difficulties and high promise. Ours is a peculiarly personal science. There may be impersonal medicine, but there cannot be impersonal psychiatry. However "biologically oriented" in our work the *person* is central to our trade. Meaning is not an asterisk and after-thought but is at the very heart of what we do. Medicine may have gotten into its present difficulties by failing to distinguish between disease and illness (97). Psychiatry brooks no such distinction. It is a specialty as well as a "generality," a vast continent of a discipline, extending from the deeply molecular to the deeply human. Bridging such realms of knowledge is quite a task. Psychiatry has always forged alliances with other disciplines, and no discipline which has worked with psychiatry has failed to be enriched by contact with us. Whether it be genetics and neurobiology or developmental, experimental and social psychology, anthropology, the social sciences, or linguistics, the gain has always gone both ways. Psychiatry poses obstinate questions at the very core of medical practice. Some twenty-five years ago, when I was invited to take up my post at Johns Hopkins, I wrote a memorandum to the search committee outlining my hopes for our field (98). Looking at this meeting in 1989, I am comforted by progress. I submit that what psychiatry is today will be very relevant to the medicine of tomorrow.

In dealing with disorders of communication, psychiatry has provided the outlines of an understanding of the role of information transfer in psychosomatic exchange. It has done so at the molecular, the inter-organ, and the symbolic level. It has addressed the individual, the dyad, and the group. It has delved into the evolution of values and belief systems and contributed to our understanding of their beneficent function in coping and healing. It has even begun to address the biological origins, correlates, and role of spiritual elements in life and the arts as potential agents of healing. The ancient functions of the physician as a teacher and a facilitator of hope are beginning to make a great deal of biological sense. Indeed, we may be witnessing a profound revolution of which modern psychiatry may be the forerunner. It has been called the information revolution, or Infomedicine (99). The concept of single-cause disease is giving place to causes seen in *context*. Analytical thinking is being incorporated into a cybernetic model in which the study of the whole and the part are inexorably linked. More and more the society within the skin appears to have its congruences and correlates without.

I suggest, in the light of the foregoing, that modern psychiatry already provides us with a more complete and comprehensive description of the body-mind connection than any other branch of medicine, and that it can help us to insights concerning the inner mechanisms of recovery and healing which may only be on the peripheral field of vision of conventional medicine. It already excels at fashioning molecular models of mental disorder. Its models of illness, however, are broader. Person, meaning, coherence (100), coping and competence are at the very core of its work. To the biophysical model, it now adds an attitudinal ("spiritual") element, and is ready to inquire into these aspects of healing by accepted methods of biomedical research. Its models of illness inexorably lead it to models of health; the techniques which have given it an understanding of the negative emotions stand ready to be applied to the study of positive states of being. Psychiatry, in trying to comprehend, is a truly comprehensive kind of medicine. I submit that, even as it is today, its peculiar amalgam of disciplines provides the best introduction to human biology that we have.

I suggest that it is time to consider how we can best put this new knowledge to the service of medicine and society. We must begin with ourselves, our own profession, and the professionals who are our colleagues. We must also recall that a powerful democratization of knowledge is afoot, especially through the media. The American public seems to be going to medical school. In our field, it behoves us to exercise quality control and ensure that the information is sound, up-to-date, and above all, useful. Within the scope of this paper I can only indicate some possible trends, and illustrate them with a few examples out of my own experience.

The New Biobehavioral Sciences; Their Role in Humanizing Medical Education

Humanizing medical education has been a recurrent "cri de coeur" echoing through reports on medical education reform for the past fifty years (101,102,103,104). Those of us who have participated in the paste and scissors operation of curricular reform know how hard it is to merge the clinical and human element into an overcrowded, overworked curriculum. Far reaching experiments in self directed learning are attempting to weave preclinical sciences into experiential, clinical practice (105,106,107,108). I suggest that the new knowledge concerning body-mind communication provides an excellent teaching "spine" for an introduction to medicine. It also enhances a student's awareness of himself/herself as a fascinating portable biological laboratory, and it can help the student put his or her knowledge to use in the great laboratory of everyday life. It is important that such exposure occur early in the curriculum. I refer particularly to the pioneering experiments initiated in Rochester by George Engel and his colleagues (107,108); and I can tell you a little about two experiments which my colleagues and I began, one at Hopkins some twenty years ago and one more recent one, still in progress in Louisville, Kentucky.

In 1964, Dr. Richard Chase, a group of colleagues, and I initiated an introductory Behavioral Science course at Hopkins, taught in the second year (109). Four themes recurred through the course: Human Development, Human Learning, Human Communication and The Social Field. Biology--psychobiology--was related to each. We tried to make it both theoretical and clinically applied; both didactic and experiential. A major feature of the course was that three departmental chairmen, of the Department of Pediatrics, Obstetrics and Gynecology, and myself, and several senior teachers from the departments of medicine and surgery participated in the course. As Dr. Engel, Dr. Reiser and Dr. Rosen had done (108), we tried to make it interdisciplinary, clinically relevant and symbiotic, demonstrating, we hoped, the pervasive influence of psychiatry in modern medical practice. The course was well received, and I was delighted to learn that it has provided a template for a more contemporary and advanced version under the inspired leadership of Dr. Paul McHugh.

At Hopkins I had the good fortune to meet Dr. Caroline Thomas who, in following a cohort of 1,337 medical students over 16 years, had developed her famous Precursors Study (110) on the basis of psychological profiles and had identified certain predictive risk factors in medical students for stress related disorders, including hypertension, coronary heart disease, depression and cancer. It occurred to me at the time that an intervention *preceding* those stressful years might be worth trying. The opportunity arose in Louisville when I had the good fortune to meet Dr. Leah Dickstein, Associate Dean of Students in that School of Medicine. Again, the Department of Psychiatry, with Dr. John Schwab's unwavering help and support, became the sponsor of what has now become known as "The Louisville Experiment (111)."

The idea is really very simple. It is a week-long event, known as the "Health Awareness Workshop," offered to medical students during the week *preceding* their official enrolment in August. Last year, out of a class of 124, 122 students, plus spouses and some eight children, attended this offering. The exercise is staffed by faculty and student volunteers. These act as "health tutors" and student mentor-colleagues in subsequent years.

The idea is to communicate to students the practical reality of the body-mind connection and to provide them with coping skills to master the competitive obstacle race which awaits them in their training. The exercise is partly didactic and partly small-group experiential. It includes overviews of the psychobiology of stress and coping, attention to nutrition, exercise, relaxation, time management, study skills, listening skills, spouse and sexual problems, substance abuse, medical ethics, and the place of faith, hope and humor in healing. We judge the experiential element to be very important. The health check and health risk appraisal is carried out by the students themselves. (We have, incidentally, discovered several early hypertensives in each of our classes.) Nutrition is taught through the preparation and serving of nutritional meals and through a student-authored cookbook. Relaxation is taught and time management and exam tips are presented by senior students. The sense of learning and sharing in joy and in fun permeates the whole exercise. Staff and students wear identical T-Shirts embossed with an attractive "Ways to Health" logo. As behooves our field, the arts are very much in evidence. By the time the Dean greets them in welcome on the last day of the exercise, social support groups have gathered spontaneously and networks have formed. No student is a stranger to colleagues or to staff. We believe that we have in the exercise the makings of an important epidemiological health laboratory for the physician-in-training. We try to convey the idea to the student that within his or her own skin there is a magnificent bodymind laboratory, that every day can be an experiment, and that a training of awareness is a key element to living a good life, one day at a time.

I have furnished these two examples. Others could be added from the literature to illustrate the catalytic role which psychiatry can and should play in shaping attitudes and patterns of care in the medicine of the future. It is not accidental that an offering such as we put together in our Behavioral Science course and in the Health Awareness program should emanate from a department of psychiatry. So far, only psychiatry, among medical disciplines, spans a coherent body of knowledge extending from mind to body, from the molecular to the symbolic, from disease to recovery, coping, and wellbeing. I suggest that we have not even begun to exercise our full influence in the training of physicians, in the planning of a humane health care system, or in bringing our knowledge into the vast, pervasive laboratory of everyday life. For far too long we have spoken only when spoken to.

I hope you have noted that the arguments and models I have put before you, while conjectural, have a distinctly practical side. Explained to the average person--to *any* patient--such communication about body-mind can carry a powerful rationale for enhancing personal initiative and coping. Our place is then to participate with our clinical colleagues in joint practice and research and to explain, and to train people who could explain what we know, to plan treatment facilities which would "do it" better and differently; and to fashion approaches which take us beyond disease into prevention, and thus lay the groundwork for a science not only of illness but of wellbeing.

We must become more active in care and education and go beyond well meant consulting-liaison work. Mode of life is emerging as the major pathogen in our society; fear, surely, is a mighty propellant. Behavioral factors are emerging as *the* risk factors in the plagues of our time, from alcoholism and AIDS to hypertension, cardiovascular disease, and possibly cancer. We must take our place firmly alongside and even ahead of other specialties in treatment, research and prevention. We must enter into joint major enterprises with our colleagues, into joint Grand Rounds, into major research and educational programs, particularly in relation to the stress related disorders: substance abuse, AIDS, adolescent disorders, and chronic diseases. We need good studies to test the cost effectiveness of the interventions we offer in terms of hard dollars, particularly on mobilizing self efficacy and speeding recovery. I submit that industry is ready to provide these dollars: But we--not others, but *we*--must take the initiative. Third party carriers are still mean in recognizing the value of our services. We must make money talk. Our hard-won body of knowledge can be put to practical use. If we are too busy to serve as educator-doctors, we should give thought to the training of professionals who could function as "explainers" to mobilize a patient's physical and psychological resources to optimize and speed recovery. There are many nurses, counselors and social workers who innately and intuitively possess these qualities and exercise them when given a chance. But I do not know of any training anywhere which offers the peculiar mix of a strong and modern theoretical foundation and applied practical experience which I would call adequate. I have named such professionals, provisionally, "explainers" or "attitudinal counselors", and the branch of medicine which they would represent, "Attitudinal Medicine." Don't misunderstand me. I do not see them as robust, rosy-cheeked Mrs. Cheerfuls, sweeping into the sickroom to spread light and laughter. Warmth, to be sure, is a requisite, but with it should come maturity, high intelligence, and the ability to master the varied body of new knowledge now forming. Also required are toughness and resilience in facing suffering, the ability to share and to communicate with others (from physicians and colleagues to patient's families, work settings and friends), and, above all, an ability to sustain a realistic optimism in the face of disappointment. Some years ago my former wife, Charmian Elkes, began at Hopkins a program for training mental health counselors. The program, drawing upon the native abilities of mature lay people coming from different backgrounds, trained them into highly successful professionals (89) who subsequently won high acceptance in the Maryland Mental Health community. A Masters degree in Mental Health Counseling was offered. Attitudinal counselors who explain as they encourage, and encourage as they explain, could be powerful factors in raising patient morale, not through exhortation but through participation, understanding, and insight. It may be worth trying.

I believe that by applying the principles of communication which are at the heart of our field we can provide leadership in the transformation of the medical environment, fashioning a true partnership between provider and consumer, reducing apprehension and fear, and enhancing hope. Could waiting areas be Learning Centers? Could the media in patients' rooms be arranged to provide choice of channels to include relevant technical information in lay languages, or offerings enhancing positive attitudes through information, through art, through humor? Could all that we know about groups be put to use in *medical* wards to speed recovery? Could all that we know about families become the therapeutic rule rather than the exception in an emergency? And moving to the outpatient setting, could a referral to a psychiatrist be robbed of its stigma, and accepted as part of a well explained, comprehensive therapeutic plan? When, long before HMOs or group health were "in," we started on a prepaid system of medical care in Columbia, Maryland (112), psychiatry was seen as a *primary* care giver, together with Pediatrics, Medicine, and Obstetrics and Gynecology. The offices were adjoining. A modest sliding fee scale limited to 10 sessions ensured acceptance. These thoughts are offered in the hope of a diffusion of what we know into the body of general medicine. Psychiatry should have the courage to use its knowledge and use it comprehensively.

Psychological Medicine, Behavioral Medicine, Attitudinal Medicine, all imply the application of what we already know in modern psychiatry to the ills endemic in modern society. There is a need for hospices for the living as well as for the dying. Modern psychiatry knows enough to help in their design.

Towards a Science of Wellbeing - The Person in the Laboratory of Everyday Life

As we move to the role of Psychological medicine in the arena of everyday life, we detect a costly paradox. For, while leading health planners are calling for a recognition of attitudinal/behavioral interventions as factors in reducing health cost (113) and in diminishing the incidence of disease, and while industry is making major capital investments to change life habits in the workplace and is already reaping clear financial return on its investment (114,115), we in medicine still stand at the periphery--preoccupied, hesitating, and "awaiting," as we say, "the evidence." Neither our curriculum nor our practice reflects these urgent societal needs. Modern psychiatry is already broad enough and strong enough to be in the lead. For the very methods and sciences which have given us medicine's advances and have led us to precise diagnoses and rational therapeutics now stand ready to be applied to the much less well mapped terrain of personal competence and wellbeing. To the ward and clinic and long term care facility we now add the laboratory of everyday life. It is beginning to prove an immensely rewarding area of investigation.

I suggest that modern psychiatry must go public with its knowledge, and that the public is ready and eager to learn what we already know. The success of media events like the PBS series on the Brain and Mind, where leading psychiatrists participated; the enormous sales of books on the Mind/Body/Brain connection; the emergence of powerful advocacy groups like the Schizophrenia Foundation, the Alliance of the Medically Ill, N.A.R.S.A.; the near catastrophic pressures put on our state health services by recent laws; these all serve to build both negative and positive pressures to move the needs of our field into the public awareness. We have an opportunity to create an informed constituency. I am amazed by the timeliness, sense of newness and power, and appeal of our work; work which, in our parochial way, we have been taking totally for granted.

I recall meeting recently with a prominent person to discuss needs for public support. "The bloom is off the medical rose. We have heard, and heard, and heard about diseases," he said. "But the Mind/Brain/Body connection--that is new, fascinating stuff. It applies to disease as it does to health. You fellows must tell the public what you know already; communicate about communication--molecular, verbal, symbolic, social; about inside the skin and out. Their eyes will light up!"

We would do well to take note of my friend's advice.

REFERENCES

1. Ayd FJ, Blackwell B: (Eds.) Discoveries in biological psychiatry. Philadelphia: J.B. Lipincott, 1970
2. Meyer A: The purpose of the psychiatric clinic. Am. J. Insanity, 1913, 69, 835-860
3. Meyer A: Psychobiology, A Science of Man. Springfield, IL: Charles

C. Thomas, 1957
4. Elkes J: Behavioral pharmacology in relation to psychiatry. In: Gruhle HW, Jung R, Mayer-Gross W, and Muller M (eds.) Psychiatrie der Gegenwart. Berlin: Springer-Verlag, 1962, pp. 929-1036
5. Elkes J: Subjective and objective observation in psychiatry. The Harvey Lectures, Series 57. New York: Academic Press, 1963, pp. 63-92
6. Elkes J: Epilogue and foreglimpse: Letter to a young colleague considering a career in psychopharmacology. In: Clark WG and de Guidice J (Eds.). Principles of Psychopharmacology. New York: Academic Press, 1978, pp. 741-53
7. Elkes J: Towards a science of health: Thoughts on brain, behavior, and wellbeing. Paper read at Symposium "Optimum Utilization of Knowledge in Service of Health" at AAAS Annual Meeting titled, "Science and Engineering Toward a National Renaissance," Detroit, Michigan, May 27, 1983
8. Elkes J: On awareness and the good day. In: Ng LKY and Davis DL (Eds.). Strategies for public health: Promoting health and preventing disease. New York: Van Reinhold, 1981, pp. 71-85
9. Weiner H: The organism in health and disease: An attempt at an integrative medical model. Paper presented at the conference on "New Models of Health, Illness and Disease: Implications of Psychoneuroimmunology," Lake Arrowhead, CA, 1987
10. Rubenstein E: Disease caused by impaired commmunication among cells. Sci Amer, 1988, 242, 102-121
11. Edelman GM: Topobiology: An introduction to molecular embryology. New York: Basic Books, 1988
12. Jerne NK: The generative grammar of the immune system. Nobel Lecture. Bioscience Reports 1985, *5*, 439-51
13. Spector NH: Interactions among the nervous, endocrine and immune systems. In: Frederickson RCA, Hendrie HC, Hingtgen JN and Aprison MH (Eds.) Neuroregulation of Autonomic, Endocrine and Immune Systems. Boston: Martinus Nijhoff Publishing, Inc., 1986, pp.329-41
14. MacLean PD: The limbic system ("visceral brain") in relation to the central gray and reticulum of the brain stem. Psychosomatic Med 1955, 17, 355
15. Nauta WJH: Hippocampal projections and related neural pathways to the midbrain in the cat. Brain 1958, 81, 319
16. Craik KJW: The nature of explanation. London: Cambridge University Press, 1952
17. Head H: Aphasia and kindred disorders of speech. London: Cambridge University Press, 1926
18. Miller NE: Learning visceral and glandular responses. Science.

1969, 163, 434-45

19. Edelman GM, Mountcastle V: The mindful brain: cortical organization and the group-selective theory of higher brain function. Cambridge: MIT Press, 1978
20. Elkes J: Schizophrenic disorder in relation to levels of neural organization. In: Folch-Pi J (Ed.) The chemical pathology of the nervous system. London: Pergamon Press, 1961, pp. 648-65
21. Edelman GM: Neural darwinism: The theory of neuronal group selection. New York: Basic Books, 1987
22. Frazer JG: The new golden bough. New York: Criterion Books, 1959
23. Jung CG: Man and his symbols. Garden City NY: Doubleday, 1964
24. Campbell J: Historical atlas of world mythology. New York: Harper and Row, 1987
25. Grof S: Beyond the brain. New York: State University of New York Press, 1985
26. Amkraut A, Solomon GS: From symbolic stimulus to pathophysiologic response. Internat J Psychia in Med. 1975, 5, 134-56
27. Ader R: Psychoneuroimmunology. New York: Academic Press, 1981
28. Nossal GJV: Current concepts: Immunology. New Eng J Med. 1987, 316, 1320-25
29. Locke SE, Colligan D: The healer within. New York: E.P. Dutton, 1987
30. Nossal GJV: Loc. Cit., p. 1320
31. Blalock JE: The Immune system as a sensory organ. J Immunol. 1983, 132, 1067-70
32. Hall NR, McGillis JP, Spangelo BL, Goldstein AL: Evidence that thymosins and other biological response modifiers can function as neuroactive immunotransmitters. J Immunol. 1985, 136, 806-11
33. Keller SE, Stein M, Camerino MS, Schleifer SJ, Sherman J: Suppression of lymphocyte stimulation by anterior hypothalamic lesions in the guinea pig. Cell Immunol, 1980, *52*, 334-40
34. Felten DL, Felten SY, Carlson SL, Olschowka JA, Livnat S: Noradrenergic and peptidergic innervation of lymphoid tissue. J Immunol. 1985, 135, 755-65
35. Bulloch K, More RY: Innervation of the thymus gland by brainstem and spinal cord in mouse and Rat. Am J Anat. 1982, 162, 157-66
36. Ader R, Cohen N: Behaviorally conditioned immunosuppression. Psychosom Med. 1975, 37, 333-340
37. Kiecolt-Glaser JK, Garner W, Speicher C, Penn GM, Holliday J, Glaser R: Psychosocial modifiers of immunocompetence in medical students. Psychosom Med. 1984, 46, 7-14
38. Locke SE, Kraus L, Leserman J, Hurst MW, Heisel S, Williams RM: Lifestress changes, psychiatric symptoms and natural killer cell

activity. Psychosom Med., 1984, 46, 441-453
39. Linn BS, Linn MW, Jensen J: Degree of depression and immune responsiveness. Psychosom Med, 1982: 44, 128
40. Stein M, Schleifer SJ, Keller SS: Stress, depression and immunity. In: Frederickson CA, Hendrie HC, Hingtgen JN and Aprison MH (Eds.) Neuroregulation of autonomic, endocrine and immune systems. Boston: Martinus Nijhoff Publishing, Inc., 1986, pp.329-41
41. Riley V, Fitzmaurice MA, Spackman DM: Psychoneuroimmunologic factors in neoplasia studies in animals. In: Ader R (Ed.). Psychoneuroimmunology, New York: Academic Press, 1981
42. Levy S: Host differences in neoplastic risk behavioral and social contributors to disease. Health Psychol, 1983, 2, 21-44
43. Lloyd R: Possible mechanisms of psychoneuroimmunological interactions. Advances, 1984, 1, 43-49
44. Levy SM (Ed): Biological mediators of behavior and disease: neoplasia. New York: Elsevier Sciences Publishing, 1982
45. Heath RG, Krupp IM: Schizophrenia as an immunologic disorder. Arch Gen Psychia, 1967, 16, 1-9
46. Solomon GF: Immunologic abnormalities in mental illness. In: Ader R. Psychoneuroimmunology, New York, Academic Press, 1981
47. Sherrington CS: Man on his nature. Cambridge (Engl.): Cambridge University Press, 1951, p. 104
48. Feldberg W, Vogt M: Acetycholine synthesis in different regions of the central nervous system. J Physiol (London), 1948, 107, 372
49. Bradley PB, Elkes J: The effect of atropine, hyoscyamine, physostigimine and neostigimine on the electrical activity of the brain of the conscious cat. J Physiol (London), 1953, 120, p. 14
50. Bradley PB, Elkes J: The effects of some drugs on the electrical activity of the brain. Brain, 1967, 80, 77-117
51. Elkes J: Drug effects in relation to receptor specificity within the brain: Some evidence and provisional formulations. In: Wolstenholme GEW and O'Connor CM (Eds.) Neurological basis of behavior. CIBA Foundation Symposium, London, 1957. London: J & A Churchill, 1958, p.303
52. Bradley PB, Elkes J: The effects of some drugs on the electrical activity of the brain. Op. Cit., pp 113-14
53. Schmitt FO: Molecular regulation of brain function: A new view. Neuroscience, 1984, 13, 991-1001
54. Keiss W, Hall NR: Psychoneuroimmunology and endocrine mediated evolution of the immune system. In: Hesch D (Ed.) Handbook of Endocrinology. Munich, West Germany: Urban and Schwarzenberg, 1989
55. Bulbring E: The action of adrenaline on transmission in the superior cervical ganglion. J. Physiol. 1944, 103, 55-67

56. Kandel ER: Cellular mechanisms of learning. In: Kandel ER and Schwartz JM (Eds.) Principles of neuroscience. New York: Elsevier Sciences Publishing, 1985
57. Reite M, Field T: Psychobiology of attachment and separation. Orlando: Academic Press, 1985
58. Hanin I, Usdin E: Animal models in psychiatry and neurology. New York: Pergamon Press, 1977
59. Evonink GE, Kuhn CM, Schanberg SM: The effect of tactile stimulation on serum growth hormone and tissue ornithine decarboxylase activity during maternal deprivation in rat pups. Communic Psychopharmacol. 1979, *3*, 363-70
60. McGaugh J: Preserving the presence of the past: Hormonal influences on memory storage. Am Psychologist, 1983, 38, 161-73
61. Black IK, Adler JE, Dreyfus CF, Friedman WJ, LaGama EF, Roach AH: Experience, neurotransmitters plasticity and behavior. In: Meltzer H (Ed.). Psychopharmacology: The third generation of progress, New York: Raven Press, 1987, pp. 463-70
62. Pert CB: Neuropeptides, the emotions and bodymind. Noetic Sci Rev, 1987, 2, 8-13
63. Nienwenhuys R: Chemoarchitecture of the brain. New York: Springer Verlag, 1985
64. Cantin M, Genest J: The heart as an endocrine gland. Sci Amer, 1986, 25r(2), 76-81
65. Selye H: History and present status of the stress concept. In: Goldberger L and Breznitz S (Eds.). Handbook of Stress, New York: McMillan, 1982, pp. 7-20
66. Rossi E: From Mind to molecule: A theory of mind body healing. Advances, 1987, 4, 46-60
67. Rossi E: The psychobiology of mind-body healing. New York: W.W. Norton, 1986
68. Overton D: Major theories of state-dependent learning. In: Ho B, Richards D and Chute D (Eds.). Drug discrimination and state-dependent learning. New York: Academic Press, 1978, pp. 283-318
69. Becker RO, Selden G: The body electric: electromagnetism and the foundation of life. New York: William Morrow, 1985
70. Bakan D: Disease, pain and sacrifice. Chicago: University of Chicago Press, 1968
71. Cunningham AJ: Information and health in many levels of man. Advances, 1986, 3, 32-45
72. Snyder SH: A marriage of molecules, mind and medicine. In: Ray OS, Wilkes-Ray D (Eds.). American College of Neuropsychopharmacology, Anniversary Anthology. Nashville, TN: ACNP Publication, 1986, pp. 153-57

73. Bloom FE: Are pharmaceutical futures necessarily a prophetless commodity. In: Ray OS, Wilkes-Ray D (Eds.). American College of Neuropsychopharmacology, Anniversary Anthology. Nashville, TN: ACNP Publication, 1986, pp.141-45
74. Meltzer HY (Ed.): Psychopharmacology: The third generation of progress. New York: Raven Press, 1987
75. Barchas JD: Considerations for a future psychopharmacology. In: Ray OS, Wilkes-Ray D (Eds.) American College of Neuropsychopharmacology, Anniversary Anthology. Nashville, TN: ACNP Publication, 1986, pp. 135-39
76. Chomsky N: Language and mind. New York: Harcourt, Brace and World, 1968
77. Whorf BJ: Language, thought and reality. New York: Wiley, 1956
78. James W: Principles of psychology, New York: Henry Holt, 1890. Reprinted by Dover Publications, New York, 1950, Vol. 1, p. 255
79. Frank J: Persuasion and healing (2nd Edition), Baltimore, Johns Hopkins University Press, 1974
80. Frank JD: Psychotherapy, the transformations of meanings. J Royal Soc Med, 1986, 79, 341-46
81. Frank JD: Psychotherapy, rhetoric and hermeneutics: Implications for practice and research. Psychotherapy, 1987, 24, 293-301
82. McHugh PR, Slavney PR: The perspectives of psychiatry, Baltimore: Johns Hopkins Press, 1983, pp. 1-26 and 125-34
83. Beck A: Cognitive therapy and the emotional disorders. New York: International Universities Press, 1976
84. Yalom ID: The theory and practice of group psychotherapy, Second Edition, New York: Basic books, Inc., 1975
85. Rhodes J, Foard T, Dickstein L: Professional peer group counseling in the management of rheumatoid arthritis: a clinical trial. In: Hall RCW (Ed.) Recent advances in psychiatric medicine, Orlando, FL: Ryandic Publishing, 1989
86. Reich W: Character analysis, New York: Orgone Institute, 1949.
87. Singer JL, Pope KS: The power of the human imagination: new methods in psychotherapy. New York: Plenum Press, 1978
88. Hiatt JF: Spirituality, medicine and healing. Sourthern Med J, 1986, 79, 736-43
89. Mental health counselor program, pilot project. Public Health Series, Publication No. 1254. Washington: DHEW, 1971
90. Spingte R, Droh R: Music in medicine. Basel, Editiones Roche, 1985
91. Jackendoff R, Lerdahl F: Grammatical parallel between music and language. In: Clynes M (Ed.). Music, mind and brain. New York: Plenum Press, 1982, pp. 83-118
92. Shehhati-Chafai G, Kau G: Comparative study of the anxiolytic

effects of diazepam and music in patients during operations in regional anaesthesia. In: Spingte R and Droh R. Loc Cit., pp. 231-236

93. Tanioka F, Takazawa T, Kamata S, Kudo M, Matsuki A, Oyama T: Hormonal effect of anxiolytic music in patients during surgical operations under epidural anaesthesia. In: Spingte R and Droh R. Loc Cit., pp. 285-291
94. Clynes M: Sentics: The touch of emotions. New York: Doubleday (Anchor), 1977
95. Adamson E: Art as healing. York Beach (Maine): Nicholas-Hays, 1984
96. Kuhn CC: A Spiritual inventory for the medically ill patient. Psychiatric Medicine, 1988, 6, 89-100
97. Kleinman A: Patients and healers in the context of culture, Berkeley and Los Angeles, University of California Press, 1980
98. Elkes J: Self regulation and behavioral medicine: Early beginnings. Psychiatric Annals, 1981, 11, 2, p. 54/27
99. Foss, L, Rothenberg K: The second medical revolution--from biomedicine to infoMedicine. Boston, Shambala Publications, 1988
100. Antonowsky A: Health, stress and coping. San Francisco, Jossey Bass, 1980
101. Rappleye WC: Medical education: Final report of the commission on medical education. AAME Commission on Medical Education., Washington, DC: Association of American Medical Colleges, 1932
102. Cope D (Ed): Man, mind and medicine--The doctor's education, a chairman's view of the swampscott study in behavioral science in medicine, 23 Oct - 4 Nov, 1986. Philadelphia, J.B. Lippincott, 1968
103. Physicians for the twenty-first Century. The GPEP report, Washington DC: Association of American Medical Colleges, 1984
104. Cousins N: Physician as a humanist. In: Reiser, DE and Rose, DH. Medicine as a human experience. Baltimore, University Park Press, 1984, p. ix
105. Neufeld VR, Barrows HS: The McMaster philosophy and approach to medical education. J. Med. Ed., 1974, 49, 1040-1050
106. Prywes M: The beer sheva experience: Integration of medical care and medical education. Isr J Med Sci, 1983, 19, 775-79
107. Engel GL: The need for a new medical model: A challenge for biomedicine. Science, 1977, 196, 129-36
108. Reiser DE, Rosen DH: Medicine as a human experience. Baltimore, University Park Press, 1984
109. Elkes J: On meeting psychiatry: A note on the student's first year. Am. J. Psychia., 1965, August, 121-8
110. Thomas CB: What becomes of medical students: The dark side. Johns

Hopkins Med. J., 1976, 138, 185-95
111. Dickstein LJ, Elkes J: Health awareness and the medical student: A preliminary experiment. Advances, 1987, 4, 11-23
112. Stone EM, Greenblatt M: The columbia plan: An interview with Joel and Charmian Elkes. Semin in Psychiatry, 1971, 3, 199-206
113. Knowles JH (Ed.): Doing better and feeling worse: Health in the United States. New York: W. W. Norton and Co., 1977
114. Fielding JH: Corporate health management. New York, Addison-Wesley, 1984
115. Pelletier KR: Health people in unhealthy places: Stress and fitness at work. New York, Delacorte Press, 1984

chapter 6

Clinical Issues In Food Ingestion And Body Weight Maintenance

Paul R. McHugh, M.D., F.A.P.A.

INTRODUCTION

The alliance between clinician and basic scientist in the study of food ingestion and body weight control has been a sometime thing! Clinicians, in particular, concerned with management of obesity and anorexia nervosa wax and wane in their patience with progress in basic science. Most opt for simple symptomatic treatments of such patients--dieting for the obese and renourishment for the anorexic--recognizing that the identification of the causes of these disorders and, thus, rational treatment and prevention is far from achieved. Basic scientists on the other hand intermittently look to the human resources of the clinician with enthusiasm, finding great interest in the "animal who talks," only eventually to return to laboratory animals when faced with the complicated problems of the "animal that deceives, denies and distorts."

The purpose of this brief essay is to lay out the natural linkages and some highlights of achievement of this alliance. I do this, as have others, in part to encourage what can be a faltering relationship but also to direct attention to distinctly different scientific domains in each of which clinicians and basic scientists can cooperate in the search for the causes of human disorders. It will be my point that it is the mutual responsibility of members of this alliance to appreciate that at present two rather distinct lines of investigation exist that can be culled to reveal details of causation in different human disorders. Eventually, a union of these lines will be achieved but this is not imminent, partly because both lines of investigation are still immature. An appreciation, though, of what each has proposed in the past and a focus on prototypic examples of contemporary study should reassure anyone that the clinical-basic science alliance remains lively

Published 1990 by Elsevier Science Publishing Co., Inc.
Psychiatry: Past Reflections–Future Visions
B.T. Taylor and I.J. Taylor, Editors

and its future full of opportunity.

I can be more specific. Human feeding and weight control, like all the issues that rest upon motivated behaviors, can be appreciated as having proximate and ultimate causes. The proximate or immediate causes of food intake and its control emerge from *experiments* revealing basic, regulatory physiology with its diversity of hierarchically organized mechanisms in the body comprehensible from the organismal to the molecular levels. Investigations to explain some feeding disorders have in the past and do in the present reveal how crucial aspects of these proximate controls can be injured. An important "two way trade" between bedside and laboratory bench exists right now in this study.

On the other hand, the ultimate causes of any motivated behavior such as food intake and some of its uniquely human problems rest upon progressively species-specific formative elements of the organism, that is, the human genome, its shaping over time by natural selection, and the successful emergence of a developmental program that depends on the interaction between the genetic instructions and the staged experiences imposed by the environment. As an ecological process, this program leads to the phenotypic expression of the genotypic direction. It is human epidemiology, the *prospective surveillance* of naturally occurring events, rather than experiment, that can bring to light the play of ultimate factors in the construction of some human disorders of food intake and weight control. This epidemiological perspective broadly construed to grasp ethological, ecological, and genetic considerations has revealed equally intriguing results as have experimental investigations into pathophysiology. It is the perspective that promises a synthesis of causation that may bring rational treatment and prevention together for many human disorders of body weight control.

Finally, to be still more specific and to introduce particular issues and our contemporary knowledge of them, human disorders of food intake and body weight control fall into two great and, at least at the moment, distinctive categories. One is based on crude pathology within the individual organism disrupting the normal functioning of the apparatus that controls the behavior. What might be called "spanner in the works" conditions. These represent the most natural and immediate sites for cooperation between clinicians and laboratory scientists. In the second category are those distortions or deviations in food intake and weight control specific to mankind emerging with development and its capacity to direct, reinforce or hinder behavioral expression. Such issues as genetic differences across populations, schedules of maturation, and variations in sociocultural processes that interact with intrapersonal factors, all offer information to explain disorders of this second type and again represent opportunities for coordination of the work of clinicians and behavioral scientists.

PROXIMATE OR IMMEDIATE FACTOR COLLABORATION BETWEEN CLINICIANS AND BASIC SCIENTISTS

Hypothalamic Obesity

The main reason for beginning with the proximate factors is that here successful collaboration between clinicians and basic scientists in the study of food intake and weight control first occurred. The very first recognition of an association between pathological lesions at the base of the brain and abnormal obesity was made in man by Frohlich (1,2,3), and was promptly followed up by Erdheim in 1904 (4) who announced that it was injury to the hypothalamus and not to the pituitary gland that produced such obesity. These remarkable observations from the clinic can be considered the opening events in the collaboration of clinicians and basic scientists in obesity because they prompted Hetherington and Ranson (1940) (5) to ask what specific structures in the hypothalamus must be destroyed to produce these effects. This question could best be addressed in animals and at the laboratory bench, and required the redeployment of the Horsley-Clarke instrument for precise placement of lesions. The success at reproducibly evoking obesity with strategically placed lesions in the ventral and medial hypothalamus of the rat was a landmark discovery in every sense of the word. On the one hand, it promoted an enthusiasm for the Horsley-Clarke instrument throughout physiological psychology and, on the other, a sharp focus on the hypothalumus and obesity that led to Brobeck's (1943) (6) demonstration that the obesity was associated with overeating and not simply to passive metabolic factors turning calories into fat (3,4,5). The relationship of the overeating to autonomic imbalances and to the metabolic and endocrine responses provoked by the brain lesion is now the active focus of research (7,8,9) and is illuminated in other essays in this volume.

It is not appropriate in this essay to go into more detail about this great achievement as I wish primarily to point it out as the classic example of work on the proximate or immediate causes in the control of food intake and body weight, where clinicians and basic scientists continue to collaborate to advantage. Suffice it to say that it has cultivated the general appreciation of the existence of physiological controls on body weight that generate their effects through behavior. The particular role of the hypothalamus itself remains to be enunciated. The preliminary view of "centers" for feeding and satiety has been replaced with concepts of a more dynamic character that offer promise in comprehending the stages in the behavioral responses of hypothalamic hyperphagia and obesity that rest on control theory. As well, an appreciation of an interactive role between the brain and the physiology and metabolism of the peripheral body has emerged. The concepts of transmitter-specific neural paths converging within the hypothalamus have opened a view that the behavioral outcomes from lesions depend on injury to both intrinsic hypothalamic mechanisms and fibers of passage. Hypothalamic obesity remains still an issue for clinicians and for bench scientists to study but its pathophysiology is emerging and the stimulus its discovery gave to the alliance remains powerful.

In fact, the ongoing examination of hypothalamic hyperphagia reveals the complicated interaction of behavioral, autonomic and metabolic issues in the production of obesity. For example, with increasing obesity fat cells become less responsive to insulin, an event that can be protective because it will tend to limit triglyceride synthesis and further fat deposition. However, if provocations to overeat persist, a vicious cycle will appear as more and more insulin is secreted to overcome the cellular resistance. The increasing insulin levels will enhance the other stimuli to hyperphagia. It is this interplay of behavioral and metabolic factors that often makes a confident analysis of the mechanisms behind an obese state complicated. The obvious clinical corollary is that the treatment of any form of obesity is likely to be difficult and subject to relapse if a primary lesion cannot be eliminated.

Cancer Anorexia

If hypothalamic obesity is the classic example of collaboration between clinicians and basic scientists over a proximate factor in the control of food intake, then cancer anorexia and cachexia are the contemporary issues that reveal the intrinsic liveliness in this collaboration.

What more clear example of the "spanner in the works" view is there than the behavioral and physiological effects of cancer? The patient with cancer may have a change in his food appetite as the very first sign of his disease. A prompt improvement in appetite may be the best indicator of successful oncologic treatment even before other objective evidence of tumor regression is apparent. The dramatic nature of this anorexia as it abruptly interrupts the eating patterns of a lifetime often before any other sign of neoplasm is noted, the significant role that the anorexia and associated wasting of body fat and lean body mass plays in the survival of the patient (often leading to death long before the local or metastatic aspects of tumor growth would have done), and the poor quality of the survival period with the anorexia-and-cachexia-induced malaise and distress have focused and sustained clinical attention on this condition.

The early assumptions that the explanation for this anorexia/cachexia might be sought from the growth characteristics of cancer, with functional or anatomical derangements to the gastrointestinal tract, cerebral metastases with increased intracranial pressure, pain-induced anorexia, or simply increased metabolic requirements from tumor growth soon led to the appreciation that these factors, though active in some patients, were not common in the majority. In fact, the incidence and severity of anorexia and weight loss bore no precise relation to the size, site, stage or histology of the neoplasm (10).

What did seem clear was that inadequate food intake was a partial explanation. Secondary features tied to being a cancer patient such as depression of mood, surgical experience or a side effect of chemotherapy did not explain this anorexia in more than a small minority. However, there have been relatively few attempts to measure the food intake of cancer patients or their energy expenditure. What data are available show that a mean daily caloric intake of 1150-1550 kcal is customary in adult weight-losing cancer patients (11,12) and that 75% of cancer patients are normo- or hypo-metabolic (13). An adequate interpretation of these data is hindered by a lack of associated information needed to evaluate their importance, such as the time course of weight loss and the premorbid food intake of the same patients.

These inadequacies in the study of human cancer patients led to the sense that cancer anorexia/cachexia is a complex outcome of a multiplicity of factors, no one of them adequate to explain much of the phenomenon. Yet it is the dramatic nature of the syndrome in humans that sustains attention on the issue. It is tailor-made for investigation in the laboratory.

In the study of tumor-bearing experimental animals, it was readily possible to demonstrate the phenomena of anorexia and cachexia with the induction of cancer. Again, the condition was not explained by the simple effects of the tumor, and although such standard laboratory approaches as seeking out learned food aversions have offered occasional demonstrations of a role in cancer anorexia, they have not held up with further study (14).

The most useful results from the behavioral studies in the laboratory were the clear signs that some circulating factor, either from the neoplasm or from the host, was active in cancer anorexia. The best indication was from parabiotic rats in which a tumor in one of the parabiotic pair induced anorexia and profound weight loss in both, without the spread of cancer to the other rat (15). The evidence that diminished food intake and body weight depended upon the area postrema in tumor-bearing rats (16) was another indication that some circulating factor noticed by the chemosensitive trigger zone of the brain was active in cancer anorexia.

It was with these suggestions that an intriguing set of discoveries has opened up inquiries into the biology of anorexia and of cancer itself. Cerami and coworkers (17,18) in efforts to determine the cause of endotoxin-induced hypertriglyceridemia in infected animals identified a circulating factor that suppressed the synthesis of lipoprotein lipase, the enzyme that promotes lipogensis in adipocytes. This factor was produced by the macrophages of the animals and could be garnered from cell cultures. It is one of the cytokines synthesized and released by blood monocytes and tissue macrophages in response to inflammation (Tracey, Lowry and Cerami, 1987) (19). These investigators, reasoning that this factor may be involved in the pathophysiology of progressive bodily wasting in disease, designated this factor as "cachectin" and have demonstrated that the tissue loss it provokes is quite different from that seen in simple caloric restriction and starvation (20).

Simultaneously, other workers (Carswell, Old, Kassel, et al, 1975) (21) had demonstrated that an anti-tumor factor could be induced in mice by bacterial endotoxin, an idea prompted in part by a set of clinical observations of tumor regression after infection by a New York surgeon made almost a century ago (Coley in 1893 and 1906) (22a,b). This factor, which killed a variety of murine and human tumor cells *in vitro* and *in vivo*, was also produced by hematopoietic mononuclear cells including macrophages. This factor was designated "tumor necrosis factor" (TNF). Many investigators working with cachectin and TNF demonstrated their comparable molecular weight. Beutler and associates (23) documented recently that purified cachectin has a tumor necrosis factor activity *in vitro*, and established from inspection of the amino acid sequences and molecular clones of TNF and cachectin that they are homologs of one protein, referred to now as "TNF/cachectin" (23).

Recombinant TNF/cachectin is now available and many laboratories have helped to uncover a long list of biological activities affected by TNF/cachectin (24,25). Crucial to the interest in body weight regulation is the demonstration that the factor suppresses the *in vitro* activity of several enzymes that contribute to lipogenesis in adipocytes. It is the suppression of these and other anabolic enzymes that gives the factor its ability to deplete body lipid stores and provokes peripheral protein wasting irrespective of caloric intake. Along with its other activities such as stimulation of interleukin-1 secretion, this may provide insight into an aspect of its tumor killing capacity.

It is, however, also clear that TNF/cachectin does lead to reduced food intake, a phenomenon that is revealed best with intraperitoneal delivery of TNF/cachectin in animals. In a similar way, anorexia is observed in humans given TNF/cachectin as an oncologic therapy (26). Thus, with the discovery of this factor we have come around to new opportunities to appreciate many of the features represented by cancer anorexia and cachexia. This host-derived factor can mediate and provoke many of the metabolic changes associated with cachexia as well as lead to reduced caloric intake in many cancers. The weight loss is likely due to a combination of these two aspects of TNF/cachectin's actions, and thus we understand the rather frequent observation of examples of cancer patients with cachexia in whom the degree of weight loss exceeds what would be expected from the reduction in caloric intake. As well, we can understand the appearance of anorexia in some patients early in their course of illness when their tumor is small and site-restricted. The anorexia may be a direct or indirect result of this circulating factor but probably depends in part on the biochemical activation of area postrema cells.

Many obvious questions remain to be answered in this new and emerging aspect of control on body weight and food intake. But the overriding question is how to make sense out of this combination of activities tied to a common factor released into the circulation by the body in response to a wide-range of assaults, from bacterial and parasitic infection to neoplasia. Are the anorexic and cachexic features simply unfortunate side effects of a factor that offers the host some means of eliminating a tumor, or is there some biological utility to the suppression of caloric intake simultaneously with an attack on the tumor itself? It has been long known that caloric restriction in animals with advanced tumors will inhibit tumor growth and reduce the incidence of spontaneous malignancies in laboratory animals. As well, the metabolic factors that lead to depletion of tissue protein may lead to the preservation of hepatic protein, a phenomenon that is usually found during an acute illness and may have survival value but can be inappropriately sustained with continuing neoplasia.

There is much more to come in addressing the ultimate fitness of this combination of features, metabolic changes associated with cachexia and reduced caloric intake, in TNF/cachectin. It offers great opportunities for investigation to students of food intake and of disease of all kinds. Agonists and antagonists for this hormone/factor are presently being sought (Oliff, 1988) (25) and will certainly prove useful to clinician-scientists concerned with nutritional abnormalities in general and cancer anorexia in particular. The entire realm of biology from genetic mechanisms to neural transmission has been opened up by this effort to study a remarkable behavioral phenomenon, cancer anorexia and cachexia, that links body weight control to disease.

In this section, I have chosen to discuss two research examples in food intake and weight control, one classic and the second new and emerging that showed the lively interaction between clinicians and basic scientists evoked by recognition of pathological states ("spanner in the works"). These reveal both the excitement and the kind of steady progress that emerges from an appreciation of the proximate or immediate factors tied to the body's machinery that can evoke particular behavioral patterns. The analysis, prompted by human syndromes, quickly turned to basic experimental studies, moving along physiological and biochemical lines. The great advantages to this work on proximate mechanisms are not restricted to the disease focus that provoked the initial studies to illuminate pathophysiology, but also lie in the revelation of the need to comprehend the normal mechanisms of physiological controls that are the paths to the homeostasis in health represented by day-to-day regulations of behavior. This work, thus, naturally draws together scientists whose interest is on breakdown of the body and its relief with those whose fascination is found in the recognition of the "wisdom of the body" that must rest on homeostatic principles and integrative actions of biology. Disease as an "experiment of nature," like all experiments, opens much of life to study.

ULTIMATE OR DISTAL FACTOR COLLABORATION AMONG CLINICIANS AND BASIC SCIENTISTS

It is my contention that not all human disorders of food intake are rooted in disease. Some are maladaptions. The search for the causes of maladaptive human behaviors leads us in other directions--away from the laboratory and the experiment and towards prospective surveys of naturally occurring events in human populations. This is a shift of focus, at least temporarily, from the study of the specific controls on food intake to a way of revealing how a misfit between these controls and emerging life situations can lead to disorder. An appreciation of factors more distal than a broken part within the bodily mechanisms can derive from epidemiological surveys broadly construed to include genetics.

"Simple" or Idiopathic Obesity

As with the previous section, so we begin this section with a classic line of research and focus on obesity first. Epidemiology, which looks at the distribution of disorders in populations and their associated risk factors, is fundamentally important in human studies and has its linkages to genetics, ethology, ecology and behavioral science. The particular focus here is not on the "epidemics" of disease from which it got its name but upon behavior within a population, the behavior of food intake.

Body weight in mankind when not affected by some clear pathology of the body, as in hypothalamic disease, actually seems a smoothly distributed characteristic much as is height. There may be some extra numbers on the high side of the curve, but individuals are often called obese when they deviate to some arbitrary degree above the mean. The acceptance of the Body Mass Index (BMI, weight (kg)/height (m) squared) as the best anthropometric indicator of obesity has eliminated some of the arbitrariness of definition because it both de-emphasizes the effect of height on weight and correlates quite well with other measures of adiposity such as skinfold thickness. Body Mass Index is a graded, bell-shaped characteristic in the USA population (with perhaps some excess on the right hand side), with obesity defined as a BMI greater than 27 (kgs/square meter) for men and 25 for women.

The first indication that obesity has a crucial sociocultural aspect came from the epidemiological Midtown Manhattan Study of mental disorders in the community (27,28). This study showed a clear relation between social class and obesity. Obesity was much more prevalent among the lower classes. It seemed avoided for some reason by the upper classes. The fascinating point that subsequently emerged was that this class distinction is a feature of developed societies. Just the reverse relation is found in underdeveloped nations where the well-to-do tend to obesity and the poor, perhaps because of caloric starvation, are thin often to the point of emaciation. These observations have held up in many studies and beyond themselves offer intriguing speculations about the meaning of weight regulation across classes and cultures. Such sociocultural interactions with food intake include a sign of wealthy status if one is plump in a culture or country where food calories are scarce, and an opposite social meaning of thinness ("A woman cannot be too rich or too thin") in cultures where calories are abundant and evidence of the control of their consumption is valued. An intriguing sociocultural obesity and its complications has been identified when a race of people who survived in famine are transported to or emerge in a calorie-rich world. These last, exemplifed best by the Pima Indians of the USA, may develop obesity and its complications because of a "thrifty genotype rendered detrimental by progress" (29)--that is, a genetic endowment for fat storage that would have the survival value of reducing the expenditure of energy during times of shortage but would overstore energy as fat when food became and remained plentiful. There is a considerable amount of evidence (30,31,32) that many obese people do have a reduced energy expenditure as indicated by their metabolic rate at rest. This low 24-hour energy expenditure is a clear risk factor for obesity, it appears to be a familial trait, and it directs attention to the search for a genetic basis for human obesity.

A.J. Stunkard has provided two important studies that indicate a strong influence of heredity on human obesity by employing two standard techniques for revealing a genetic element, an adoption study and a comparison of monozygotic and dizygotic twins. The Danish adoption study (33) used the birth and health history registers available in that country. Stunkard and colleagues demonstrated a clear correlation (using Body Mass Index) between the weight of adoptees and their natural parents but no correlation with the weight of the adoptive parents.

In his twin study, Stunkard's group (1986) (34) demonstrated a much higher correlation of BMI in monozygotic than in dizygotic twins. In fact, the implications of these data are that as much as 80% of the variance in BMI can be accounted for in some way by the genetic makeup. This is a remarkable figure and, as he points out, contrasts with data from twin studies in conditions assumed previously to be more strictly tied to heredity such as hypertension (57%) and epilepsy (50%).

The epidemiological question that is emerging now in the study of human obesity is how to put these observations together--that is the clear evidence of environmental and sociocultural influences on obesity with the equally clear evidence of a genetic contribution. Once again the nature-nurture issue seems to beset us. However, as in every behavior-based disorder (and obesity at its root depends at least in part on the behavior of food consumption), the ultimate and crucial issue to comprehend is not the genes alone, nor the environment alone, but the interaction of the two factors. "The action is in the interaction" says Stunkard, and he bases his opinion directly on his understanding of the heritability concept derived from monozygotic and dizygotic twin comparisons. This method, intended to discriminate the environmental factors that dizygotic and monozygotic twins share from the genetic factors that render monozygotic twins identical, has the disadvantage of placing all the interactive causal factors of genes and environment into the genetic compartment and thus overestimates its contribution.

With behavior-driven disorders such as obesity, it is very likely that not only are there genetic controls on the basic metabolism (and those genes can and should be discovered), but also that there are genetic controls on the actions of individuals in a given environment. Thus, genes may influence such things as the individual's search for calories within the environment, the avoidance of protective activities such as exercise, and a preference for such sedentary behaviors as reading, writing or viewing television.

Much of the excitement in obesity research today is in seeking major genes that can interact with the environment in this way. The simplest example is the intriguing genetic differences in sweetness tasting (Bartoshuk, 1979) (35). People differ in their "sweet worlds;" some live in a "vivid and bright" sweet world because their capacity to appreciate sweetness is genetically enhanced. Others without this amplified capacity live in a "pastel" sweet world (these are Linda Bartoshuk's felicitous metaphors). The potential for consumption to be influenced by the faculty for taste interacting with environments that differ in the availability of refined sugar seems obvious.

Thus, it is the capacity for genetic analysis right down to the molecular level that has increased our explanatory power. As well, though, the ultimate explanations for obesity in given individuals and populations will be found in the interplay of genetic constitution with the reinforcing environment that is itself susceptible to change over time. These explanations will emerge from epidemiologically based studies and then join up with laboratory studies to illuminate multiple behavioral and metabolic features that lead to obesity.

Anorexia Nervosa

If obesity research is emerging into the daylight, the study of anorexia nervosa remains in the shadows. On first blush this seems surprising, given that obesity seems a "constitutional" issue defined simply by a deviation above the population mean for body weight, whereas anorexia nervosa seems to have a more categorical nature with symptomatic criteria like a disease. One might expect that a search for proximate causes and mechanisms would have been more successful in anorexia nervosa than has proven true.

There remains, despite a degree of diagnostic agreement, not only great ignorance about the fundamental cause of this condition, but real doubts about certain defining features, such as whether there are distinctly separate entities of abnormal weight control, restrictive anorexia nervosa and binging bulimia nervosa, or whether these are simply variants of the same disorder. It is even debatable whether the food restricting, perception-altered, emaciated anorexic patient is to be seen as an individual deviating quantitatively to an extreme in a commitment to the food fads and body weight consciousness of our society or whether she suffers from a clear qualitative aberration from normal as a syndromic definition tends to imply (36). There are champions for each of these points of view, and there are also those who would merge the differences by proposing that anorexia nervosa has both quantitative and qualitative aspects when viewed over its natural history. These fundamental disagreements, though, identify our ignorance about this condition. It is possible, however, to lay out the established information in a fashion that holds promise for future research and eventual comprehension.

To begin with, I think that the most useful criteria of anorexia nervosa are those of Russell (37) (see Table). They are simple, derived from a long personal clinical experience with a broad range of patients, and indicate that whatever may be the cause for the condition, behavior is basic to it.

Whereas in obesity the increased body weight emerges gradually over the course of development due to some insensible imbalance between food intake and energy consumption, in anorexia nervosa the patient is conscious of a struggle to achieve a reduction in her body weight. This struggle is represented by her active efforts to avoid or eliminate caloric intake. This behavior and its sustaining mental state (the overvalued idea in Russell's terms) can often be given a clear onset in time and even an initiating stimulus. The search for the explanation of this behavior--the stubborn rejection of nourishment based on a resolve to be very thin--that could reveal its cause, explain what sustains its course

Russell Criteria (Russell, 1979) for Anorexia Nervosa

1. **Self-induced loss of weight (resulting mainly from the studied avoidance of foods considered by the patient to be fattening).**

2. **A characteristic psychopathology consisting of an overvalued idea that fatness is a dreadful state.**

3. **A specific endocrine disorder which in the postpubertal girl causes the cessation of menstruation, or a delay of events of puberty in the prepubertal or early pubertal female.**

and its variants, and might bring about its rational rather than symptomatic treatment has so far been unsuccessful.

Thus, for example, the last decades have seen a good deal of physiological, metabolic and endocrine research in anorexia nervosa, prompted in part by the view embedded in Russell's criteria that there is a "specific endocrine disorder" in these patients. This research has attempted to identify bodily derangements that might represent either predispositions or precipitants to the behavior. These studies, often construed as attempts to reveal a proximate pathophysiology at the root of anorexia nervosa and thus to identify it as another disease expressing itself in behavior, include assessment of such hypothalamically derived functions as gonadotropin levels and body temperature responses, but also extend to peripheral physiology in evaluations of gastrointestinal motility and changes in ovarian anatomy.

Every observation of a deviation of these features from normal in anorexia nervosa has proven on follow-up after refeeding to be a symptom of the food restricted and starved state, and thus likely to be a result rather than a cause or even a predisposing feature of the behavior. All anomalies disappear with renourishment and restoration of body weight. Even the underlying suspicion that anorexia nervosa represents a form of the lateral hypothalamic syndrome proved on careful examination to be unlikely (Stricker and Andersen, 1980) (38).

From the physiological point of view, anorexia nervosa has so far provided a model of human starvation and its consequences. This is not a trivial matter for the clinician because many of the features of chronic starvation are important to identify when a course of treatment and explanations for distressing symptoms of the disorder are offered to the anorexic patient. Thus, it is helpful to be able to identify the early sense of fullness and even nausea during refeeding as a complication of reduced gastric emptying (39). Information that there is a need for extra body weight recovery to restore normal menses and complete reproductive capacity (40) is critical in defining for the patient the goal weight sought by the treatment team. Other discoveries such as the sonographic identification of ovarian atrophy and its restoration with refeeding have permitted a definition of stages of recovery (41).

However, if the aim of research is the discovery of cause, these pathophysiological studies have revealed only the symptoms and consequences of the behavior of food restriction, and little of its generation. We are still left with the question, what can lie behind this resolve--this drive to be thin--this insistent rejection of nourishment and its natural effects on the body? One turns to seek ultimate factors in frustration from the failures to find proximate ones.

For this reason, an epidemiological approach with its potential to identify common factors that differentiate these patients from normals in broader terms than pathophysiology is promising and gives a sense of direction to contemporary studies. The time-place-person triad of epidemiology brings out several unique facts that may come to illuminate the syndromic criteria. These can be briefly summarized.

Anorexia nervosa is a behavioral disorder that primarily affects (1) youthful females of the (2) upper classes in (3) developed nations in the (4) contemporary era. This is the major set of features, the ones that deserve most attention, and whose limits are to be appreciated.

First is the female sex of the afflicted. This is not an absolute exclusion, but since females outnumber males 10 to 1 in anorexia nervosa, we certainly should devote attention to aspects of women's lives and to see the male examples as anomalous and offering perhaps some opportunity to identify a feature that might point up an element provoking or sustaining the behavior in females. The high incidence of homosexuality (42) among the males with anorexia nervosa suggests, for example, an extra strength for concerns about sexuality at the heart of anorexia nervosa.

That it is youthful females, primarily those emerging from puberty, rather than an even distribution of the disorder across all ages promotes a focus of attention on the events of puberty and its immediate aftermath in women, not on all of the other psychosocial features that distinguish the lives of women from men across the lifespan. These events of puberty include the establishment of a cyclical program of gonadotropin release, and the emergence of a female bodily contour tied to the capability and sustenance of procreation. These bodily changes in women are more than simply biological events since they both influence the self attitude of a young woman and draw attention to her as an individual emerging from girlhood into the phase where her attractiveness and suitability for marriage are being considered. The increased incidence of anorexia nervosa in young women who are in occupations where their appearance is a premium such as ballet students and fashion models tends to secure a view that a risk factor for the condition is attention to bodily appearance.

There is evidence that those who succumb to anorexia nervosa, though, have some constitutional vulnerability that makes these interpersonal and cultural features particularly burdensome to them. This evidence has emerged both from the epidemiological and clinical studies. Thus, a genetic contribution to anorexia nervosa is secure. It rests on an increased concordance in monozygotic as compared to dyzygotic twins and upon a higher rate of anorexia nervosa among sisters (43). Exactly how this genetic contribution may function is uncertain, but it may emerge indirectly through the personality characteristics that derive in part from genetic instructions. As I shall discuss, the restricting anorexic tends to have a personality of introversion and self-reflection, and these features may enhance the influence of sociocultural pressures that provoke concerns about appearance.

Finally, the condition is increasing in its incidence. The evidence for a sharp rise in anorexia nervosa includes the observations of Theander (1970) (44) who noted a five-fold increase in Malmo, Sweden between the 1930s and 1950s, of Jones et al (1980) (45) who demonstrated a doubling of incidence in Monroe County in New York State, and Szmukler (1985) (46) who documented a rise in the annual incidence from 1.6 to 4.1 per 100,000 population in Northeast Scotland between the late 1960s and the early 1980s. In fact, as many as 1 in 250 schoolgirls in England (Crisp, Palmer and Kalucy, 1976) (47) have the condition, although many fewer suffer from it to the degree of needing hospitalization. All these studies of incidence considered and rejected the possibility that these increases might be more apparent than real and dependent on the increased diagnostic interest of physicians in anorexia nervosa or on families seeking medical attention for their daughters prompted by an enhanced awareness of the disorder gained through the media.

Along with this increased incidence, there is also evidence for a recent spread of the disorder outside its prime targets. Females both younger and older than the original 14 to 25 year-old range are now being reported. The appearance of anorexia nervosa in prepubescent girls can stunt bodily growth and development. Older women are often examples of relapses, but all specialists in anorexia nervosa can now report the initial appearance of the disorder in an occasional case over age 30.

There is clear evidence that anorexia nervosa is spreading beyond the confines of the upper classes of developed nations. Several examples have been reported in American blacks from impoverished backgrounds, and as well amongst women in the upper classes of the "third world" nations (48). There is even a suggestion that there is an increased incidence of anorexia nervosa in males. Certainly, most anorexia nervosa services now regularly have at least one male patient in the hospital at any time, a rare phenomenon a decade ago. The appearance of the apparent new disorder, bulimia nervosa (37), in which the weight loss is less and the morbid fear of fatness is associated with the behavior of gorging and purging, rather than calorie restricting, suggests that whatever is provoking anorexia nervosa, it is spreading to engage other behavioral activities tied to maintaining a low body weight.

These then are the epidemiological observations. The next question is how to use them to approach the cause or causes of anorexia nervosa. Thus, they do not suggest that this condition is a result of some bodily disease or internal chemical imbalance. At least no such disorder can be proposed for such a relatively circumscribed group of victims embraced by class and culture. As with obesity, it is probable that internal physiological consequences of the nutritional state may sustain the behavior or encourage it once it becomes established.

But why should a behavior provoking a state of starvation break out amongst young women who live in the midst of plenty? The pathophysiological consequences do not explain the initiation. We, thus, turn to interpret this behavior by identifying goals promoted by the contemporary culture that attract particular individuals.

A plausible formulation of the epidemiological data is to see this behavior as incited by a set of sociocultural attitudes that rains down on all in this era. Its effect is to pick out a vulnerable minority, mostly women, to induce, cultivate, and sustain a response that can vary in its strength depending upon a number of other provocative or protective features only some of which we have identified.

The sociocultural force most often mentioned is the emerging and persisting enthusiasm for thinness as an ideal bodily shape. This enthusiasm certainly can be tied to the fear of fatness of anorexia nervosa patients and perhaps verified as a provocative factor by the increased incidence of the disorder amongst occupations where thinness is demanded. However, essentially synchronous with the emerging cultural enthusiasm for thinness has been an increasing sexualization of adolescence in the last several decades. A preoccupation with bodily appearance, shape and size, is a natural response to this influence. Anorexia nervosa may be for some young women a way of reacting to and even defending against the complicated nexus of choice and demand imposed upon them at this time as they develop out of girlhood. This would be to view anorexia nervosa as a female ascetic response to the broadly construed sexual engrossments of this period.

Any construal that a cultural force induces a maladaptive behavior, though, must propose that there is some particular vulnerability in the people who respond to this pressure since cultural forces act upon all members of the society, only some of whom display the behavior in question. As has been mentioned above, anorexia nervosa appears much more frequently amongst individuals with an introverted temperament. That is, they often have the kind of affective constitution that tends to the self-reflections and sustained moods that generate concerns about the future.

A social setting that draws attention to her changing bodily appearance and may include some inklings about sexuality can be experienced more powerfully by an introverted than an extroverted young woman as a challenge to her self-management. It may be met by a stance of restriction and a resolve to sustain thinness as a kind of conflicted search for control in her situation. Once fasting and restriction are established then the physiological and physical changes that emerge, and even the bodily sensations associated with them, can aid and sustain the resolve by giving the individual evidence of success. These successive phenomena may enhance other reinforcements such as peer support to shift her from simply a weight consciousness that is almost universal in contemporary women into attitudes powerful enough to sustain a persisting, recurrent and even life-threatening behavior.

This view of anorexia nervosa as a spiral of behavioral responses with the initial food restriction prompted by sociocultural pressures striking on the vulnerable and then being reinforced by consequences that encourage more restriction in a self-perpetuating fashion matches some of the clinician's experience with this condition and particularly the clear clinical observation that early interruption of restriction is the best treatment for the disorder (49). As well, this view of an interactive process can explain the increasing incidence of the behavior as the cultural pressures continue, become locally amplified as in certain families or institutions, and through suggestion and example draw in individuals who are not so obviously predisposed as the initial victims.

Thus, the epidemiological evidence can be combined with the clinical evidence to propose that anorexia nervosa is a maladaptive response based ultimately upon the characteristics of human beings to see implications in life circumstances. This would fit the clinical opinion of Russell that anorexic patients have an "overvalued idea," i.e. a morbid devotion to an opinion shared by many others, but provocative of disorder when it becomes a ruling passion.

Thus, most of the clinical and epidemiological data suggest that the cause of anorexia nervosa is embedded in the combination of vulnerable personalities conflicted over the values of this era and adapting to them with a behavior that can become self engrossing and self sustaining. This formulation leaves several unanswered questions. Among them: why *are* women so much more vulnerable to this disorder than men? What is the distortion of perception that can blind anorexics to their thinness? Why is it so hard to treat? These questions and others remain as provocative issues for further research to confirm or reject the meaningful interpretation set forward here. At the moment, however, it seems the best account we have for this strange condition.

In summary, from the consideration of both idiopathic obesity and anorexia nervosa, we can propose that disruptions in human feeding do not always derive from bodily disease and the injury to normal controls, but rather can emerge from more ultimate factors such as human genetic variation, reinforcing life events, and the role of meaning tied to culturally based values that shape the expression of behaviors in our species. Although we might all agree that eventually these ultimate influences must work through the bodily mechanisms discerned by experiment, it is also clear that these superimposed anomalies of feeding are not so easily duplicated by animal models nor adequately assessed at a tissue level. They seem tied to the biopsychology issues unique to mankind: a species with its own genetic endowment that has evoked a capacity to imagine a future, to represent it with an idea, and to find therein a meaning for behavior. These anomalies are illuminated by methods derived from epidemiology that permit a multiplicity of causes and sustaining mechanisms to be glimpsed, perhaps first as disconnected risk factors and only with further careful, often cross cultural study, put together into coherent, testable explanations formulated as the outcome of constitutional factors, life experience, and shared values.

CONCLUSION

It was not my major aim in this essay to give an encyclopedic account of the human disorders of feeding and weight control. Such an achievement was not only outside my charge, it is outside my scope. Rather, I wished to emphasize a natural separation among these disorders seen in the clinic, and the different contemporary logics which are being applied to their study. I hoped to impart the view that there are two major lines of investigation, on the one hand laboratory-based emphasizing biochemical and physiologic experiment, and on the other epidemiologically-based emphasizing surveillance of human populations distinguished by genetic and sociocultural variations. These lines can be distinguished as the search for proximate and ultimate causal factors. There is, I believe, emerging a greater contact between these two lines of research but they remain, by their nature, relatively separate and distinct. They evoke different questions and must be approached by experts in quite different methods.

However, it is the concept of motivated behaviors, directed towards goals tied to the vital needs of the organism, based on psychoneural systems that function to organize activity and its commerce with surrounds, that holds this work together. These systems are subject to pathological change from within the organism and to deviant influences from without. In this essay I have looked at feeding behavior and some of its disorders; it should be obvious that a similar approach is also to be applied to disorders in any of the other motivated behaviors of mankind.

ACKNOWLEDGMENTS

I want to thank Marie Killilea, Timothy Moran, and James Wirth for very helpful criticisms and suggestions of earlier drafts of this essay.

This work was supported by National Institute of Diabetes and Digestive and Kidney Diseases (DK-19302).

REFERENCES

1. Frohlich A: Ein fall von tumor der hypophysis cerebri ohne akromegalie. Wien klin. Rundschau 15:883-886; 906-908, 1901
2. Bruch H: Progress in Pediatrics. The frohlich syndrome. Am. J. Dis. Child 58:1282-89, 1939
3. Fulton JF: Introduction: Historical Resume. In: The hypothalamus and central levels of autonomic function. Research Publications, Association for Research in Nervous and Mental Disease, 20:xiii-xxx, 1939, Baltimore, The Williams and Wilkins Company, 1940
4. Erdheim J: Ueber hypopysenganggeschwulste und hirncholestratome. Sitzungsb. d. Akad. d. Wissensch. Math.-naturw Kl 113:537-726, 1904
5. Hetherington AW and Ranson SW: Hypothalamic lesions and adiposity in the Rat. Anat. Rec. 78:149-172, 1940
6. Brobeck JR, Tepperman J, and Long CNH: Experimental hypothalamic hyperphagia in the albino rat. Yale J. Biol. & Med. 15:831-853, 1943

7. Bray GA and York DA: Hypothalamic and genetic obesity in experimental animals: An autonomic and endocrine hypothesis. Physiol. Rev. 59:719-809, 1979
8. Friedman MI and Stricker EM: The physiological psychology of hunger: A physiological perspective. Psychol. Rev. 83:409-431, 1976
9. Powley TL: The ventromedial hypothalamic syndrome, satiety, and a cephalic phase hypothesis. Psychol. Rev. 84:89-126, 1977
10. Holroyde CP and Reichard GA: General metabolic abnormalities in cancer patients: Anorexia and cachexia. Surgical Clinics of N. America, 66:947-956, 1986
11. Moloney M, Moriarty M and Daly L: Controlled studies of nutritional intake in patients with malignant disease undergoing treatment. Hum. Nutr. Appl. Nutr, 37A:30-35, 1983
12. Walsh TD, Bowman KB and Jackson GP: Dietary intake of advanced cancer patients. Hum. Nutr. Appl. Nutr., 37A:41-45, 1983
13. Kwox LS, Crosky LO, Feurer ID, et al: Energy expenditure in malnourished cancer patients. Ann. Surg., 197:152-162, 1983
14. Levine JA and Emory PW: The significance of learned food aversions in the aetiology of anorexia associated with cancer. Br. J. Cancer, 56:73-78, 1987
15. Norton JA, Moley JF, Green MV, Carson RE and Morrison SD: Parabiotic transfer of cancer anorexia/cachexia in male rats. Cancer Res., 45:5547-5552, 1985
16. Bernstein IL, Treneer CM, Kott JN: Area postrema mediates tumor effects on food intake, body weight, and learned aversions. Am. J. Physiol., 249:R296-R300, 1985
17. Cerami A, Ikeda Y, Le Trang N, Hotez PJ and Beutler B: Weight loss associated with an endotoxin-induced mediator from peritoneal macrophages: The role of cachectin (Tumor Necrosis Factor). Immunology Letters, 11:173-177, 1985
18. Rouzer CA and Cerami A: Hypertriglyceridemia associated with trypanosoma brucei brucei infection in rabbits. Mol. Biochem. Parasitol., 2:31-38, 1980
19. Tracey KJ, Lowry SF, and Cerami A: Physiological-responses to cachectin. In: Ciba Foundation Symposium, No. 131, 1987, Wiley, New York, pp. 88-108
20. Fong Y, Moldawer LL, Marano M, Manogue K, Tracey KJ, Wei H, Kuo G, Fischman DA, Cerami A and Lowry SF: Chronic cachectin/TNF or IL-la administration induces cachexia with redistribution of body proteins and decreased myofibrillar protein mRNA levels. Am. J. Physiol., (in press)
21. Carswell EA, Old LJ, Kassel RL, Green S, Fiore N, Williamson B: An endotoxin-induced serum factor that causes necrosis of tumors. Proc. Natl. Acad. Sci. USA, 72: 3666-3670, 1975

22a. Coley WB: The treatment of malignant tumors by repeated inoculations of erysipelas: With a report of ten original cases. Am. J. Med. Sci., 105:487-511, 1893
22b. Coley WB: Late results of the treatment of inoperable sarcoma by the mixed toxins of erysipelas and bacillus prodigiosus. Am. J. Med. Sci., 131:375-430, 1906
23a. Beutler B, Greenwald D, Hulmes JD, Chang M, Pan Y-CE, Mathison J, Ulevitch R, and Cerami A: Identity of tumour necrosis factor and the macrophage-secreted factor cachectin. Nature, 316:552-554, 1985
23b. Beutler B and Cerami A: Cachectin and tumour necrosis factor as two sides of the same biological coin. Nature, 320:584-588, 1986
24. Beutler B and Cerami A: Cachectin: More than a tumor necrosis factor. The New Engl. J. Med., 316:379-385, 1987
25. Oliff A: The role of tumor necrosis factor (Cachectin) in cachexia. Cell, 54:141-142, 1988
26. Sherman ML, Spriggs DR, Arthur KA, Imamura K, Frei E and Kufe DW: Recombinant human tumor necrosis factor administered as a five day continuous infusion in cancer patients: Phase I toxicity and effects on lipid metabolism. J. Clin. Oncol., 6:344-350, 1988
27. Srole L, Langner TS, Michael ST: Mental health in the metropolis: The midtown manhattan study. McGraw-Hill, New York, 1962
28. Langner TS and Michael ST: Life stress and mental health. Free Press, Glencoe, Illinois, 1963
29. Neel JV: Diabetes Mellitus: A "thrifty" genotype rendered detrimental by "progress"? Am. J. Hum. Gen., 14:353-362, 1962
30. Leibel RL and Hirsch J: Diminished energy requirement in reduced-obese patients. Metabolism, 33:164-170, 1984
31. Ravussin E, Lillioja S, Knowler WC, Christin L, FreymondD,Abbott WGH, Boyce V, Howard BV and Bogardus C: Reduced rate of energy expenditure as a risk factor for body weight gain. New Engl. J. Med., 318:467-472, 1988
32. Roberts SB, Savage J, Coward WA, Chew B and Lucas A: Energy expenditure and intake in infants born to lean and overweight mothers. New Engl. J. Med., 318:461-466, 1988
33. Stunkard AJ, Sorenson TIA, Hanis C, Teasdale TW, Chakraborty R, Schull WJ and Schulsinger F: An adoption study of human obesity. New Engl. J. Med., 314:193-198, 1986
34. Stunkard AJ, Foch TT and Hrubec Z: A twin study of human obesity. JAMA, 256:51-54, 1986
35. Bartoshuk LM: Bitter taste of saccharin related to the genetic ability to taste the bitter substance 6-n-Propylthiouracil. Science, 205:934-935, 1979

36. Garner DM, Olmsted MP and Garfinkel PE: Does anorexia nervosa occur on a continuum? Int'l J. Eating Disorders, 2:11-20, 1983
37. Russell GFM: Bulimia nervosa: An ominous variant of anorexia nervosa Psychol. Med., 9:429-448, 1979
38. Stricker EM and Andersen AE: The lateral hypothalamic syndrome: Comparison with the syndrome of anorexia nervosa. Life Sciences, 26: 1927-1934, 1980
39. Robinson PH, McHugh PR, Moran TH and Stephenson JD: Gastric control of food intake. J. Psychosomatic Res., 32:593-606, 1988
40. Frisch RE: Fatness, menarche and female fertility. Perspectives in Biol. and Med., 28:611-633, 1985
41. Treasure JL, Gordon PA, King EA, Wheeler M and Russell GF: Cystic ovaries: A phase of anorexia nervosa. Lancet, 2:1379-1382, 1985
42. Herzog DB, Norman DK, Gordon C and Pepose M: Sexual conflict and males. Am. J. Psychiat., 141:989-990, 1984
43. Strober M, Morrell W, Burroughs J, Salkin B and Jacobs C: A controlled family study of anorexia nervosa. J. Psychiat. Res., 19:239-246, 1985
44. Theander S: Anorexia nervosa: A psychiatric investigation of 94 female patients. Acta Psychiat. Scand. Suppl., 214:1-194, 1970
45. Jones DJ, Fox MM, Babigan HM and Hutton HE: Epidemiology of anorexia nervosa in Monroe County. Psychosom. Med., 42:551-558, 1980
46. Szmukler GI: The epidemiology of anorexia nervosa and bulimia. J. Psychiat. Res., 19:143-153, 1985
47. Crisp AH, Palmer RL and Kalucy RS: How common is anorexia nervosa? A prevalence study. Brit. J. Psychiat., 128:549-554, 1976
48. Buhrich N: Frequency of presentation of anorexia nervosa in Malaysia. Aust. N. Z. J. Psychiat., 15:153-155, 1981
49. Szmukler GI and Eisler I: The implications of anorexia nervosa in a ballet school. J. Psychiat. Res., 19:177-181, 1985

This article was printed in the Handbook of Behavioral Neurobiology, Volume 10, E.M. Stricker, ed., Plenum Press. Reprinted by permission.

chapter 7

Child Psychiatry: Where Have We Been And Where Are We Going?

Leon Eisenberg, M.D., F.A.P.A.

In 1897, Paul Gauguin painted a masterpiece of post-Impressionist art, *Where Do We Come From? What Are We? Where Are We Going?*, now on display at the Boston Museum of Fine Arts. With the magic of art, he tried to convey the alpha and omega of human existence by means of:

> "Color! This profound mysterious language, language of the dream." (1)

My task, fortunately, is far more modest. No masterpiece is expected. I have been assigned Guaguin's questions; the answers called for are not mankind's origins and destiny, but only the past and future of child psychiatry. Because I have lived through a substantial part of where child psychiatry has been, its first American textbook having appeared as recently as 1935 (2), my memory is in good part that past. Having almost become history myself, I am freed from the likelihood of living long enough to see my speculations about its future proved wrong.

This being the age of full disclosure, I must caution you that my vision of past and future has been focused by the psychobiological lens crafted at Hopkins by Adolf Meyer. To calibrate for the optical characteristics of that lens, recall that Meyer (3) rejected:

> "the neurologizing tautology; [that is, the belief]...that only those facts are scientific which can be reduced to terms of nerve cells"

and was equally disdainful (4) of the messianic claims for psychoanalysis as:

> "the exclusive way to salvation."

What was the state of the art when I began my training in 1952?

As to theory, psychoanalysis was just about the only game in town. The alternative was what Lief (5) termed the "commonsense psychi-

Psychiatry: Past Reflections–Future Visions
B.T. Taylor and I.J. Taylor, Editors

atry" of Adolf Meyer. Though Leo Kanner reminded those willing to listen just how uncommon a commodity common sense is, it hardly seemed enough justification for a claim of expertise. Unable to live with uncertainty (6), the best and the brightest embraced analytic theory fervently. Mastery of its arcane symbols and recondite language demanded a long and costly apprenticeship. The acolyte emerged with a set of concepts that defied common sense. *Ad hominem* arguments enabled adherents to dismiss objections rather icily on the grounds that they arose from the unanalyzed unconscious of the objectors. If analytic candidates raised questions about the validity of theory, those questions were interpreted as resistance rather than legitimate intellectual issues (7).

Child psychiatrists of the '50s viewed the infant as a *tabula rasa* on which experience was to write the script for personality, cognition and behavior. Zealous to counter prevailing superstitions about prenatal "impressions," most of us dismissed propositions that alcohol ingestion during pregnancy influenced fetal development as misguided moralism. Having just emerged from a war against racial ideology, we became so adroit at pointing out the many methodological flaws in existing genetic studies of schizophrenia that few took arguments about hereditary contributions to psychopathology seriously. In the optimistic spirit that had led Victor Hugo to proclaim that the opening of each new school meant the closing of a prison (whereas history was to show that school and prison populations grew *pari passu*), it was an article of faith that the control of mental illness could be attained *if only* there were to be a sufficiency of child guidance clinics, properly educated parents, and appropriately trained school teachers. It was a faith on which stubborn facts had yet to intrude (8).

Little attention was paid to diagnosis; when it was addressed, the positions set forth were as likely as not to be misleading. Eminent psychoanalysts maintained, on theoretical grounds, that neither affective disorder (9) nor schizophrenia (10) could occur in childhood because the necessary mental structures were missing. Diagnosis *was* irrelevant for the practitioner; treatment was by psychotherapy; it was centered on the idiosyncracies of family dynamics rather than on symptom patterns. True, the first effective drug, amphetamine, had been introduced by Bradley in 1937 (11), but there was little else in the formulary. Indeed, when the "tranquilizing" drugs, which were said to have "revolutionized" adult psychiatry, were first applied to treating children with behavior disorders, controlled clinical trials revealed more toxicity than benefits (12).

This brief sketch of the field in the '50s is admittedly a cartoon. There were, to be sure, countervailing forces. I was fortunate in having a teacher, Leo Kanner, who disputed the conventional wisdom (13). Perhaps because I never recovered from an Oppositional Disorder (DSM-III

313.81), several of my early publications dealt with brain and behavior (14,15). Those among us who had matured beyond the oral stage of psychosexual development balked at swallowing psychoanalytic doctrine whole (7). Still, these bold strokes convey the main trends in child psychiatry 40 years ago.

If that in brief is where we *were*, where we *are* began with Leo Kanner's 1943 report of a unique psychiatric disorder of the first years of life: early infantile autism (16). His original paper proposed that the syndrome represented an "*inborn* autistic disturbance of affective contact." His hypothesis was so far out of fashion with the times, however, that it dropped from sight even in his own later papers (17). Some 30 years were to pass before mounting evidence made evident both the heterogeneity of the autistic phenotype and its roots in CNS abnormality: such evidence as autistic syndromes in children with congenital rubella (18), greater concordance among identical than fraternal twins (19), abnormalities in the vermix of the cerebellum (20), and differences in cerebral metabolism (21). The point I emphasize here is that Kanner's designation of a clinical entity unique to childhood served to establish the importance of diagnostic differentiation. Today, its legitimacy is reflected in the operational criteria for diagnosis incorporated in DSM-III-R (22) and in standardized methods for patient evaluation such as the Diagnostic Interview Schedule for Children (23), the Children's Depression Scale, the Children's Depression Inventory (24) and the Child Behavior Checklist (25). The result has been greater reliability in diagnosis; establishing validity remains a task for future research (26).

A second challenge to the conventional wisdom appeared in 1958 with the publications of Lee Robins and her colleagues (27,28). The St. Louis investigators, with remarkable skill, uncovered the life course of more than 90% of some 500 children who had been seen for behavior problems 30 years earlier and contrasted their outcomes with those of a suitably chosen control group. The highest concentration of adult psychopathology was found among the youngsters with antisocial behavior; contrary to expectation, the 28 destined to become schizophrenic had been characterized by aggression, incorrigibility, paranoid ideation and running away from home rather than by shy, withdrawn schizoid personalities. In the annual review article on child psychiatry for 1958 in The American Journal of Psychiatry (29), I wrote:

> "These findings should spur a reexamination of our preoccupation with treating the neurotic child to the exclusion...of the antisocial child, since it appears to be the latter who constitutes the greatest risk for later personal and social decom-

pensation."

Professor Robins' studies of adult outcomes of child psychiatric patients were to change the field (30).

Confidence in the efficacy of child guidance was further upset by the findings of the Cambridge Somerville Delinquency Prevention Project (31). Although the case workers "treating" the youngsters had been confident that their clients benefitted from their care, a quantitative comparison of outcome for experimentals and controls, based on the number of court appearances and the number of offenses, demonstrated no significant between-group differences. Indeed, a long term follow-up by McCord in 1978 (32) was later to suggest that the "treated" youngsters were somewhat worse off than the controls. Although one study we carried out (33) did provide evidence in favor of short term psychotherapy, most investigators reported little difference when treated children were contrasted with those on a waiting list or those designated as controls (34). Two decades later, there is stronger, if still incomplete, evidence for the effectiveness of psychotherapeutic interventions (35). However, we still do not know *how much* of *what kind* of psychotherapy *for which* patients is likely to be most beneficial.

A third major force for change was the impetus provided by epidemiologic field studies. Lilienfeld and Pasamanick introduced the concept of a "continuum of reproductive casualty" extending from miscarriage and stillbirth at the one extreme, through cerebral palsy and epilepsy, to learning problems and behavior disorders at the other (36,37). Michael Rutter and his colleagues at The Maudsley provided the first systematic data on the distribution of disorders of behavior and academic attainment among school children as a function of age, gender, health status, residence and family environment (38,39). The late David Smith and his colleagues at the University of Washington (40,41) called to attention the fetal alcohol syndrome resulting from the teratogenic and behavioral effects of maternal alcohol consumption, particularly during the first trimester of pregnancy (42). By now, it is abundantly clear that low birth weight is a major determinant of neonatal and infant mortality and of morbidity among survivors and that low birth weight itself is a function of maternal age, smoking during pregnancy, maternal nutrition, and the adequacy of prenatal care (43). Indeed, if all pregnant women in the U.S. began their prenatal care in the first trimester and continued to receive care through delivery, current rates of low birth weight could be reduced by 15% among whites and 12% among blacks (44). Unfortunately, because of huge gaps in the "safety net," the proportion of women not receiving care until the third trimester, or no care at all, has remained unchanged for the last decade.

A fourth new note was sounded by the studies of Chess, Thomas and Birch (45,46) which heralded the importance of individual differences in infant temperament, already evident by the third month of life. With their work, the conceptual model of the infant was transformed; it was no longer an inert and passive recipient of care; it began to be seen as an active participant in the family drama. Three decades ago, psychiatric discourse on the cause of behavior disorders began with a slogan familiar to detective story fans: *cherchez la femme.* Today, we acknowledge the existence of fathers and the possibility of match or mismatch between characteristics of infants and parents (47,48).

Finally, genetics, once banished from respectable company, has reemerged with new charisma. Seymour Kety, David Rosenthal and Paul Wender developed an elegant conceptual scheme and a meticulous clinical methodology which enabled them to demonstrate that schizophrenia was transmitted from biological parents to their offspring even when the offspring had been adopted away in infancy (49). Although it was not until 1956 that cytologists were able to establish an accurate count of the human chromosome number (50), within three years, Lejeune (51) had discovered trisomy 21 as the chromosomal basis for sporadic cases of Down's Syndrome. Two decades later, the fragile X syndrome was identified as the leading hereditary cause of mental retardation in males (52,53) and as a predisposing factor for other forms of psychopathology in males (54) and in female "carriers" (55). With the development of new tools for the dissection of the chromosome with restriction fragment length polymorphisms (RFLPs), explanations for abnormal behavior in terms of inherited brain dysfunction have grown apace.

The wheel has come full turn. When I began my training, the brain, as far as psychiatrists were concerned, might just as well have been ballast inside the skull to keep it from floating off into space. Today, many of my colleagues view it as an organ that secretes thoughts and feelings much as endocrine glands secrete hormones (56). The renaissance of biological reductionism carries with it the danger of trading a brainless psychiatry for a mindless psychiatry (57). But it has forced the reexamination of hitherto neglected issues. The still unmet challenge is to integrate concepts from the biological sciences with those from the social sciences to enlarge and enrich our understanding of human personality and development.

All of this is heady stuff and brings us to the last theme in the title of this address: where are we going? In my view, that future will in large part be determined by investigations stemming from two distinct but interpenetrating fields: genetics and epidemiology. Progress in genetics permits greater precision in the analysis of the relevant environment; environmental change highlights the role of heredity. Permit me a brief digression into tropical disease to illustrate the complementarity of the two methods of investigation.

Vivax malaria is found only in individuals whose red cells are parasitized by *Plasmodium vivax*, an infectious agent transmitted by mosquitos. On the basis of this information, vivax malaria is classified as a parasitic disease.

It is also the case, however, that vivax malaria is found only in persons who are positive for the Duffy blood group (58). Duffy blood group status is genetically determined. Since only Duffy positives have vivax malaria, vivax malaria can as well be classified as a genetic disease.

The resolution of the apparent paradox lies in the fact that *P. vivax* is able to penetrate the red cells of Duffy positive individuals by attaching to the Duffy antigen (or a structurally related receptor) on the red cell surface (59). Duffy negative persons are invulnerable to *P. vivax* infections because the parasite is unable to penetrate their red cells. Thus, the vivax malaria phenotype demands *both* genetic susceptibility *and* exposure to an inoculum of the parasite. Neither necessary condition is sufficient; both "causes" must be present at one and the same time. This conjunction has had important evolutionary consequences. West African blacks who inhabit a geographic area where *P. vivax* and its mosquito vector are endemic are almost entirely Duffy negative as the result of selection against the susceptible genotype (60).

With this example in mind, let us now turn to an analysis of the interaction between nature and nurture in the genesis of psychopathology. In a recent essay, Plomin and Daniels (61) underscore the irony that data from human behavioral genetics provide the strongest evidence for the role of environmental determinants in psychopathology, although such determinants are found in a somewhat unexpected quarter. In the authors' words:

> "Behavioral genetic research in personality, psychopathology and cognition...leads to the conclusion that the most important source of environmental variance is *non-shared* environment."

To rehearse their thesis briefly, quantitative genetic theory uses the covariance among relatives on normally distributed traits to estimate the role of heredity. However, because closely related individuals ordinarily share family environment as well as heredity, family resemblances can stem from either or both sources. To circumvent this conflation of effects, two major research designs are employed: adoption studies and twin studies.

If genetically related individuals are adopted apart and reared in uncorrelated environments, the resemblances found among them must be due to genetic factors alone. In contrast, if genetically unrelated individuals are adopted together into the same family, they will resemble each other only for reasons of shared environment. When relatives reared together are no more similar on a given trait than relatives reared apart, it is evident that growing up together (that is, *shared* environment) does not explain the observed variance in the trait; the effect of environmental influences must be *non-shared.* For example, familial concordance rates for schizophrenia among first degree relatives are the same whether the relatives are reared at home or adopted away. That is, sharing the same home with a schizophrenic relative does not appear to increase the risk for manifest disease despite the presence of a familial predisposition.

Twin design compares resemblances of identical with those of same-sexed fraternal twins, the coefficient of genetic relationship for the former being 1.0 and for the latter 0.5, on average. To the extent that heredity affects a given trait, correlations would be expected to be about twice as great for identical as for fraternal twins. In fact, the concordance for schizophrenia among fraternal twins is about 10% (the same as that reported for first degree relatives) whereas average concordance rates in studies of identical twins is about 45% (62). This difference in concordance points to the power of genetic determinants of schizophrenia; simultaneously, the observation that half of the variance among monozygous twins is unexplained directs attention to environmental determinants. Because genetically identical twins reared in the same family exhibit different outcomes, those determinants are not shared.

What might such non-shared influences be? The first obvious set are those that are distributed more or less by chance: prenatal events, birth injuries, CNS infections, brain trauma and so on. "By chance" does not accurately describe their distribution because we know that misfortune aggregates in some families, that it is related to social class, and that personality traits, such as risk-taking, influence their likelihood. A second set of factors include those that determine the child's role in the family: birth order, gender, sibling interactions, and differential parental treatment of one offspring as against another. Third, there is the world outside the family, the world of peer groups, schools, employment, neighbors and so on. Finally, the psychological relevance of environmental experiences for a given child is colored by the way those events are perceived by that child.

As the result of the new genetics, I anticipate far greater precision in the way we think about, and therefore greater ability to intervene to alter, the social determinants of mental development. This statement will not surprise those familiar with what I have said and written before. Some may take it for senile perseveration. Others may be inclined to dismiss it as mere wishful thinking. After all, if there is any strand that typifies what has been exciting about psychiatric research in the last decades of this century, it is the double strand of the DNA helix; that is, the quite extraordinary progress, and the promise of much more to come, in characterizing the hereditary determinants of psychopathology. It is that very progress, I contend, which will open the door for new developments in social psychiatry. Let me try to explain the ostensible paradox first by considering the converse: the ways in which social change has abetted genetic research.

Rickets, resulting from the conjunction of dietary inadequacy with limited exposure to sunlight, was once endemic in northern climates. With an increased standard of living and consequent improvement in diet, the disorder has become relatively uncommon. It was after this change that investigators began to recognize patients who exhibited rickets despite an adequate diet, a condition Albright et al. (63) termed vitamin D-resistant rickets. The distribution of D-resistant rickets was shown to be familial (64). The familial disorder was shown to be X-linked with virtually complete generation-to-generation transmission (65). Further dissection by the methods of clinical genetics revealed a subgroup who respond to sizable doses of vitamin D and who exhibit an autosomal recessive mode of inheritance (66). More recently, Scriver et al. (67) described another variant: osteomalacia without rickets, a positive therapeutic response to 1,25-$(OH)_2D_3$ and autosomal dominant inheritance. Still other variants have been described as the tale continues to unfold; they need not be detailed here.

To take an example closer to home for psychiatry, the four "d's" of pellagra (dermatitis, diarrhea, dementia and death) were matters of much concern in the first decade of this century, particularly to psychiatrists responsible for institutionalized populations (68). Whereas familial aggregation led some clinicians to suspect that pellagra was hereditary and some that it was infectious, others invoked a toxin produced by a fungus and still others a nutritional deficiency because of its association with low social class and a diet consisting largely of maize. Goldberger's (69) heroic research proved that pellagra is a dietary disease, traced two decades later to niacin deficiency. By the end of World War II, pellagra had receded as a major public health problem in the U.S.; economic progress ended the dependence of Southern tenant farmers on milled corn as a dietary staple (70). This change in figure/ground relationship made possible the recognition of Hartnup's disease, a clinical disorder manifested by a pellagra-like rash, cerebellar ataxia and psychiatric symptoms, arising from homozygosity for a rare autosomal allele, which results in impaired tryptophan uptake (71,72,73). Examples can be multiplied but these two must suffice here.

I do not argue that vitamin D-resistant and vitamin D-dependent rickets, Hartnup's disease and a host of other inherited metabolic disorders would never have been discovered, had the "noise" of environmentally determined disease not been reduced, but merely that they were made more evident, and therefore more likely to be identified, because a prepotent source of variance had been removed. When improved living standards or medical progress diminishes the extrinsic causes of a particular clinical condition, without eliminating that condition altogether, the residual cases manifest a net increase in heritability (74).

Now let us switch figure and ground, the ground now being genetic variation and the figure environmental effects. The more precisely we can specify offspring at risk for a given psychiatric disorder because of an inherited diathesis, the greater the possibility of detecting features of the environment which precipitate overt disease in some descendants--and may produce phenocopies in others. There is, by now, persuasive evidence from family studies and population studies (75,76,77,78,79) that children of parents with affective disorder are at considerably greater risk for depression in childhood as well as for other psychiatric disorders. The demonstration of this clustering of cases in families with a history of affective disorder in one or both parents makes it possible to undertake controlled clinical trials of plausible interventions to reduce the development of overt disease in offspring (80). Given the relatively low rate at which depression occurs before adolescence, samples drawn from the general population would have had to be prohibitively large to detect the effects of intervention, were it not for the new capability of targeting "risk-enriched" populations.

The increasing evidence for genetic heterogeneity in affective disorders promises greater precision to come. Egeland and co-workers (81) have recently identified a locus for bipolar disease on chromosome 11 in an Old Amish kindred; however, no such association was found in Icelandic (82) and non-Amish American kindreds (83) characterized by autosomal dominant transmission. At about the same time, Baron et al. (84) noted a linkage between bipolar disorder and the X-chromosome markers for color blindness and glucose-6-dehydrogenase deficiency in three Israeli kindreds. Furthermore, Sherrington and his coworkers (85) have reported cosegregation of schizophrenia with an RFLP on chromosome 5 in seven Icelandic and British families, although a similar search in a Swedish pedigree proved fruitless (86). Whether the Sherrington study will prove to be a false lead or a rare marker cannot now be ascertained. These studies, exciting as they are, have only begun the analysis of heterogeneity, made possible by the use of RFLPs to identify members at risk in informative families. It may prove to be the case that the nature and the extent of the requisite environmental precipitants varies from one genetic "species" to another.

Thus far, I have argued for a research strategy, one in which students of the environment employ genetics to add to the power of their own research methods and geneticists use environmental variation to bring hereditary factors into sharper relief. Such strategies will not eliminate and perhaps not even reduce disputes about the relative importance of nature and nurture in the genesis of behavior. At the extremes of nature and nurture, that is, lethal mutants or lethal environments, there is little room for disagreement. However, in an "expectable" range of environments (that is, those which species ordinarily encounter and in which selection has operated) parsing out relative contributions of nature and nurture in the development of complex behaviors becomes far more difficult. What we all too easily overlook is that the young of every species inherit, along with their genes, their parents and the ontogenetic niche they inhabit (89).

The second strand in the genome of contemporary research that will influence the phenotype of psychiatry in the next century is epidemiology: the study of the distribution of disease in populations by time, place and person and the study of the factors that influence that distribution (88). At the descriptive level, epidemiology seeks to provide an accurate tally of the kind and the extent of the disease burden, key to effective public health planning. More than that, it provides data essential for testing the causal hypotheses derived from clinical work, hypotheses often flawed by the skewness of patient samples. Beyond both, epidemiology makes possible the generation of new causal hypotheses by detecting associations between disease and demographic variables. Finally, it provides a crucial test of the effectiveness of interventions applied in routine medical practice as distinct from their efficacy as demonstrated in experimental protocols. In Wade Hampton Frost's words (88):

> "Epidemiology at any given time is something more than the total of its established facts. It includes their orderly arrangement into chains of inference which extend more or less beyond the bounds of direct observation."

Population-based studies have provided, for the first time, reliable data on the prevalence of mental disorders in children (89). There remain unresolved questions about validity, about the explanation for site-specific differences in ascertained prevalence, and about the relationship between disorder, impairment and the use of mental health services. But it is not these findings, valuable as they are, that I stress here. As I see it, the future of our field will be influenced more by data on causes of mortality which are not traditionally viewed as "psychiatric."

Epidemiologic surveillance highlights a major public health issue: the disproportionate and morally indefensible toll from violence among black Americans. Mortality rates from homicide are 5.9 times higher among black males and 3.9 times higher among black females than for their white counterparts. The rate for black males peaks at 99.6 per 100,000 for those 25 through 29 years of age in 1984 (90). Multivariate analysis of the demographic statistics indicates that a substantial part of the racial differential is accounted for by socioeconomic status (91). But even if money is *the* specific remedy for poverty, it is not likely in the current political climate to be made available in the amounts needed. To what extent is it possible, based on what is known about the relationship between life circumstances and violent behavior, to design public health interventions in schools, churches and other community settings to reduce this carnage?

Lee Robins (92) has demonstrated, with several independent replications, that three factors are robust predictors of adult antisocial behavior: sociopathy in parents, school truancy and antisocial behaviors during school years. This defines an appropriate target for preventive intervention. It is not that all antisocial youngsters become antisocial adults (though about half do) but that antisocial behavior in adult life rarely appears in the absence of childhood precursors. The elementary school interventions currently under study by Comer (93) in New Haven and by Kellam and his colleagues in Baltimore give promise of improving academic attainment and reducing behavior problems among disadvantaged children. The challenge is to build on these early findings. Delinquency prevention must be high on the agenda of 21st century pediatrics and psychiatry.

In his recent Salmon Lecture, Mickey Stunkard (94), whose academic career spans the same time period as mine, provided an eloquent statement of where we have been and where we are going in general psychiatry:

> "American psychiatric thinking [in the 1950's]...was informed by a very general psychoanalytic theory of human behavior... much prized by practitioners...because of the assurance that it conveyed....The theory was already hardening into ideology.... It tried to explain too much too soon. It was impatient with the modest, low level kind of inquiry more appropriate to our field....The major development of the past thirty years...[has] been the rise of... modest clinical inquiry....We are still far from the kind of grand synthesis envisaged by psychoanalysis....We have only glimpses of what we seek. But they are intriguing glimpses that are leading us to an

ever better understanding."

To bring my account of once and future child psychiatry to completion on an historic note, let me remind you of an interchange that took place almost 60 years ago. In 1931 a leading pediatrician of the day, Joseph Brenneman (95), attacked child psychiatry in a paper angrily entitled: "The Menace of Psychiatry." He decried the armchair speculations, the indifference to empirical data and the *ex cathedra* theories of development that bewildered pediatricians and made parents guilty. James Plant's (96) response was published under the gentler title: "The Promise of Psychiatry." His remarks were prescient:

> "We are, as a people, going through great changes in the matter of human relationships. Whether you like it or not, the families which are your clientele are finding themselves face to face with new and profound social problems. These matters affect the conduct and health of the patients...because every family is having to adjust itself to these changes. You cannot escape these problems by deprecating them....The promise of psychiatry is the promise that if the pediatrician will address himself to these problems he will face a vista of rare challenge...."

Plant was clearly right about the pace of change in family life and the problems it poses for child health and development (96). I am equally convinced he was right about a vista of rare challenge. Will we meet that challenge? I promise to answer that question if you will invite me to the next symposium 50 years from now.

REFERENCES

1. Brettell R, Cachin F, Freches-Thory C, Stuckey CF: The Art of Paul Gauguin. Washington, National Gallery of Art, p. 393. 1988
2. Kanner L: Child Psychiatry. Springfield, Ill., C.C. Thomas. 1935
3. Meyer A: Conditions for a home of psychology in the medical curriculum. J. Abn. Psychol. 7:313-325, 1912
4. Meyer A: Psychobiology: A Science of Man. (The 1931 Salmon Lectures.) Springfield, Ill., C.C. Thomas, p. 105. 1957
5. Lief A: (ed.). The Commonsense Psychiatry of Dr. Adolf Meyer. New York, McGraw-Hill. 1948
6. Whitehorn JC: Education for uncertainty. N. Eng. J. Med. 265:301-309, 1964
7. Eisenberg L: If not now, when? Am.J. Orthopsychiat. 32:781-793,

1962a
8. Eisenberg L: Preventive psychiatry. Ann. Rev. Med. 13:343-360, 1962b
9. Rochlin G: The loss complex. J. Am. Psychoanalyt. Assoc. 1:299-316, 1959
10. Katan M: Structural aspects of a case of schizophrenia. Psychoanalyt. Stud. Child 5:175-211, 1950
11. Bradley C: Behavior of children receiving amphetamine. Am. J. Psychiat. 94:577-585, 1937
12. Cytryn L, Gilbert A, Eisenberg L: The effectiveness of tranquilizing drug plus supportive psychotherapy in treating behavior disorders of children. Am. J. Orthopsychiat. 30:113-129, 1960
13. Eisenberg L: In Memoriam: Leon Kanner 1894-1981. Am. J.Psychiat. 138:1122-1124, 1981
14. Eisenberg L: Psychiatric aspects of brain damage in children. Psychiat. Quart. 31:72-92, 1957
15. Eisenberg L: Conceptual problems in relating brain and behavior. Am. J. Orthopsychiat. 30:37-48, 1960
16. Kanner L: Autistic disturbances of affective contact. Nerv. Child 2:217-250, 1943
17. Kanner L: Problems of nosology and psychodynamics of early infantile autism. Am. J. Orthopsychiat. 19:416-426, 1949
18. Chess S: Autism in children with congenital rubella. J. Autism Child Schiz. 1:33-47, 1971
19. Folstein S, Rutter M: Infantile autism: a genetic study of 21 twin pairs. J. Child Psychol. Psychiat. 18:297-321, 1977
20. Courchesne E, Yeung-Courchesne R, Press C, Hesselink J, Jernigan P: Hypoplasia of cerebellar vermal lobules VI and VII in autism. N. Eng. J. Med. 318:1349-1354, 1988
21. Horwitz B, Rumsey JM, Grady CL, Rapoport SI. The cerebral metabolic landscape in autism. Arch. Neurol. 45:749-755, 1988
22. DSM-III-R: Diagnostic and Statistical Manual of Mental Disorders. Washington, American Psychiatric Association, 1987
23. Gutterman EM, O'Brien JD, Young JG: Structured diagnostic interviews for children and adolescents: current status and future directions. J. Am. Acad. Child Adol. Psychiat. 26:621-630, 1987
24. Knight D, Hensley VR, Waters B: Validation of the children's depression scale and the children's depression inventory in a prepubertal sample. J. Child Psychol. Psychiat. 29:853-863, 1988
25. Achenbach TM: Assessment and Taxonomy of Child and Adolescent Psychopathology. Newbury Park, CA. Sage. 1985
26. Rutter M, Shaffer D: DSM-III: A step forward or back in terms of the classification of child psychiatric disorders? J. Amer. Acad. Child Psychiat. 19:371-394, 1980

27. O'Neal P, Robins LN: The relation of childhood behavior problems to adult psychiatric status. Am. J. Psychiat. 114:961-969, 1958a
28. O'Neal P, Robins LN: Childhood patterns predictive of adult schizophrenia: a 30 year follow-up study. Am. J. Psychiat. 115:385-391, 1958b
29. Kanner L, Eisenberg L: Review of psychiatric progress: child psychiatry and mental deficiency. Am. J. Psychiat. 115:608-610, 1959
30. Robins LN: Deviant Children Grown Up. Baltimore, Williams & Wilkins. 1966
31. Teuber HL, Powers E: Evaluating therapy in a delinquency prevention program. Proc. Assn. Res. Nerv. Ment. Dis. 31:138-147, 1955
32. McCord J: A thirty-year follow-up of treatment effects. Am. Psychol. 33:284-289, 1978
33. Eisenberg L, Conners CK, Sharpe L: A controlled study of the differential application of outpatient psychiatric treatment for children. Jap. J. Child Psychiat. 6:125-132, 1965
34. Eisenberg L: Child psychiatry: the past quarter century. Am. J. Orthopsychiat. 39:389-401, 1969
35. Kolvin I, Garside RG, Nicol AR, Macmillan A, Wolstenholme F, Leitch LM: Help Starts Here: The Maladjusted Child in the Ordinary School. London, Tavistock Publications. 1981
36. Lilienfeld AM, Pasamanick B: The association of maternal and fetal factors with the development of cerebral palsy and epilepsy. Am. J. Obstet. Gynecol. 70:93-101, 1955
37. Pasamanick B, Knobloch H: Retrospective studies on the epidemiology of reproductive casualty. Merrill-Palmer Quart. Behav. Dev. 12:743, 1966
38. Rutter M, Cox A, Tupling C, Berger M, Yule W: Attainment and adjustment in two geographic areas: I. The prevalence of psychiatric disorder. Brit. J. Psychiat. 126:493-509, 1975
39. Rutter M, Tizard J, Yule W, Graham P, Whitmore K: Research report: Isle of Wight studies, 1964-1974. Psychol. Med. 6:313-332, 1976
40. Jones KL, Smith, DW, Ulleland CN, Streissguth AP: Pattern of malformation in offspring of chronic alcoholic mothers. Lancet i:1267-1271, 1973
41. Streissguth AP, Landesman-Dwyer S, Martin JC, Smith DW: Teratogenic effects of alcohol in humans and laboratory animals. Science 209:353-361, 1980
42. Streissguth AP, Barr HM, Sampson PD, Parish-Johnson JC, Kirchner GL, Martin JC: Attention, distraction and reaction time at age 7 years and prenatal alcohol exposure. Neurobehav. Tox. Teratol. 8:717-725, 1986
43. McCormick MC: The contribution of low birth weight to infant mortality and childhood morbidity. N. Eng. J. Med. 312:82-90. 1985

44. Institute of Medicine. Preventing Low Birth Weight. Washington, D.C., National Academy Press, 1985
45. Thomas A, Chess A, Birch HG, Hertzig ME, Korn S: Behavioral Individuality in Early Childhood. New York, New York University Press. 1963
46. Thomas A, Chess A, Birch HG: Temperament and Behavioral Disorders in Children. New York, New York University Press. 1968
47. Chess S: Mal de mere. Am. J. Orthopsychiat. 34:613-614, 1964
48. Chess S: Developmental theory revisited. Canad. J. Psychiat. 24:101-112, 1979
49. Kety SS: The significance of genetic factors in the etiology of schizophrenia: results from the national study of adoptees in Denmark. J. Psychiat. Res. 21:423-429, 1987
50. Tjio JH, Levan A: The chromosome number in man. Hereditas 42:1, 1956
51. Lejeune J, Gautier M, Turpin R: Le mongolisme, premier exemple d'aberration autosomique humaine. Compt. Rend. 248:1721-1722, 1959
52. Jacobs PA, Glover T, Mayer M, Fox P, Gerrard J, Dunn H, Herbst D: X-linked mental retardation: a study of 7 families. Am. J. Human Genet. 7:471-489, 1980
53. Sutherland G, Hecht F: Fragile Sites on Human Chromosomes. Oxford, Oxford University Press. 1985
54. Bregman JD, Leckman JF, Ort SI: Fragile X syndrome: genetic predisposition to psychopathology. J. Autism Dev. Disord. 18:343-354, 1988
55. Reiss AL, Hagerman RJ, Vinogradov S, Abrams M, King RJ: Psychiatric disability in female carriers of the fragile X chromosome. Arch. Gen. Psychiatry. 45:25-30, 1988
56. Andreasen NC: Brain imaging: applications in psychiatry. Science 239:1381-1388, 1988
57. Eisenberg L: Mindlessness and brainlessness in psychiatry. Brit. J. Psychiat. 148:497-508, 1986
58. Miller LH, Mason SJ, Clyde DF, McGinnis MH: The resistance factor to Plasmodium vivax in blacks. The Duffy blood group phenotype F_yFy. N. Eng. J. Med. 295:302-304, 1976
59. Miller LH, Mason SJ, Dvorak JA, McGinnis MH, Rothman IK: Erythrocyte receptors for Plasmodium knowlesi malaria. Science 189:561-563, 1975
60. Bodmer WF, Cavalli-Sforza LL: Genetics, Evolution and Man. San Francisco, W.H. Freeman and Company, pp. 405-407, 1976
61. Plomin R, Daniels D: Why are children in the same family so different from one another? Behav. Brain Sci. 10:1-16, 1987
62. Gottesman II, Shields J: Schizophrenia: The Epigenetic Puzzle.

Cambridge University Press, Cambridge, United Kingdom. 1982

63. Albright F, Butler AM, Bloomberg E: Rickets resistant to vitamin D therapy. Amer. J. Dis. Child. 54:529-547, 1937
64. Christensen JF: Three familial cases of atypical late rickets. Acta Paediatr. Scand. 28:247-270, 1940-41
65. Winters RW, Graham JB, Williams TF, McFalls VW, Burnett CH: A genetic study of familial hypophosphatemia and vitamin D-resistant rickets. Trans. Assoc. Am. Physicians 70:234-242, 1957
66. Fraser D, Salter RB: The diagnosis and management of the various types of rickets. Pediat. Clin. North Amer. 5:417-441, 1958
67. Scriver CR, McDonald W, Reade T, Glorieux FH, Nogrady B: Hypophosphatemic nonrachitic bone disease. Am. J. Med. Genet. 1:101-117, 1977
68. Singer HD: Mental and nervous disorders associated with pellagra. Arch. Int. Med. 15:121-146, 1915
69. Goldberger J, Waring CH, Willets DG: The prevention of pellagra: a test of diet among institutional inmates. Public Health Reports 30:3117-3131, 1915
70. Sydenstricker VP: The history of pellagra, its recognition as a disorder of nutrition, and its conquest. Am. J. Clin. Nutrition 6:409-414, 1958
71. Hersov LA: A case of childhood pellagra with psychosis. J. Ment. Sci. 101:478-483, 1955
72. Baron DN, Dent CE, Harris H, Hart EW, Jepson JB: Hereditary pellagra-like skin rash with temporary cerebellar ataxia, constant renal amino aciduria, and other bizarre biochemical features. Lancet ii:421, 1956
73. Jepson JB: Hartnup Disease. In: Stanbury JB, Wyngaarden JB, Frederickson DS: The Metabolic Basis of Inherited Disease. 4th edition. New York, McGraw-Hill, pp. 1563-1577, 1978
74. Scriver CR: Window panes of eternity: health, disease and inherited risk. Yale J. Biol. Med. 55:487-513, 1982
75. Beardslee WR, Keller MB, Klerman GL: Children of parents with affective disorder. Int. J. Fam. Psychiat. 6:283-299, 1985
76. Beardslee WR: Conceptual and clinical issues in the design of a preventive intervention for adolescents of parents with serious affective disorders. Unpublished manuscript, 1988
77. Weissman MM, Leckman JF, Merikangas KR, Gammon GD, Prusoff BA: Depression and anxiety disorders in parents and children: results from the Yale Family Study. Arch. Gen. Psych. 41:845-852, 1984
78. Weissman MM, Prusoff BA, Gammon GD, Merikangas KR, Leckman JF, Kidd KK: Psychopathology in the children (ages 6-18) of depressed and normal parents. J. Amer. Acad. Child Psychiat. 23:78-

84, 1984

79. Welner Z, Rice J: School-aged children of depressed parents: a blind and controlled study. J. Affect. Disorders 15:291-302, 1988
80. Beardslee WR, Keller MB, Lavori PW, Klerman GK, Dorer DJ, Samuelson H: Psychiatric disorder in adolescent offspring of parents with affective disorders in a non-referred sample. J. Affective Disorders 15:313-322, 1988
81. Egeland JA, Gerhard DS, Pauls DL, Sussex JN, Kidd KK, Allen CR, Hostetter AM, Housman DE: Bipolar affective disorders linked to DNA markers on chromosome 11. Nature 325:783-787, 1987
82. Hodgkinson S, Sherrington R, Gurling H, Marchbanks R, Reeders S, Mallet J, McInnis M, Petursson H, Brynjolfsson J: Molecular genetic evidence for heterogeneity in manic depression. Nature 325:805-806, 1987
83. Detera-Wadleigh SD, Berrettini WH, Goldin LR, Boorman D, Anderson S, Gershon ES: Close linkage of c-Harvey-ras-1 and the insulin gene to affective disorder is ruled out in three North American pedigrees. Nature 325:806-808, 1987
84. Baron M, Risch N, Hamburger R, Mandel B, Kushner S, Newman M, Drumer D, Belmaker RH: Genetic linkage between X-chromosome markers and bipolar affective illness. Nature 326:289-292, 1987
85. Sherrington R, Byrnjolfsson J, Petursson H, Potter M, Dudleston K, Barraclough B, Wasmuth J, Dobbs M, Gurling H: Localization of a susceptibility locus for schizophrenia on chromosome 5. Nature 336:164-167, 1988
86. Kennedy JL, Giuffra LA, Moises HW, Cavalli-Sforza LL, Pakstis AJ, Kidd JR, Castiglione CM, Sjogren B, Wetterberg L, Kidd KK: Evidence against linkage of schizophrenia to markers on chromosome 5 in a Northern Swedish pedigree. Nature 336:167-170, 1988
87. West MJ, King AP: Settling nature and nurture into an ontogenetic niche. Dev. Psychobiol. 20:549-562, 1987
88. Lilienfeld AM, Lilienfeld DE: Foundations of Epidemiology. 2nd edition. New York, Oxford University Press, Chapter I, pp. 3-22, 1980
89. Costello EJ: Developments in child psychiatric epidemiology. J. Am. Acad. Child Adol. Psychiat. Vol. 28, pp. 836-841, 1989
90. Gulaid JA, Onwuachi-Saunders EC, Sacks JJ, Roberts, DR: Differences in death rates due to injury among blacks and whites, 1984. Morb. Mort. Wkly. Rep. 37SS3:25-31, 1988
91. Williams KR: Economic sources of homicide: estimating the effects of poverty and inequality. Amer. Soc. Rev. 49:283-289, 1984
92. Robins LN: Sturdy childhood predictors of adult antisocial behavior. Psychol. Med. 8:611-622, 1978
93. Comer JP: The Yale-New Haven primary prevention project: a

follow-up study. J. Amer. Acad. Child Psych. 24:154-160, 1985
94. Stunkard AJ: The Salmon Lecture: Perspectives on human obesity. Bull. N.Y. Acad. Med. 64:902-940, 1988
95. Brenneman J: The menace of psychiatry. Am. J. Dis. Child 42:376-402, 1931
96. Plant J: The promise of psychiatry. Am. J. Dis. Child 44:1308-1320, 1932
97. Eisenberg L: Preventive pediatrics: the promise and the peril. Pediat. 80:415-422, 1987

chapter 8

Changing Concepts And Treatment Of Schizophrenia

Heinz E. Lehmann, M.D., L.F.A.P.A.

We have effective treatments of schizophrenia today but do we have valid concepts? One of the distinguished speakers at this conference published a paper a few years ago on "The Impossible Concept of Schizophrenia" (1), and another well known researcher on schizophrenia recently wrote that he "cannot see the concept of schizophrenia abandoned for a long time to come" (2). There is indeed a troubling uncertainty abroad about the existence of the very concept of schizophrenia.

By definition, a concept is an abstract general representation of an entity. But is schizophrenia really a (nosological) entity? Bleuler referred to it as "the group of schizophrenias" and everybody today seems to agree that there are several heterogeneous groups involved. Is schizophrenia, rather than a nosological entity, a disease, an assembly of discrete diseases, or a syndrome like the organic brain syndrome or the dementias? In that case, rather than a concept, schizophrenia should be called a construct, an arbitrary representation. Hardnosed scientists would probably prefer this term since there is as yet no biological criterion for schizophrenia. It all depends on one's personal perspective which, by definition, is a limited viewpoint. Most clinicians prefer to refer to schizophrenia as an entity, a concept, confident that sooner or later biological markers will prove them right.

When I was a spectator as a medical student and then a clinician-actor in the fascinating scenario of schizophrenia in the early thirties, we had quiet and scholarly discussions on the phenomenology of schizophrenia, on some of its psychodynamics, on its bizarre symptoms, on the differences between Kraepelin's and Bleuler's concepts. Our treatments, however, were limited to protectionist constraint in institutions and symptomatic control of agitation with sedatives.

Psychiatry: Past Reflections–Future Visions
B.T. Taylor and I.J. Taylor, Editors

Today, there is no longer discussion about schizophrenia in a scholarly, calm atmosphere, but an avalanche, a pandemonium of continuously changing new observations, new imagery, new research data, new

TABLE 1

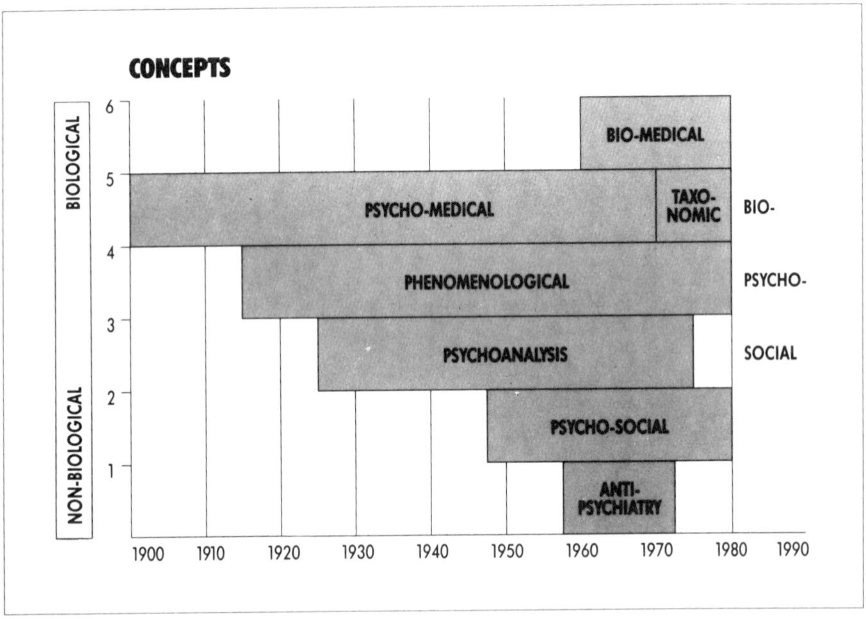

hypotheses, new notions coming not only from psychiatry but from a multitude of more or less related disciplines. For somebody who is nostalgically thinking of the old days it may seem like having crossed from a quiet library into a disco, filled with din and stroboscopic flashes, where everybody dances to his own tune and conversation is no longer possible. Yet if you close the door to the exciting scene, schizophrenia still is almost as elusive and mysterious as it ever was. We do not know its cause nor how to cure it nor how to prevent it.

PSYCHOMEDICAL CONCEPT

In 1899, Kraepelin stated: "The nature of dementia praecox leaves little doubt that it involves heredity and a tangible affection of the brain, probably damage or destruction of cortical cells due to autointoxication, which is the result of chemical disturbances that in some way may be associated with a disorder of the gonads" (3).

Seventeen years later, in 1916, Bleuler said: "One must acknowledge that at least the great majority of clinical pictures which are now collected under the name of dementia praecox rests on some toxic action or anatomical process which arises independently of psychic illness.... The principal group, in my opinion, is certainly caused by organic changes" (4).

Since then, some observers have veered into the strictly medical perspective and some have split off into the strictly psychological viewpoint, but the majority still hold at least a dual view.

Today, my own definition of schizophrenia is: a mental illness with a still-unknown physical substrate, involving possibly a genetically-determined susceptibility to an error of metabolism that affects the brain at a certain age and leads to social withdrawal and psychotic experiences and behavior, often terminating in permanently impaired social functioning.

In the last fifteen years, the psychomedical model has been overlaid by the new taxonomic model which focuses entirely on operational definitions of symptoms and syndromes and about which I shall say more later.

PHENOMENOLOGICAL CONCEPT

The phenomenological concept was formulated by Jaspers in Europe, where it came to be generally accepted by the early 192Os. It is a difficult concept for many scientifically oriented North Americans to grasp, particularly those who have welcomed DMS-III with open arms.

In Jaspers' words: "Phenomenology's task is to intuitively grasp the mental state which the patient experiences as image-like reality" (5).

This approach is almost the exact opposite of that of DSM-III which actually distances the patient from the examiner. It means sensing personally the individual's state of existence, not measuring, labeling, evaluating or selecting specific indications for treatment of specific homogeneous subgroups of patients. It is, in Wings' words, a "limpid exposition of the individual patient--extending into the treatment period" (2). It means entering the world of the sick person through empathy which in its radical extreme has found expression in the "praecox feeling," which the Dutch psychiatrist Rumke proposed as an essential diagnostic criterion for schizophrenia (6).

PSYCHOANALYTIC CONCEPT

By the late 1920s and early 1930s psychoanalysis had developed to a stage where, particularly in North America, it was considered to have theoretical and therapeutic potential for a more or less specific approach to schizophrenia.

Freud had originally considered schizophrenia to be a narcissistic neurosis which was untreatable with psychoanalytic techniques because the nature of the disease prohibited the development of transference between patient and therapist. But in the 1930s some analysts found that it was indeed possible to produce transference in schizophrenic patients, although the transference turned out to be extremely fragile and even potentially explosive. A more recent psychoanalytic concept of schizophrenia might be described as follows: "schizophrenia is a primary disturbance of object relations and interpersonal relationships due to intrapsychic conflicts, infantile trauma and a decathexis of mental representations of objects and drives." But with the advent of effective biological therapy in the 1950s, psychoanalysis could no longer be considered the exclusive, theoretical mainframe for schizophrenia and it lost the virtual, conceptual monopoly which it had held, at least in the U.S., for about two decades.

PSYCHOSOCIAL CONCEPT

The psychosocial concept was the next to appear on the scene, at the end of World War II, in the wake of several investigations of the social roots of schizophrenia. Leading the attack on older concepts was Goffman in his study of the influence of institutionalization on psychiatric patients (7). Goffman coined the term "total institutionalization" and claimed that it produced a great deal of regression, leading to a social breakdown syndrome. He pointed out that dehumanizing exploitation of patients was occurring in mental hospitals and that devastating iatrogenic symptomatology was being created.

A few years earlier Faris and Dunham had published their findings of the cluster phenomenon of schizophrenia in city slums (8), and a little later Hollingshead and Redlich reported on the influence of socio-economic strata on the distribution of schizophrenia (9), followed by Morrison and Goldberg's studies on schizophrenic downward mobility and the breeder vs. drifter hypothesis (10).

At that time, British and American hospitals were turning to an open door policy and a sweeping new Kennedy era. Camelot optimism was taking hold throughout the field of psychiatry. Community Mental Health Centers were being created as a "quick fix" for the centuries old riddle of schizophrenia.

Neither Goffman's horror picture--based on a study of one hospital half a century ago--nor the Polyanna-ish expectations of limitless benefits from deinstitutionalization are valid generalizations today. However, the psychosocial concept remains with us today and almost surely will continue to stay with us in the foreseeable future as a part of the management of schizophrenia.

ANTIPSYCHIATRIC CONCEPT

The antipsychiatric concept raised its iconoclastic head in the late 1950s, as it had in less systematic form from time to time in previous years, as long as 100 years ago.

There were three main streams in the antipsychiatric movement:

The first might be called the label model, proposed by sociologists who considered schizophrenia to be a label for people whose deviant behavior is not acceptable to society. A diagnosis of schizophrenia, they believed, was merely a convenient way to remove undesirables from the community.

A second model, with sinister undertones, is the "myth" model created by Szasz, a professor of psychiatry at Syracuse University (11). Szasz proposed that functional mental disorders, such as schizophrenia, are simply myths or metaphors that allow psychiatrists with vested interests to benefit financially from and exercise power over a helpless minority.

Third, there is the more benevolent "developmental crisis" model proposed by Laing, Cooper and others (12). They see schizophrenia as an altered state of consciousness, in response to an intolerable social and family situation, that finally results in a break which, with proper management, can lead to personality growth and enhanced functioning.

All of these concepts grasped the imagination of many intellectuals and students in the rebellious 1960s and created considerable turbulence in psychiatric thinking until the mid 1970s.

BIOMEDICAL CONCEPT

The biomedical concept is not very different from the psychomedical concept, except for its emphasis on schizophrenia as a biological disease. The concept was ushered in by the serendipitous discovery of the unexpected effectiveness of antipsychotic drugs in the treatment of acute schizophrenia in the 1950s (13). The fact that physical agents were dramatically and specifically effective in suppressing schizophrenic symptoms in one stroke invalidated the psychoanalytic claim that there was no point in looking for biological factors in schizophrenia. It also created a compelling need to look for the mechanisms of action of these drugs. What did they do to the brain and why were they so specifically effective in eliminating specific experiential and behavioral manifestations, thus changing the phenomenological picture of schizophrenia? This search rapidly led to a spate of new discoveries about neurotransmitters, neuronal receptors, neuropeptides, major developments in the imaging of the brain structure, its metabolism and its vascular physiology--all new and amazing discoveries in the living brains of animals and humans.

New discoveries in molecular biology opened doors to investigations of genetics and cerebral processes that had been undreamed of only 20 years before. What had started out quite modestly as an attempt to understand why antipsychotic drugs worked in schizophrenia has by now become a gigantic development of a new discipline; i.e., neurobiology and the neurosciences, so gigantic that, as some psychiatrists believe, it has diverted too much attention to its specific achievements and lost most of its links with clinical concepts of schizophrenia.

An interesting new perspective has recently been introduced by Zubin with his vulnerability model. He proposes to abandon the concept of schizophrenia as a progressive disease and introduce the concept of a vulnerable personality suffering repeated breakdowns when exposed to psychosocial stresses. He thus exchanges the perspective of an ongoing disease with remissions for that of a healthy, but vulnerable, individual with episodic breaks (14).

TAXONOMIC CONCEPT

The newest newcomer of concepts is the taxonomic. This is really a special development of the psycomedical concept, but it fascinates those psychiatric clinicians worldwide who were feeling dissatisfied with a too-subjective and therefore unscientific way of making psychiatric diagnoses. The new movement started in the 1970s with the goal of operationalizing the diagnostic criteria of schizophrenic and other mental disorders, thus freeing clinicians from the theoretical and speculative notions on etiology and meaning. With such a new approach, communication between clinics and investigators was much facilitated. Through a sequence of proposed diagnostic systems from the Feighner approach (15) to The Research Diagnostic Criteria (16) and finally to DSM-III and its latest revision (17), a new focus of interest was created, along with a reconceptionalization of the psychomedical concept. This is sometimes referred to as the neo-Kraepelinian approach. Where Bleuler and Kraepelin had differed was in the fact that Bleuler both changed the name from Dementia Praecox to Schizophrenia in order to redirect the clinicians' attention from a deteriorating process to a characteristic syndrome and expanded the concept of schizophrenia beyond that of Kraepelin. One consequence of this tendency to widen the concept of schizophrenia was the overdiagnosis of this disease in North America when compared to the prevailing mode of diagnosis in the United Kingdom, a phenomenon that was demonstrated by the convincing U.S.-U.K. research project in the 1960s.

Since even the most sophisticated neurobiological developments in the biomedical sphere have not succeeded in producing a biological marker for schizophrenia that would once and for all put diagnostic uncertainties to rest, more diagnostic systems of subgrouping schizophrenia are currently being created or reconsidered. In DSM-III-R some new categories that are related to schizophrenia have been introduced; e.g., schizophreniform psychosis, schizoaffective disorder and schizotypal personality disorder. Reexamined today is also the diagnostic application of Schneider's 12 first-rank symptoms of schizophrenia (18) and Leonhards' 16 systematic schizophrenic subgroupings and 4 non-systematic groups (19).

The latest addition to schizophrenic subgroupings has been Crow's interesting Type I and Type II distinction (20). These are, of course, in addition to the older groupings, such as nuclear schizophrenia, paranoid vs. nonparanoid, good prognosis vs. bad prognosis, and process vs. reactive schizophrenia.

It is not my assignment to discuss critically these diagnostic efforts which currently absorb much clinical and research interest. As part of the psychomedical concept, and in the absence of a biological diagnostic criterion, unanswered taxonomic questions will, of course, continue into the future.

We must not forget, however, that in psychiatric diagnosis, more than in the diagnosis of physical disease, the idea that the whole is greater than the sum of its parts applies. The DSM-III approach, scientifically sound as it may be, in the area of the psychomedical approach to the diagnosis of schizophrenia lacks the image or gestalt-oriented input of personal experience and empathy that characterizes the phenomenological approach. It resembles more the putting together of a jig-saw puzzle than the systematic exploration of a psychological phenomenon.

BIO-PSYCHO-SOCIAL CONCEPT AND TREATMENT

In recent years it has been increasingly realized that whatever concept is used in our thinking about schizophrenia and whatever

TABLE 2

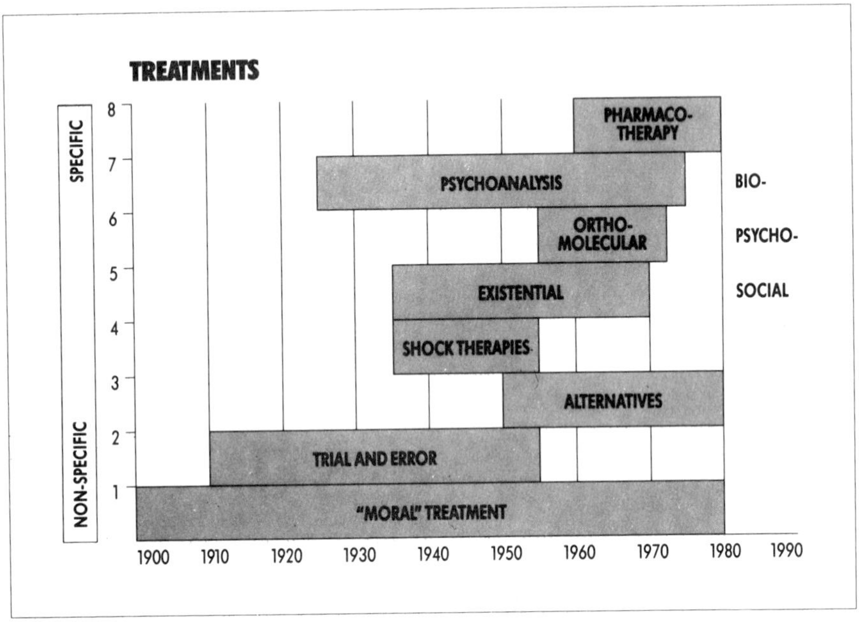

treatment is applied to it, there is an urgent need for integration of all the different concepts and treatment methods. This integration, which aims at unifying separate approaches, is referred to as the bio-psycho-social theoretical and pragmatic approach to schizophrenia. What this means, of course, is simply that biological, psychological and social factors all have to be considered on an equal footing in both intellectual and pragmatic approaches to any mental disorder, including schizophrenia.

The idea of a three-way integration may really be only wishful thinking. It is no more possible to think of intricate biological mechanisms at the same time as complex psychological activities and an idiosyncratic social context in one singular view than it is to see the two appearances of a reversible figure at once. This triple-headed synthesizing concept is really hardly more than an *aide-memoire*, a rapid checklist to remind us that the well-being and the health or disease of all human beings are anchored in these three essentials.

MORAL TREATMENT

At the time of the French Revolution, Pinel liberated mental patients from their chains and, for the first time, clearly took responsibility for such patients as a physician. Before Pinel this responsibility had been left to the church, the police and various government agencies. Pinel, and his disciple Esquirol, then wrote the first medical textbooks on psychiatry and introduced the first very general, but highly effective, therapeutic method of "moral treatment."

In the first half of the 19th century, tremendous successes were claimed for this non-specific and non-biologically oriented treatment which at that time comprised, as an important part, custodialism or asylum. However, toward the end of the 19th century mental hospitals had become so crowded that the true sense of moral treatment as being protective and supportive was almost completely lost.

Moral treatment is no longer known under this name but is now referred to as psychosocial, alternative, milieu, occupational, recreational or rehabilitation therapy. It comprises all, not primarily medical, but humane and rational treatments of psychiatric patients. This kind of amorphous treatment will, I hope, continue indefinitely in the therapeutic management of schizophrenia.

TRIAL AND ERROR

Trial and error characterized the next era of treatment and was a forerunner of biomedical therapy. It consisted of a wide array of almost randomly chosen and often very aggressive biological interventions, such as artificially-produced fever, intoxications, prolonged sleep, early vitamin treatment, skin irritation and heroic measures to produce leucocytosis; e.g., by means of injecting oil of turpentine into the abdominal wall. This resulted in a huge sterile abscess, that had to be surgically opened under sterile conditions, in an operating room. Also on the surgical plane, removal of "focal infections" was carried out by the surgical removal of a considerable length of intestines. None of these far-fetched treatments was based on anything but the most arbitrary speculations of those who undertook them and, needless to say, none of these treatments worked.

One exception was Klaesis' prolonged sleep treatment introduced in the 1920s which often produced temporary improvement of schizophrenic symptoms (21). This was, however, a costly, time-consuming and rather hazardous treatment at that time. Many patients, heavily sedated with barbiturates for a period of weeks, would develop pneumonia, at a time when we had no antibiotics to deal with this complication.

The trial-and-error era came to a definite end with the introduction of antipsychotic drugs in the 1950s.

PSYCHOANALYTIC THERAPY

Psychoanalytic therapy was the first specific approach to the treatment of schizophrenia based on psychoanalytic theory. Its more systematic beginnings I somewhat arbitrarily put into the mid 1930s. It flourished, particularly in the U.S., until its relative ineffectiveness in the treatment of schizophrenia was demonstrated in the 1970s.

Although Freud had considered schizophrenia to be untreatable with psychoanalytic techniques, a few special therapists and clinics, like Chestnut Lodge where Frieda Fromm-Reichmann (22) did her heroic work, were able to demonstrate some temporary therapeutic success with extremely intense and rather idiosyncratic psychoanalytic techniques. The serious problem with the psychoanalytic treatment of schizophrenia was that there were never sufficient therapists for the time-consuming procedure. Also, the special personality traits required of therapists were rarely available. Treatment was reserved for a few wealthy people who, unfortunately, often relapsed as soon as treatment stopped. There were long waiting lists and improvement had a short half-life.

By the 1970s psychoanalysis had lost its popularity as a desirable treatment for schizophrenia, and in the early 1980s a carefully designed 2-year study in Boston, carried out by senior, experienced therapists, showed clearly that psychoanalytic, insight-oriented therapy was not superior to general, supportive and reality-oriented psychotherapy (23).

EXISTENTIAL THERAPY

Existential therapy grew out of the confluence of psychoanalysis and phenomenological concepts (24). It involves the frequent and intense contact between therapist and patient that characterized psychoanalytic therapy, but far from taking the passive, mostly non-responsive attitude of analysis, existential therapy depends on intensive, ongoing interaction between therapist and patient. It aims not at reinforcing the schizophrenic patient's isolation in his world but at building bridges to relationships with others. Existential explanations of the patient's behavior and experiences are grounded in observation, empathy and understanding rather than in interpretations. This kind of treatment involves such concepts as "encounter," a specific, unpredictable, but very important empathic meeting of the minds of therapists and patients, and such other non-analytical and non-biological notions as *kairos*, meaning the usually unpredictable, favorable time for therapeutic intervention, as well as the concepts of spatiality and temporality of the world in which the individual patient lives, which are phenomenological more than psychological categories.

I think that this form of therapy as a main approach to schizophrenia, mostly practiced in Europe, probably came to an end in the mid 1970s when the importance of psychoanalysis lost its impact.

INSULIN AND SHOCK TREATMENT

The first revolutionary breakthrough in the treatment of schizophrenia came in the mid 1930s, with Sakel's insulin-induced hypoglycemic coma therapy (25) and von Meduna's convulsive therapy (26). There had never before been any therapeutic results in schizophrenia lasting more than a few hours, for instance, that followed the injection of sodium amytal or the inhalation of CO_2. But now, acute schizophrenic patients would go into lasting remission within a few weeks. True, patients who had been ill with schizophrenia for more than six months did not respond very well to insulin coma therapy, and Meduna's metrazol-treated patients who had lost their symptoms in most cases relapsed within two or three weeks. But, at least, psychiatrists were no longer completely helpless, simply diagnosing an incurable disease.

Working in the insulin ward in that era was a tremendously exciting, and often terrifying, adventure that consisted in bringing patients close to the threshold of death and then dramatically reviving them. Clinicians in the "insulin ward" worked in a pungent sea of sweating bodies, and sticky sucrose was everywhere. There was always the danger of producing an irreversible coma and a fatal outcome.

Convulsive therapy was at first based on the injection of camphor in oil intramuscularly, then on the injection of metrazol intravenously, and finally developed by Cerletti and Bini to electro-convulsive treatment (27). Metrazol convulsions took about 20-30 seconds to develop after the injection started, and during that time, until the convulsion-producing concentration of metrazol had reached the brain, the patient underwent unspeakable anxiety and panic. As just one example of the darker side of this treatment, one of our schizophrenic patients committed suicide the day before his scheduled metrazol injection. He left a note saying that he could not go through another treatment. The introduction of electricity to induce a seizure eliminated these problems, simplifying treatment and improving its safety.

ALTERNATIVES

Running concurrently with the psycho-social concept was treatment by alternatives to institutionalization and strictly medical treatment. It consisted in mass deinstitutionalization which saw the U.S. institutional population plummet from 500,000 in the early 1950s to fewer than 150,000 in the late 1970s. It led to rapid growth of psychiatric outpatient clinics, the development of new social resources, such as supervised residences, drop-in centers, mobile crisis units, individual and group supportive psychotherapy, behavioral social skills training, self-help groups, case management (28) etc., along with similar non-institutionalized, non-medical adjuncts, one of the newer and most effective alternative approaches being family psychoeducation (29).

But for the most part, alternative therapies unfortunately produced a cart-before-the-horse situation. For not yet completely understood, politically flavored reasons, the big institutions were depopulated, and "liberated" patients, many still very ill, flooded the streets before there were even halfway adequate resources to help them survive in the community.

The most effective alternative therapies should, of course, continue indefinitely.

ORTHOMOLECULAR (MEGAVITAMIN) TREATMENT

Orthomolecular, or megavitamin, treatment was a curious interlude that lasted from the mid 1950s to the mid 1970s. It was based on Hoffers' reported clinical observations that huge doses of certain vitamin B factors as well as vitamin C and some others (also trace minerals) would cure acute as well as chronic schizophrenia (30).

Pauling, a chemist and two-time Nobel Laureate, developed a theory of orthomolecular therapy which stated simply that mental disease was due to the wrong mix of molecules in the brain which needed to be corrected (31). There was much public response to this kind of therapy which even took on political overtones. But systematic and well-controlled efforts to duplicate earlier findings in order to establish the effectiveness of this kind of treatment failed (32).

PHARMACOTHERAPY

With the early 1950s came the first effective antipsychotic drugs: the phenothiazines and reserpine. Reserpine was not used for long but the phenothiazines, first introduced into psychiatry by the French clinicians Deniker and Delay, are still the mainstay of antipsychotic pharmacotherapy (33). For some time it was thought that this class of drugs had specific antischizophrenic properties and thus might lead to a cure of schizophrenia, but it soon became clear that the drugs were capable only of suppressing psychotic symptoms, of whatever origin, for as long as an adequate blood level was maintained.

Today, the most intensive research in the therapy of schizophrenia is in the field of pharmacotherapy. There is a steady stream of new derivatives of the old, conventional drugs, and there is a constant search for new neurochemical and pharmacological models to be used for the development of novel antipsychotic agents that are not based entirely on the by now time-honored but somewhat simplistic model of inhibition of cerebral dopaminergic activity.

One thing, however, is certain. In just about every effective, present approach to the treatment of schizophrenia there is a pharmacological component, around which all alternative therapies are assembled, be they psychotherapy, family education or behavioral modification focused on social skills training.

CONCLUSION

Looking back over our tables of changing concepts and treatments, we note that both terminate in the bio-psycho-social model, reminding us that the concepts that are still with us are the psychomedical, the phenomenological, the psychosocial and the biomedical. Of the various treatments, we have retained the always valid moral treatment, that is the humane component of every single therapy, the psychosocial alternatives and the pharmacotherapies. These are the concepts and treatments that are either so universal that they have stood the test of time or are so effective that we will continue to need them for the foreseeable future. It would be progress if we had achieved nothing else but to have weeded out ineffective, unproductive ideas or treatments of schizophrenia over the last 50 years. But we have done much more: we have created some new approaches to our thinking and treatment that may promise even more rapid progress in the years to come. Schizophrenia as we know it today may in the future go by another name as we learn more, perhaps N.A.D.D., which would stand for Nucleus Accumbens Dopamine Dysergia.

REFERENCES

1. van Praag HM: About the impossible concept of schizophrenia. Comprehensive Psychiatry, Vol. 17, No. 4 pp. 481-497, 1976
2. Wing JR: in: Search for the causes of schizophrenia. (ed.) Häfner, Gattarz WF, Tanzarik W, Berlin, Springer, 1987
3. Kraepelin E: Psychiatrie. ein lehrbuch für studierende und aerzte. Leipzig: JA Barth, 1899, vol. 2
4. Bleuler E: Physisch und psychisch in der pathologie. Z. Neurol. Psychiatr. 30:426-475, 1916
5. Jaspers K: Allgemeine Psychopathologie. Siebente Auflage. Berlin-Göttingen-Heidelberg. Springer (1959), page 47. (Authors' Translation)
6. Rümke HC: Über die schizophrenie; in: Rümke HC (ed.). Eine blühende psychiatrie in gefahr. Berlin, Springer, 1967
7. Goffman E: Characteristics of total institutions, in: Symposium on prevention and social psychiatry, Washington, D.C. U.S. Government Printing Office, 1958
8. Faris REL, Dunham HW: Mental disorders in urban areas, Chicago, University of Chicago Press 1939
9. Hollingshead AB, Redlich FG: Social class and mental illness, New York, John Wiley, 1958
10. Goldberg EM, Morrison SL: Schizophrenia and social class, Brit. J. Psychiat. 109:785-802, 1963
11. Szasz TS: Commitment of the mentally ill: "Treatment" or Social Restraint? J. Nerv. and Ment. Dis. 125,293. 1957
12. Laing R, Cooper D: Reason and violence, New York, Vintage, 1971
13. Delay, J, Deniker P, Harl JM: Traitement des états d'excitation et d'agitation par une méthode médicamenteuse dérivee de l'hibernotherapie. Ann. Méd. psychol. 110:267-273, 1952
14. Zubin J, Magaziner J, Steinbauer SR: The metamorphosis of schizophrenia: From chronicity to vulnerability. Psychological Medicine. 13:551-571, 1983
15. Feighner JP, Robins E, Guze SB et al: Diagnostic criteria for use in psychiatric research. Arch. Gen. Psychiatry, 26:57, 1972
16. Spitzer RL, Endicott J, Robins E: Research diagnostic criteria. New

York State Department of Mental Hygiène, New York, 1975
17. DSM-III-R, The American Psychiatric Association, Washington, 1987
18. Schneider K: Wesen und erfassung der schizophrenen. Zeitschrift ges. Neurol. Psychiat. 99:542, 1925
19. Leonhard K: Die atypischen psychosen und kleist's lehre von den endogenen psychosen. In: Psychiatrie der Gegenwart, (ed.) H.W. Grule vol.1, Berlin, Springer, 1960
20. Crow TJ, Cross AJ, Johnstone EC, Owne F: Two syndromes in schizophrenia and their pathogenesis. In: FA Henn and HA Nasrallah (eds.), Schizophrenia as a brain disease. New York: Oxford University Press, 1982, pp. 196-234
21. Kläsi J: Über die therapeuteische anwendung der "Dauermarkose" mittels somnifens bei schizophrenen. Z. Neurol. Psychiatr. 74:557-592, 1922
22. Fromm-Reichmann, F: Principles of intensive psychotherapy. Chicago, The University of Chicago Press, 1950
23. Gunderson TG, Frank AF, Katz HM, et al: Effects of psychotherapy in schizophrenia. Comparative outcome of two forms of treatment, Schizophrenia Bulletin, Vol.10, No.4, 1984, 564-584. National Institute of Mental Health
24. Binswanger L: The case of Ellen West, in: May R, Angel E, Ellenberger HF eds. Existence, New York, Basic Books, 1958
25. Sakel M, Dussik KT: Ergebnisse der hypoglykämieschockbehandlung der schizophrenie. Z. Neurol. Psychiatr. 155:351, 1936
26. von Meduna L: Versuche uber die biologische beinflussung des ablaufes der schizophrenie. Z. Neurol. Psychiatr. 152:235-262, 1935
27. Cerletti U, Bini L: L'Elettroshock. Arch. Gen. Neurol. Psychiatr. Psicoanal. 19:266, 1938
28. Kiesler GA: Mental hospitals and alternative care, Noninstitutionalization as potential public policy for mental patients. American Psychologist, Vol.37, No. 4,349, 1982
29. Anderson GM: A Psychoeducational Program for families of patients with schizophrenia. In: MacFarlane WR (ed.) Family therapy in schizophrenia, pp. 99-116. New York, Guilford Press, 1983
30. Hoffer A, Osmond H, Callbeck MJ, Kahan I: Treatment of schizophrenia with nicotinic acid and nicotinamide. J. Clin. Exper. Psychopathol. 18:131-158, 1957
31. Pauling L: Orthomolecular psychiatry. Science 160:265-271, 1968
32. Ban TA, Lehmann HE: Nicotinic acid in the treatment of schizophrenias. Canadian Mental Health Association Collaborative Study. Progress Report II. Can. Psychiatr. Assn. J. 20:103-112, 1975
33. Lehmann HE, Hanrahan GE: Chlorpromazine. New inhibiting agent for psychomotor excitement and manic states. Arch. Neurol. and Psychiat. Vol.71. pp. 227-237

chapter 9

Anxiety And Depression: Past, Present And Future

Gerald L. Klerman, M.D., F.A.P.A.

"Anxiety" and "depression" are among the grant concepts of 20th century psychiatry. The relationship between these two conditions has long been the matter of intense interest, investigations and debate.

Among the issues in the debate are the relationship of normal anxiety and depression to each other, the relationship of clinical states of anxiety and depression to normal states, and the question of whether there exists a condition of mixed anxiety-depression.

THE PAST

This situation has not always been the dominant one. During the 18th and 19th century, the earliest periods of medical domination of psychiatry and its recognition as a medical subspecialty, relatively little attention was paid to conditions which we call "neurotic." The "neurotic-psychotic" distinction did not become popular among clinicians and layman until the very end of the 19th century and the first decades of the 20th century.

Our forerunners in the 18th and 19th century were mainly concerned with psychoses, their origin, nature, forms, and classification.

Patients with conditions that today we would diagnose "neurotic" or "depressive" whether by DSM-III or ICD-9 criteria, seldom came into contact with psychiatrists. The psychiatrist's main concern was with psychoses or, as they were called in those days, the "insane," and the contact between the psychiatrist and the patient would be mainly diagnostic to ascertain whether the patient was insane or psychotic and the associated decision as to whether or not hospitalization and commitment were called for.

Psychiatry: Past Reflections–Future Visions
B.T. Taylor and I.J. Taylor, Editors

This is not to say that patients with conditions which today we would call hysterical, obsessive/compulsive, phobic, or depressive did not occur. While the epidemiologic rates may have fluctuated, sufficient numbers of such cases must have existed. However, the expectations of the society have changed and it is likely that a considerable number of patients whom today we would diagnose as anxious and depressed would have regarded their condition as God's will or the vicissitudes of life rather than a medical condition worthy of professional attention and therapeutic intervention.

The situation changed dramatically in the late decades of the 19th century and the first two decades of the 20th century preceding the onset of World War I. In most large cities in Western Europe and North America, increasing numbers of middle class patients, most often female, sought assistance from medical authorities for distressing symptoms which were nonpsychotic and did not appear immediately to be life threatening. They often involved obsessions, convulsions, compulsive acts, fears, worries and other signs of nervousness. New diagnostic terms were coined to describe these patients--neurasthenia, psychasthenia.

The year 1895 stands out. In this year Freud published a paper "On Separating Anxiety Neurosis from Neurasthenia" and Kraepelin proposed manic-depressive insanity as a separate diagnostic group. It is widely recognized that many of the descriptions of neurotic conditions were first put forth by Freud, who also wrote a series of papers clarifying the criteria for separating psychoses from neuroses, criteria which rapidly became accepted by most psychiatrists, independent of their commitment to psychoanalysis.

As the number of psychiatrists outside of mental institutions grew and more and more patients came into treatment and gradually therapeutic efforts were undertaken beyond description and diagnosis. During this period, the psychoanalysts held the intellectual, scientific and professional leadership offering the only available coherent theory of causation and treatment and the promise of therapeutic success.

THE PRESENT SITUATION: DEVELOPMENT SINCE WORLD WAR II

World War II marked a major historical point in psychiatric involvement in anxiety and depression. Large numbers of psychiatrists saw military duty in the U.S., British and other services and gained extensive experience with a variety of clinical conditions. The role of combat stress as a major precipitating event and the threat of death through combat led to stress being considered a major organizing theoretical principle for many psychiatrists with extension into civilian life.

Here clinical observations were combined with the neurophysiological and endocrine studies of Selye. The terms "anxiety and depression" had gained increasing public attention. Auden had written his poem "The Age of Anxiety" which was set to music as a ballet by Bernstein, the advent of nuclear power and the struggles against totalitarianism led to wide acceptance of the term "anxiety" in general public. Recently, however, there has been a shift and attention to depression and evidence of a possible new age of melancholia, particularly among adolescents and young adults.

Scientifically, the issues under consideration included the following:

1. What is the relationship between normal anxiety and normal depression and clinical states?
2. Do the clinical states of anxiety and depression represent the symptomatic expression of a common underlined pathological process that is a single disease? We will call this the unitary theory.
3. If the unitary theory is not accepted, then what further subdivisions would one propose for classification of depressive disorders?
4. What is the relationship of anxiety to depressive disorders given the high rates of comorbidity?

The intellectual basis of this debate was mainly articulated by the English, notably the papers by Aubry Lewis who proposed that anxiety and depression be considered a single affective disorder.

This debate was a specific extension of a more general intellectual split within psychiatry between the Maierian approach and the Kraepelinian approach. Lewis described himself on numerous occasions as a disciple of Maier and in his 1930-1933 papers on melancholia he stated explicitly that his intent was to apply to the Kraepelin category of manic depressive insanity the same critique that had been earlier put forth by Maier in his psychobiological theory and his criticism of Kraepelin concept of dementia precox. Figure 1 and Figure 2 outline these issues.

These issues have been approached by a number of different methods and in this section of the paper I shall review the presently employed methods to answer these questions and clarify issues of dispute and disagreement.

These methods include:

1. Multivariate statistics.
2. Response pattern to psychopharmacologic agents.
3. Biological markers and laboratory tests.

4. Response patterns to psychological manipulations and interventions.

	ANXIETY	DEPRESSION
NORMAL AFFECT	FEAR	SADNESS GRIEF
SYMPTOM	DISEASE	DEPRESSION
SYNDROME	ANXIETY NEUROSIS PHOBIA	ENDOGNEOUS DEPRESSION

FIGURE 1. Methods of Investigating Relationship of Anxiety to Depression

Use of Multivariate Statistics

Multivariate statistics, particularly factor analysis, had been talked about for many years, but because of the extensive calculations required were considered to be too tedious and laborious. In the early 1950s, Wittenbourne and Lorr reported factor analytic results of ratings of inpatients and both reported a mixed anxiety depression factor. Two events in the 1950s led to acceleration in the use of multivariate statistics in psychopathology in general. These two events were the development of high speed electronic computers which made possible the calculations previously considered too onerous and, second, the advent of psychopharmacologic agents which created the demand for rating scales to assess the efficacy of drugs for the treatment of psychoses, anxiety and depression.

The first extensive application of these methods to the problems of the relationship of anxiety and depression were undertaken by Martin Roth and his associates in Newcastle. In a series of studies which have become landmarks in psychopathology, they applied factor analysis and multiple discriminate function analysis to data on symptoms collected from patients. They addressed two questions; one, the separation of anxiety and depressive disorders, and second, having established the psychopathological independence of these two conditions, they also use similar strategy for subtypes of depression.

As stated previously, this debate over classification was part of a larger set of issues in British and North American psychiatry. In 1954, Roth along with Maier, Gross and Slater had published the First Edition of their TEXTBOOK OF CLINICAL PSYCHIATRY which included in the introduction a resounding reaffirmation of the Kraepelinian tradition of psychiatry as a medical specialty with emphasis on discreet disorders and the importance of genetic and biological factors in causation. They were openly critical of Maierian approaches in general, and also of the impact of psychoanalysis with its emphasis on early development and intrapsychic structures.

Aubry Lewis, for many years the Director of the Institute of Psychiatry at the Maudsley Hospital, had identified himself as a protagonist of the Maier view, and the debate between Maudsley Hospital and the Newcastle group over the classification of anxiety and depression became the template for a large series of other professional and scientific issues in British psychiatry. Lewis and his associates, notably Kendall, had proposed a unitary approach in which anxiety and depression were regarded part of an affective disorder and which emphasized the continuity between normal experiences of anxiety-fear and sadness-depression and the clinical states. In contrast, Roth and his associates emphasized the discontinuity of the depressive condition from normal sadness and were vigorous proponents of a binary theory or a dualistic theory with emphasis on the distinction between endogenous and neurotic depression. Multivariate statistical techniques were used to reinforce the clinical proposition of the differentiation of depression put forth by Gillespie in 1929, which began the modern concern with endogenous depression. Subsequently, these same statistical techniques were applied, mainly to the question of the classification of depression. Factor analysis was extensively used in the 1960s and in at least seven studies the authors identified what they interpreted to be an endogenous factor.

As regards the separation of anxiety and depression, two large studies in North America, Downey and Rickles in Philadelphia and Prusoff and Klerman in New Haven applied discriminate function analysis to self-rating and found that two thirds of the patients could be separated into anxiety and depressive groups but that a significant degree of overlap existed in the range of approximately one-third of patients who could not be easily classified by the multivariate algorithm.

As shown in Figure 2, there was an interesting asymmetry in the debate. Whereas major emphasis was placed on the separation and classification within the depressive disorders, at that time relatively little attention was paid to possible revamping of the anxiety neurosis diagnosis, an issue which emerged later. At this time, Roth published a paper on the phobic depersonalization syndrome and the calamity reaction describing a group of patients who by DSM-III standards would be regarded as having panic attacks rather than generalized anxiety.

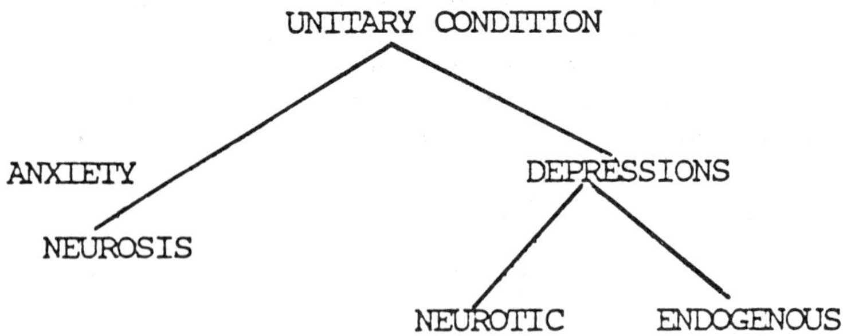

FIGURE 2. Nosology of Anxiety and Depression

In a further application of this technique, Kiloh and Garside, also associates of Roth at Newcastle, applied these statistical techniques to symptom ratings of patients being treated with tricyclic antidepressants, imipramine. Kuhn had originally described the efficacy of imipramine for endogenous depressed patients, based on clinical observation. Kiloh and Garside documented the effects on specific symptoms and demonstrated that the pattern of response to imipramine was identical to the symptom. This has laid the groundwork for the standard prediction; namely, that tricyclic antidepressants are most effective against depressions whose symptom patterns include neurovegetative signs and retardation and other features of the endogenous pattern.

Through the 1950s and 1960s as new psychopharmacologic agents became available, there was active interest in developing some framework in which to interpret the diverse action of these drugs. At first attention was given to "target symptoms," but it soon became apparent that more complex levels of psychopathologic organizations were involved and approaches based on syndromal prediction became more popular. Thus, it became clear that neuroleptic drugs were effective against psychotic syndromes, particularly schizophrenic but also paranoid and other delusional syndromes, lithium was effective against acute episodes of mania and prevention of the recurrences of both manic and depressive syndromes and bipolar illness, and the tricyclic and MAO Inhibitors were effective against depression, particularly typical or endogenous depression.

The conventional wisdom held that benzodiazepines were relatively ineffective against the core symptoms of depression but were of use in a wide range of depressive symptoms. Klein, however, made an interesting observation that patients with panic attacks do not respond to benzodiazepines but do respond to tricyclics. He also reinterpreted reports from England by Tyrer and others that patients with atypical depression and particularly with phobic anxiety responded to MAO Inhibitors. This pattern of drug response was a major source of evidence in support of the proposal to split DSM-II/ICD-8-9, Anxiety Neurosis into two forms of anxiety, Generalized Anxiety and Panic Anxiety. This separation was first embodied in the SADS RDC and then incorporated in the DSM-III and DSM-III-R.

The pattern of efficacy of the tricyclic MAO Inhibitors and benzodiazepines was a powerful source of validation for the separation of anxiety disorders from depressive disorders and furthermore for the separation within the depressive disorders of the endogenous pattern responsive to tricyclic antidepressants.

In the early 1980s, reports appeared that a new triazolabenzodiazepine, alprazolam, was effective in the treatment of panic/anxiety in addition to its demonstrated efficacy for general anxiety. The early reports were soon confirmed in large double-blind placebo-controlled studies.

The efficacy of alprazolam, a benzodiazepine, challenged the standard formula and raised questions as to its possible uniqueness. A number of hypotheses were offered. Pharmacodynamically, it was shown that in animal preparations alprazolam reduced firing in the locuscoeruleus as did imipramine and other compounds. Moreover, there were effects on the down regulation of the beta-adrenergic system. The hypothesis has been put forth that unlike other benzodiazepines, alprazolam possesses actions against the beta-adrenergic system, the CNS system implicated in many of the neuropharmacologic theories of anxiety. The other hypothesis related to pharmacokinetic aspects. It was noted that alprazolam was one of a group of high potency compounds with affinity for the BZ receptor. Another compound in this group, called adanazalan, has also been shown to have efficacy at higher doses than used previously, efficacy approximately equivalent to alprazolam. Moreover, it was noted that the dosage used in the treatment of panic anxiety (4-6 mg. per day) is considerably higher than the dose used for generalized anxiety and stress reactions. This dose would be the equivalent of 60 mgs. of diazepam per day, a dose which would be difficult for patients on diazepam to tolerate because of the degree of sedation. Surprisingly, patients on this dose of alprazolam do not report difficulties with sedation so one possibility may be that the alprazolam has a higher margin between therapeutic efficacy and sedative side effects in the dose range 4-6 mgs. or equivalent for other BZ.

Subsequently, studies with other benzodiazepines at higher than usual dosage seem to indicate that the apparent alprazolam uniqueness was related more to the vigorous dosing schedule than to any pharmacodynamic properties. Positive reports about effects similar to alprazolam at higher doses have appeared for diazepam, lorazepam and chlorazepam.

To further complicate the situation, there are a number of reports as to the value of tricyclic antidepressants in the treatment of GAD. Previously the standard treatment for GAD was considered to be benzodiazepines but recent studies have called this conclusion into question. Before the issue can be resolved, further work is needed on the diagnostic validity of GAD, topic of controversy in itself.

These pharmacologic issues also relate to the possible efficacy of alprazolam as an antidepressant. For many years there has been controversy over the value of benzodiazepines and depression in general (see review by Schatsberg and Cole and Deltito and Klerman). In ambulatory patients with mild-to-moderate forms of depression, particularly when symptoms of anxiety, agitation and insomnia predominate, alprazolam and benzodiazepines have been reported to be effective at least in the short-run, two-four weeks; however, over more prolonged periods of time, the superiority of the tricyclics appears demonstrated. There are a number of reports of the value of alprazolam and the treatment of depressives. The full consensus has not yet been reached. The pattern seems to be that ambulatory patients with Hamilton scores under 20 do quite well but that as the severity of the depression increases, particularly if there are endogenous and neurovegetative signs, the compound has less efficacy.

A methodologic issue contaminates this research. The most widely used scale for the assessment of depressive symptoms and their response to medication is the Hamilton. However, it is now apparent that a sizeable proportion of the variance attributed to change in the Hamilton Scale can be with anxiety clusters (see Figure 2). Thus, apparent reduction in the total Hamilton score should not be immediately interpreted as an antidepressant effect since the mixture of core depressive and anxiety symptoms will vary with different patient samples and at different levels of severity of the syndrome.

THE FUTURE

Therefore, the conclusion must be reached that attempts to unravel the problems in the relationship between anxiety and depressive disorders through clarification of the patterns of response to psychopharmacologic treatment agencies have not succeeded and that previously agreed upon formulae have to be rethought or perhaps even abandoned as it is shown that benzodiazepines at high dose have efficacy and panic equivalent to tricyclic and, moreover, that tricyclics are effective in the treatment of GAD.

Interest in the biology of anxiety and panic was given impetus in the early 1980s by the observation of high degrees of comorbidity of anxiety and depressive symptoms not only in generalized anxiety but also in panic anxiety symptoms. Reports appeared that a substantial percentage of patients being treated for panic disorder had coexisting depressive symptoms often meeting criteria for primary major depression or unipolar depression. Moreover, the efficacy of antidepressant drugs, particularly tricyclic and MAO Inhibitors, against panic attacks even in the absence of depression further stimulated interest in the biological relationship of anxiety and depression. The hypothesis soon emerged that biologically anxiety states and depressive states might be clinical manifestations of the same etiology or pathophysiology. A number of biological markers and laboratory tests have been investigated to answer this matter. Probably the most common single test employed is the Dexamethasone Suppression Test (DST) and the evidence is overwhelming that the pattern of response of panic patients is not that of severe depressives, but only a small fraction of panic patients are nonsuppressors and the response to dexamethasone does not support a unitary hypothesis.

Another line of investigation involves laboratory provocation of panic attacks. Earlier observations by Pits that patients with anxiety neurosis had episodes of intense anxiety and discomfort while receiving infusions of sodium lactate were replicated by Klein and associates and this initiated a series of studies of other provoking agents.

Future prospects are bright. I have not discussed family and genetic studies nor the cognitive behavioral approach. My prediction is that anxiety and depression will be further separated into complex disorders.

chapter 10

Neurobiology Of Affective Disorders: The Evolution From A Cross-Sectional Perspective To A Longitudinal Vision

Frederick K. Goodwin, M.D., F.A.P.A.[1]

This paper will weave practical, clinical suggestions into an essentially theoretical framework intended to fit into the philosophy of this symposium: Looking at the past and present in an attempt to discern future directions of research and clinical practice.

The affective disorders in many ways constitute a paradox. While the knowledge generated to treat major depression and manic-depressive illness represents modern psychiatry's most important accomplishment, these disorders nonetheless remain under-treated and often inappropriately treated. From a clinical perspective, the distance between appropriate and achievable care on the one hand, and what is known and routinely provided on the other hand, is perhaps nowhere larger than in the affective disorders.

Affective illness also is paradoxical insofar as looking toward the future requires that we look first to the past. American psychiatry needs to relearn the lessons taught by prominent 19th century European descriptive psychiatrists who observed that recurrence was fundamental to the major affective disorders. In the United States, where physicians typically treat mobile populations of patients for relatively brief periods of time, we have tended to focus on the treatment of acute episodes. Unlike our European colleagues, few American clinicians have the opportunity to see patients over their entire life course. Today, as it becomes more apparent that many of the limits of clinical practice with

[1]The concepts outlined in this chapter are drawn substantially from Manic-Depressive Illness, by F.K. Goodwin and K.R. Jamison, Oxford University Press, 1990.

Published 1990 by Elsevier Science Publishing Co., Inc.
Psychiatry: Past Reflections–Future Visions
B.T. Taylor and I.J. Taylor, Editors

these disorders reflect insufficient attention in research and practice to their long-term unfolding and recurrent nature, we should be grateful to the Europeans for reminding us that the correct approach to treating the affective disorders is that of managing a chronic illness.

In this paper, I will emphasize the fundamentally recurrent nature of the major affective disorders and will suggest reasons for our all-too-common inattention to that central feature as well as the impact that inattentiveness has had on research and clinical practice, especially in the U.S. Against that backdrop, I will consider the importance of research on bipolar illness as a means of examining the phenomenon of recurrence in major affective illness broadly. In the final sections of the paper, I will discuss three productive research strategies for elucidating mechanisms of cyclicity.

A FUNDAMENTALLY RECURRENT ILLNESS

The original Kraepelinian model of manic-depressive illness (1) encompassed all recurrent, major affective disorders--the bipolar form of the illness, which consists of both manic and depressive episodes, and the unipolar form, which manifests as recurrent major depressive episodes. Kraepelin built his observations on the work of a small group of 19th century European psychiatrists who, in their passion for ever finer distinctions, had cataloged abnormal human behavior into hundreds of classes of disorder. More than any other single individual, Kraepelin brought order and sense to this categorical profusion. He constructed a nosology based on careful description, reducing the categories of psychoses to two: manic-depressive illness and dementia praecox, later renamed *schizophrenia.*

Kraepelin's model consolidated most of the major affective disorders into one category because of their similarity in core symptoms, family history of illness, and, especially, the pattern of recurrence over the course of the patient's lifetime, with periods of remission and exacerbation and a comparatively benign outcome without significant deterioration. He saw mania as one manifestation of the illness, not as the distinguishing sign of a separate bipolar disorder, as it is in today's American diagnostic practice.

The European and American concepts of manic-depressive illness began to diverge almost immediately after Kraepelin's ideas became widespread in the early years of the 20th century. Europeans, adhering to a traditional medical disease model, emphasized the longitudinal course in both research and clinical work. Ever pragmatic, Americans wanted to treat the illness with the techniques at hand, which at that time were derived from the "moral treatment" movement in mental hospitals and the emerging dynamic therapies based on psychoanalytic theory. Research and clinical efforts in the United States thus slighted clinical description and genetics and turned instead to the psychological and social contexts in which the symptoms occurred.

The significance of the divergence of European and American perspectives became clearly evident in the 1960s when, on the continent, explorations of linkage between clinical typology and family history led to the formulation of the bipolar-unipolar distinction, by which manic-depressive patients were grouped according to the presence or absence of a prior history of mania. First proposed by a German, Karl Leonhard (2), the distinction was elaborated by other Europeans, such as Jules Angst (3) and Carlo Perris (4); it was advanced, as well, by the Washington University group in St. Louis, Missouri, neo-Kraepelinians who gave impetus to mounting concern for an etiology-free, description-based diagnostic system in the United States.

The bipolar-unipolar distinction represented a logical refinement of the already well-defined Kraepelinian model, with its emphasis on recurrence and endogeneity. As useful as it is in both research and clinical contexts, however, it proved to be problematic when applied to the much broader American conception of affective disorders. The bipolar subgroup was clearly defined, but the other component of Kraepelinian manic-depressive illness--endogenous, recurrent unipolar depression--was obscured by its confusion with other affective disorders. In American usage, *unipolar* disorder encompassed any mood disorder that was not bipolar, regardless of its severity or course. Although the third edition of the *Diagnostic and Statistical Manual of Mental Disorders* (DSM-III) (5) clarified the situation somewhat by requiring that criteria for major affective disorder be met before the bipolar-unipolar distinction is drawn, a diagnosis of unipolar disorder was still broader than the Kraepelinian concept, since it did not require a prior course of illness.

Renewed attentiveness to the importance of recurrence in major depressive disorders--and, particularly, awareness of research suggesting that recurrent unipolar disorders may have more in common with bipolar disorder than with single episode unipolar disorders--has underscored a weakness in the current *DSM-III(R)* classification (6), namely that the bipolar group is separated away from the others at the outset, giving misleading emphasis to its existence as a discrete category. In research and clinical practice, there is considerable risk associated with emphasizing polarity at the expense of recurrence and cyclicity.

CROSS-SECTIONAL VS. LONGITUDINAL RESEARCH DESIGN

Although recurrence is a fundamental characteristic of affective illness, surprisingly few of the biological and pharmacologic theories and data pertaining to the disorder have addressed the biology of recurrence. Most studies reported in the literature have tended instead to reflect a cross-sectional perspective and have consequently focused on examination of the state of being either in mania or depression (Table 1). As Mandell has noted, "Stability, the most important predictive aspect of the dynamics of complex systems; i.e., the brain, has never been a significant descriptive parameter in any formal psychopharmacologic program of basic or clinical research." (7).

TABLE 1
Conceptual Approaches to the Biology of Affective Illness

Cross-Sectional Approaches

- Biological effects of antidepressant or antimanic drugs (e.g., the amine hypotheses)
- State-dependent changes (e.g., amine metabolites)
- Contributions to clinical topology (e.g., DST)
- Predictors of treatment response (e.g., MHPG)
- Intersection of normal variance with illness (e.g., CSF 5-HIAA)

Longitudinal Approaches

- State-independent abnormalities (the biology of vulnerability)
- Biological correlates of natural course variables (e.g., age of onset, number of episodes, cycle length)
- Focus on within-patient variance
- Mechanisms of cyclicity (the biology of recurrence)
  - Effects of drugs on cycle length
  - Kindling and sensitization
  - Biological rhythms, circadian and seasonal

The original concept of the pharmacologic bridge was constructed from analogies between the *acute* effects of various drugs (such as reserpine and the antidepressants) on brain neurotransmitter amines and their clinical effects on episodes of illness. Similarly, direct studies with humans measured "snapshots" of state-dependent biological changes during depression or mania, such as amine metabolites or urine neuroendocrine function. While some interesting spinoffs developed from these cross-sectional approaches (such as the dexamethasone suppression test as a way to confirm underlying biological remission from a depressive episode) little was learned about vulnerability (so important for genetic studies) or of the inherent tendency for mania and depression to recur.

More recently, a plethora of questions answerable only through longitudinal study have begun to receive the research attention they warrant. Are patients with early onset of the illness different from those who have late-age onset? How do those with multiple episodes differ from those with fewer? There is growing acknowledgement of the need for longitudinal studies designed to address questions regarding biological correlates of natural course variables of major depressive disorders. For example, does Post's observation of increasing CSF norepinephrine levels with successive affective episodes (8) signal an increasing anxiety response as the patient anticipates the increasing disruption by the illness? Also, application of molecular genetics to studies of mental disorders implicitly calls for longitudinal approaches, especially "well-state" studies, given that the optimal usefulness of genetic markers as tools for enhancing early intervention and prevention is contingent on their presence when a patient is recovered or, ideally, before the occurrence of a first episode.

The issue of longitudinal as opposed to cross-sectional focus is not only of interest to researchers, it also has immediate and practical implications for physicians and patients, with regard to both treatment and prognosis. That is, while many treatments can dramatically alter overt symptoms, it is increasingly evident that clinical decisions about the pharmacologic management of acute episodes as well as prophylaxis must be made in the context of the tendency of the illness to recur and persist.

BIPOLAR ILLNESS: PARADIGM FOR RESEARCH ON RECURRENCE

Because in the vast majority of instances manic and depressive episodes can be predicted to revert to normal at some finite time, either spontaneously or in response to effective treatments, longitudinal studies of bipolar disorder provide invaluable opportunity to compare biological measures during the illness with the same measures in the recovered state; such studies are essential if one is to circumvent the problem of inter-individual variability. Moreover, the recurrent pattern--of recovery to "normal" and/or change to an "opposite" state--

ensures the usefulness of the bipolar form of the illness as an unsurpassed paradigm for separation of state and trait variables in mental disease. The *regularity* of recurrence in some patients permits the clinical investigator to anticipate the onset of an episode and, thus, to schedule data collection at critical points; the frequent *rapidity* of the "switch" (especially into mania) allows intensive efforts to understand the relationships between stress and biological changes in the onset of illness by looking at the temporal sequence of events, one approach to the ultimate question of causality.

While we focus here on bipolar illness, we emphasize that the pattern of recurrence in major affective illness is found in unipolar forms of the illness as well. In the *unipolar* pattern, depressive episodes occur against a backdrop of normal, symptom-free intervals that can range from a few months to years or even decades. In about 15 to 20 percent of unipolar patients, recovery is not complete; that is, the acute episode of major depression remits to a less severe state of chronic depression (9). In the *bipolar* pattern, manic or hypomanic episodes occur in addition to the depressive episodes and normal periods. Compared to the unipolar pattern, the bipolar pattern shows an earlier age of onset and is generally more recurrent; that is, has a greater overall frequency of episodes. Bipolar illness represents about 25 to 35 percent of major affective illness (10). As noted below, lower incidence estimates for bipolar illness that still appear in most textbooks are based on underestimates of the bipolar-II pattern in which *hypomania* alternates with depression.

Rates of Recurrence

Drawing on an extensive review of the literature, Zis and Goodwin (11) estimated that the true recurrence rate for major affective disorder is approximately 80 percent; that is, recurrence is the rule, and single episodes are the exception. For unipolar depression, there is enormous individual variability in number of unipolar depressive episodes, with the median appearing to fall between 5 and 7. In the bipolar form, the median number of episodes ranges from 13 to 15, again with considerable individual variability. In the subgroup of patients who seem only to experience a single episode of illness, onset tends to be later, and, often, the depression seems to be organic, rather than a true "primary" depression.

Unfortunately, textbook estimates of average recurrence rates generally are much lower, in the range of 50 to 60 percent. Upon close inspection, these estimates come from literature reviews which include many studies fraught with methodological difficulties that cause underestimations of recurrence; these include short duration of observation, a focus on hospitalized episodes (with exclusion of episodes that precede an index admission), high drop-out rates with no follow-up, inclusion of "non-recovered" patients, many of whom actually were rapidly cycling but were counted as having a single episode, and a high unipolar to bipolar patient ratio. While a few methodological problems contribute to overestimations of recurrence in the affective disorders, most lead to underestimations.

From a clinical perspective, the cost of underestimating recurrence was strikingly depicted in the NIMH Collaborative Study of Depression (12). This multi-site study followed a group of patients with major depression (predominantly unipolar) for two years; each had actually been recruited to one of five research centers studying clinical and biological aspects of major depression. Treatment was by physicians' choice. At the two year follow-up, only 43 percent were found to have recovered and stayed well, a rate well below anticipated treatment-maintained remissions which should be in the range of 65 percent. When outcomes were examined more closely, only 17 percent of the patients were found not to have recovered at all, that is, to have been truly treatment resistant. The bulk of the poor outcome group was made up of individuals who experienced an episodic course of illness (40 percent of the total sample), a pattern which was associated with a diagnosis of "double depression" (major depression superimposed on a chronic minor depression) at entry into the study. Presumably, had these patients' physicians focused on the management of recurrence as well as the management of episodes, overall outcome would have been much more favorable.

Under-Recognition of Bipolar Illness

Not only is the extent of recurrence underestimated; so too is the prevalence of bipolar illness. When hypomania and mania are accounted for, bipolar illness accounts for roughly one-third of all major depressive disorders. The lower estimates reported traditionally have been a function of the low reliability with which bipolar-II disorders are diagnosed; the difficulty reflects, in large part, the understandable failure of patients to report, or clinicians to recognize as symptoms of illness, those initially positive states associated with hypomania such as decreased need for sleep, more energy, inflated self-esteem, increased productivity, clarity of thinking, and hypersexuality. Of course, the diagnosis requires that these behaviors persist and eventuate in adverse social consequences.

On the part of patients, the failure to recall mania or hypomania is not solely attributable to cognitive problems associated with the illness, or to the phenomenon of looking backwards through the prism of the existing depression; it also appears to be a matter of selective denial. In administering the SADS-L to a sample of patients who had previously been hospitalized for mania, Tsuang (13), found that 40 percent denied having had a manic episode. Gershon et al. (14), at the NIH Clinical Center, found patients' recognition of past hypomania to be virtually non-existent, while family members or significant others were much more likely to have noted the symptomatic behaviors. Given the often severe consequences of undiagnosed bipolar illness, these findings underscore the importance of obtaining confirmatory evidence regarding prior course of illness.

Recognition of the more subtle forms of bipolar illness is facilitated by the subclassification system described by Angst (15), that subdivides bipolar illness into categories that weight the predominance of symptomatology. He subdivided bipolar patients into three categories according to their pattern of recurrence: MD, Md, and Dm.

The first, MD, represents the core illness, with both major manic and major depressive episodes requiring hospitalization; Md patients have full manic episodes, but less severe depressive episodes; i.e., not requiring hospitalization; Dm patients have been hospitalized for depression, but their manic episodes are not severe enough for hospitalization--i.e., they have histories of hypomania. Using this system, Angst determined that of his total population of bipolars (male and female), nearly half were what, in the U.S., are termed bipolar-II. His conclusion is consistent with several other studies, including Egeland's very careful study of the Old Order Amish (16), and sharply contradicts epidemiologic studies which suggest that bipolar-II disorder is only about one-half as prevalent as the bipolar-I pattern.

Although Angst did not find a male-female difference in overall rates of bipolar illness comparable to that seen in unipolar depression, (i.e., a higher frequency among women, especially among older patient cohorts) he did find that the more depressive forms of bipolar illness were more frequent among females while manic forms are more common among males (Table 2). He found, moreover, that the MD patients had the most episodes, and Dm patients the least. On the other hand, among the cohort studied in the NIMH collaborative study, the Dm (bipolar-II) patients had the most prior episodes, although the rate did not differ significantly from that of bipolar-I patients (17).

"Pseudo-Unipolar" Illness

Of special importance to clinicians are those unipolar patients whose illness may be closely related to bipolar disorder; that is, they have a bipolar family history, a "bipolar like" depressive presentation marked by excessive sleep and psychomotor retardation, an early age of onset, and a high episode frequency. What is most relevant clinically is that these "pseudo-unipolar" patients may resemble bipolar patients in their pharmacological responses; that is, they respond to prophylactic

TABLE 2
Patterns of Episodes: Frequency of Syndrome Patterns in Bipolar Disorder by Sex (95 Patients, 1,176 Episodes)

Pattern of Syndromes[a]	Males		Females		Males	Females
	N	%	N	%	%	%
D	80	18.3	194	26.3		
d	75	17.2	246	33.7	35.5	60.0
M	127	29.1	75	10.1		
m	27	6.2	26	3.5	35.3	13.6
DM	5	1.1	15	2.0		
Dm	23	5.3	66	8.9		
dM	7	1.6	4	0.5	15.3	16.6
dm	32	7.3	39	5.2		
MD	2	0.5	11	1.5		
Md	19	4.3	18	2.4		
mD	3	0.7	11	1.5	12.6	9.2
md	31	7.1	28	3.8		
Q	6	1.4	6	0.8		

The episodes, whether D, M, DM, or MD, are preceded and followed by well intervals. The percentages reflect the proportion of episodes across all patients, not the proportion of patients in which a particular pattern predominates

D = Severe depression (requiring hospitalization)
d = Mild depression (not requiring hospitalization)
M = Mania (requiring hospitalization)
m = Hypomania (not requiring hospitalization)
Q = Questionable, unknown

[a] Pattern reflects the sequence of episodes in the natural course

Adapted from Angst, 1978

lithium and tend to get hypomanic when treated with antidepressants. Because of the potential for bipolar type pharmacologic responses, it is critical that the clinician identify these patients prior to treatment decisions.

Cycle Length: The Language of Recurrence

Whether a focus on longitudinal aspects of major depressive disorders is viewed through the lens of research or clinical practice, specific terminology is necessary to describe the phenomenon of recurrence. A key descriptor of recurrence is "cycle length," the period of time extending from the beginning of one episode of illness to the beginning of the next. Unlike the ends of episodes, which often are confused by treatment effects, episode onset tends to be more clearly demarcated.

Grof and colleagues (18) have noted that episode duration has less intra-individual than inter-individual variability. The tendency of episode duration to be relatively constant within a given individual underscores the importance of knowing cycle length. If cycle length is known, one can roughly approximate the "free interval," or period of time between episodes. This measure is important, given its relevance to decisions about prophylactic treatment, for example, or in determining the advisability of a "drug holiday" in such instances as that of a patient who plans to become pregnant.

Turning again to studies of bipolar patients, aggregate data from large samples reveal an orderly pattern of initial recurrence as the illness unfolds, inter-individual variability notwithstanding. Studies from the pre-prophylactic lithium era as well as more recent ones (Figure 1), collectively reporting on some 1,200 bipolar patients followed for an average of 19 years, indicate that over the course of the first four to five episodes, average cycle length successively decreases with time, eventually reaching an apparent limit point which averages about one year, albeit with enormous inter-individual variability. As discussed in detail below, this pattern is consistent with the notion that at least some bipolar patients are poorly buffered from environmental influences and, thus, perhaps vulnerable to the imposition, by light and/or temperature, of a seasonal rhythm on the timing of episode recurrence.

Mechanisms of Cyclicity

The remainder of this chapter will consider three approaches to framing questions about the biology of recurrence. Each approach offers significant clinical insights. A first involves examining the effects of drugs (and thyroid) on cycle length. A second looks at sensitization kindling. A third looks at biological rhythms, especially seasonal rhythms.

Effects of Drugs on Cycle Length

The presence of distinct and, in many respects, opposite states in manic-depressive illness poses interesting questions regarding the mechanisms of action of drugs. Medications currently used in treatment produce six discrete clinical responses: an increase or decrease in depression; an increase or decrease in mania; and an increase or decrease in the frequency of episodes. While this discussion will focus on the two latter categories of effect, it is noteworthy that insofar as

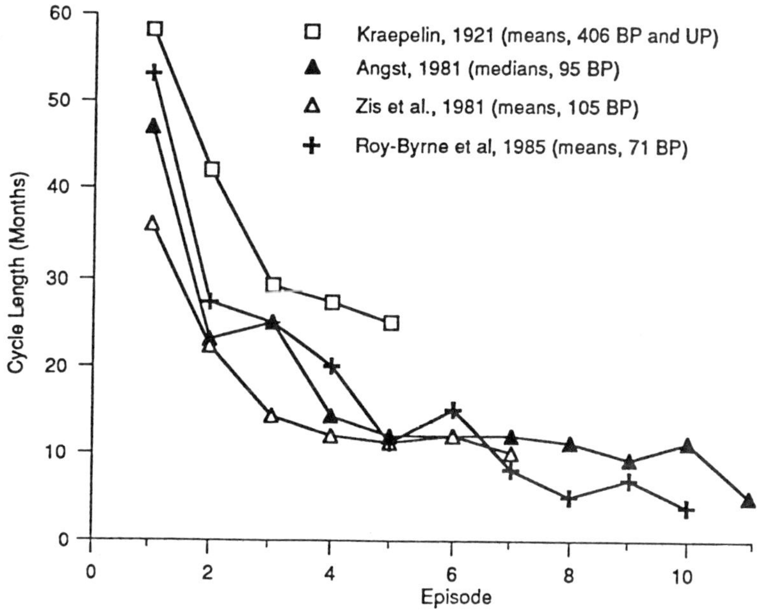

FIGURE 1. Relationship Between Cycle Length and Episode Number

this entire range of outcomes affords opportunities to observe a rich array of behavioral and pharmacologic correlations, it has served to amplify applications of the pharmacological bridge and continues to be a key factor in the maturation of modern neurobiology.

Increasing Cycle Frequency

The original psychopharmacological observation in the affective disorders, which formed the basis for the catecholamine hypothesis, was Crane's (19) 1956 observation of the effects of MAO inhibitors on depression on a 26-year old man being treated for tuberculosis. In his original report, Crane did not report simply an antidepressant effect; rather, he reported cycling. Thus, the first report of an antidepressant effect of a drug was actually a report of drug-induced cycling. In the years since, considerable evidence has accrued that antidepressants can and do increase cycle frequency in at least some patients.

An interesting approach to the question of drug-induced cycling was taken by Angst (20), who overlaid the carefully recorded switch rates of patients in his clinic over a six-decade span on a chronology of developments in clinical psychiatry. The base line switch rate during the two decades in which no treatments were available for depression was around 2 percent. With the introduction of ECT in the 1940s, the switch rate increased sharply. During the 1950s, when neuroleptics were used to treat diverse psychiatric disorders, including major depression, the switch rate declined to baseline levels. With introduction of the tricyclics in the 1960s, switch rates again increased dramatically, some four-fold over the spontaneous switch rate.

Few investigators have access to the extensive historical records or stable patient populations available to Angst. Lacking that, much contemporary research concerned with the effects of antidepressant medications on cycle length focuses on patients with rapid cycling manic-depressive illness who are estimated to account for some 15 percent of all bipolar patients (21). While demonstrating that a patient with a normal two-year cycle had converted to a one-year cycle might require 5 or 6 years of follow-up, a rapidly cycling patient averaging 4 or more episodes of illness annually would provide the necessary data in a significantly compressed period of time. Although there are important unresolved questions regarding the comparability of rapid cycling patients to those with the more common 12 to 24 month cycle lengths, it is noteworthy that family histories do not suggest the existence of a genetic subgrouping of rapid cyclers clearly differentiated from non-rapid cyclers. Moreover, some 80 percent of rapid-cycling patients had normal cycle patterns early in the course of illness and only gradually converted to rapid cycling. The presence of the typical pattern part of the time argues against rapid cycling as a separate illness.

In a systematic longitudinal study (although not controlled in the formal sense) Kukopulos et al. (22) found that while lithium typically was no more effective than placebo in rapid-cyclers, it was very effective in a group of rapid-cycling patients who never had been treated with antidepressants. The finding suggests that in people who have a propensity or vulnerability to rapid cycling, treatment with antidepressant drugs may induce cycling and, in some way, induce lithium resistance. This important study, which has never been refuted, cries out for replication.

Consistent with this report is their systematic observation of 434 bipolar patients in a clinical setting in which they noted significant differences in lithium prophylaxis as a function of episode sequence (23). The classical MDI course (normal interval, mania, depression, normal interval) was associated with the most favorable prophylactic response; the DMI (depression, mania, interval) course had significantly more patients with only partial responses; patients with the CC (continuous circular) course and short cycles (analogous to rapid cycling) showed essentially no response to lithium, while continuous cycles with long cycle lengths responded reasonably well. The best lithium responders in this study were bipolar-II patients with the classical MDI course; all of them showed at least a partial response. Although these observations are contaminated by the various supplemental antidepressants frequently administered (intermittently or continuously) along with lithium, they are nevertheless of interest since they reflect the realities of clinical practice. The relatively poor results of DMI-course patients may reflect the impact of tricyclics given to treat depression; that is, the mania following a depression may be drug-induced and such manias, according to Kukopulos, are relatively resistant to lithium treatment.

Wehr and Goodwin (24) observed bipolar inpatients at the NIMH who, although not rapid cyclers, averaged 2 to 2-1/2 episodes per year, more than double the average rate; they showed that reversible rapid cycling between mania and depression could be induced by tricyclic and MAOI antidepressants in certain patients. Wehr et al. (25) prospectively followed 51 rapid-cycling bipolar patients and observed a consistent shortening of cycle length associated with tricyclics and a consistent lengthening of cycle length when patients were off the medications; the cycling appeared to depend on the continuing administration of antidepressants in approximately half of the patients. When the investigators discontinued antidepressants and administered lithium, they obtained essentially complete remissions in 37 percent of the patients who previously had been considered refractory to treatment.

Rapid cycling has been propsed to be an extreme development of tendencies which are inherent in bipolar patients and perhaps in some unipolars as well (25). One of those natural tendencies is the increasing frequency of episodes.

Persuasive evidence that tricyclic cycle induction may not be confined to those with more frequent episodes is offered by Quitkin et al. (26), who conducted a 3-year double-blind prospective study of bipolar-I patients comparing lithium alone with lithium plus imipramine. The investigators were meticulous in balancing the two groups (e.g., in handling differential dropout rates, etc.). As shown in Table 3, results revealed the combined treatment group to have had 50 percent more total relapses than the lithium alone group; a two-and-one-half fold increase in manic relapses in bipolar patients in spite of being protected by highly competent lithium monitoring. On the other hand, the added tricyclic gave no advantage with respect to reduction in depressive relapses which were low on either drug.

In the case of unipolar patients, antidepressants obviously work; i.e., they accelerate recovery. A less certain issue--whether they also bring the next depression sooner in certain patients--has never been formally addressed in a controlled study. However, a major review of controlled prophylactic studies of bipolar and recurrent unipolar patients (27) raises an interesting question. As can be seen in Table 4, on lithium alone, the one-year relapse rates for patients of either

TABLE 3
Depressive and Manic Depressive Relapses in Bipolar Patients on Maintenance Medication: A Three-Year Prospective Study

	Lithium (N = 38)		Lithium + Imipramine (N = 37)		All Patients (N = 75)
Outcome	%	Months[a]	%	Months	%
Total Relapses (N = 20)	21		32		27
Depressive Relapses (N = 7)	10	11	8	3	9
Manic Relapses (N = 13)	10	7	24	10	17

65% of all relapses occurred within first 4 months (5 of 7 depressive, 8 of 13 manic)

[a]Months are average time to relapse

Data from Quitkin et al., 1981a

polarity decreased dramatically, with nearly identical rates for the bipolar and unipolar groups. Bipolar patients who were administered tricyclic maintenance medication had a relapse rate as high as those patients receiving placebo; the striking difference was the direction of relapse, with bipolar patients on placebo relapsing primarily to depressive episodes, while those on tricyclics relapsed to manic episodes. The one-year relapse rate among the recurrent unipolar patients treated with tricyclics was 50 percent higher than among those treated with lithium (35 percent vs 22 percent), a pattern that would be consistent with the possibility that some recurrent unipolar patients experienced more frequent episodes of illness while on tricyclics. Such a possibility requires further evaluation.

The important point about this review is that both the bipolar and unipolar groups selected for these prophylactic trials had similar average cycle lengths; that is, the unipolars as well as the bipolars had episode frequencies in the range of every year or two. Unfortunately, the major U.S. studies of prophylaxis among unipolar patients have not focused on those unipolars with a natural rate of recurrence in the typically bipolar range. The heterogeneity of the unipolar samples in the U.S. studies, as well as their tendency to confound adequate treatment of the episode (continuation treatment) with prophylaxis, may have led to misleading conclusions about the relative efficacy of lithium and the tricyclics in unipolar illness.

The studies reviewed by Schou (27) pose questions that could be addressed under the model proposed in Figure 2, which suggests that an antidepressant drug may work by accelerating the natural course of the

TABLE 4
Prevention of Manic-Depressive Illness with Lithium and with Tricyclic Antidepressants: Summary of the Controlled Trials

Diagnostic Group	Medication	Patients[a] N	Relapsing Within a Year[b] %
	Lithium vs Placebo		
Bipolar	Lithium	186	20
	Placebo	187	73
Unipolar	Lithium	76	22
	Placebo	77	65
	Antidepressants vs Placebo		
Bipolar	Antidepressants[c]	26	65
	Placebo	10	68
Unipolar	Antidepressants[d]	187	35
	Placebo	187	67

[a]Excludes patients who withdrew from trial for reason other than relapse
[b]Includes patients who withdrew from trial because of relapse
[c]10 patients received imipramine; 1 received maprotiline
[d]72 patients received imipramine; 107 received amitriptyline; 8 received maprotiline

Update of Schou, 1979b

illness. Both depressive and manic episodes tend naturally to evolve towards remission, either into a euthymic phase or into an episode of opposite polarity. An antidepressant which reverses a depressive episode has, in effect, accelerated the natural tendency of the episode towards remission. By the same token, it may accelerate the next sequence in the natural course; i.e., the onset of a manic episode. Drug-induced acceleration of a manic episode may result in the mania coinciding with the natural course of a depressive episode, resulting in a mixed-state, a not infrequent outcome of tricyclics in bipolar patients. The top portion of the illustration illustrates how the ability of antidepressants to accelerate bipolar disorder can also translate into a paradoxical (albeit controversial) observation--the antimanic effect of imipramine, as reported many years ago by Akimoto (28).

Decreasing Cycle Frequency

Questions regarding the capacity of various agents to decrease cycle frequency appear to be less controversial; at the same time, they suggest with greater clarity an important future line of neurobiological research.

Lithium, the original and primary means of treating cycling disorders, and the more recently developed anticonvulsant therapies clearly illustrate an increasing sophistication in theory concerning the mechanisms of action of drugs. The issue of lithium's acute antidepressant effects is the subject of an extensive and--given frequent misunderstanding of the time frame over which it must be measured--controversial literature. Although not addressed here in detail, the issue cannot be ignored when constructing theory. Indeed, the most interesting new theory about the mechanism of action of lithium presupposes a therapeutic effect in both manic and depressive states. Thus, Berridge (29) has demonstrated that lithium acts bi-directionally beyond the synapse and post-synaptic receptor, at the second messenger system, in effect bringing down hyperexcitable systems while enhancing a hypoexcitable system. This might provide the basis for understanding the paradox of a drug with both antidepressant and antimanic effects as well as stabilizing properties.

An analogous explanation has been proposed to explain carbamazepine's biphasic actions. It is reported that chronic treatment with

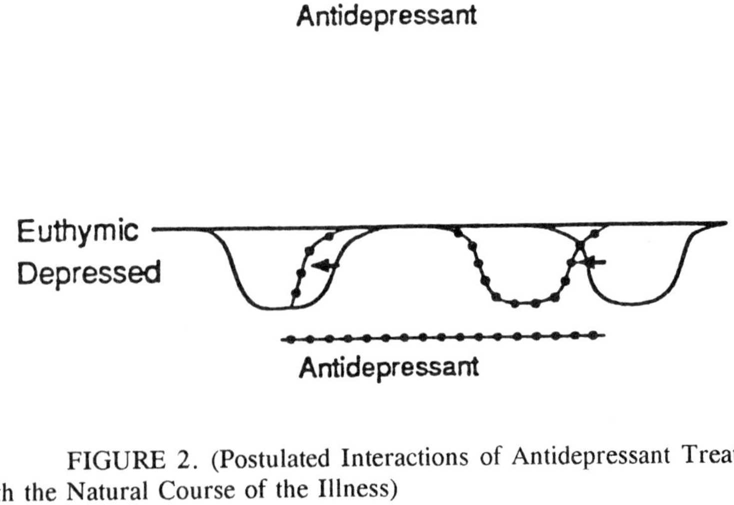

FIGURE 2. (Postulated Interactions of Antidepressant Treatment With the Natural Course of the Illness)

a wide variety of antidepressant drugs and ECT is similar to treatment with GABA-mimetic agents in their capacity to up-regulate GABA receptors (30) while down-regulating beta-adrenergic receptors. Thus, the apparent pharmacological enhancement of GABA transmission has been associated with both antimanic and antidepressant effects; this would be consistent with some mood-behavior modulating role for GABA systems and may relate to the kindling-sensitization model discussed below.

Preliminary evidence that a selective inhibitor of the "A" form of monoamine oxidase (MAO-A) may indeed be stabilizing rather than cycle-inducing raises interesting questions about differences in the neurotransmitter effects of selective MAO-A inhibitors compared to the mixed AB inhibitors that characterize all of the MAOIs currently marketed in this country. It also has been reported that among the second generation of antidepressants, serontonergic agents--e.g., fluoxetine, a serotonin-reuptake inhibitor--may be less likely to precipitate mania than traditional tricyclics. No such reactions have been reported in the controlled trials (31) although scattered case reports of mania in outpatients with moderately severe depressions who are taking fluoxetine have appeared. Whether this risk is, indeed, lower than that associated with other antidepressants remains to be seen.

Thyroid treatment of cyclic disorders is a very new field with incomplete but interesting data. Thyroid abnormalities have been associated with periodic psychotic states for many years (32) and found able to be suppressed through large doses of exogenous thyroid hormone (33). Although Cowdry et al. (34), studying patients being administered lithium (which has a subtle anti-thyroid effect that may unmask subtle thyroid pathology), found overt hypothyroidism in half of the rapid cycling patients and elevated TSH (a measure of subclinical hypothyroidism) in 93 percent of these patients, side effects and medical management complications discouraged systematic pursuit of thyroid treatment in manic-depressive illness. Recently, however, a related and more clinically feasible approach has been studied by Bauer and Whybrow (35). They found that supplemental thyroxine, in doses sufficient to produce "supranormal" T_4 levels, successfully converted 10 of 11 lithium-resistant patients with rapid cycles into lithium responders; of the four patients taken off thyroxine under double-blind conditions, three quickly relapsed. This finding is consistent with that of Hatterer (36) who has shown that low normal T-4 levels are strongly associated with relapse. It is important to note that all of the thyroid values were in the normal range, indicating that simply determining that a patient is in the normal range (which is very broad) tells one very little about subtle thyroid-mood interactions.

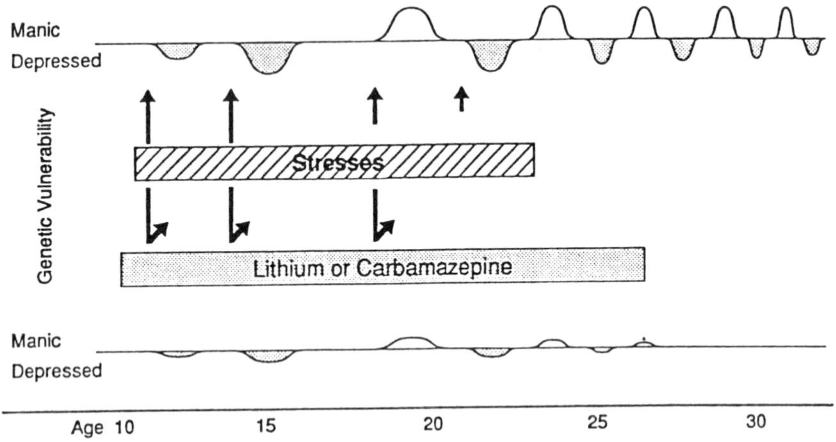

FIGURE 3. Schematic illustration of the postulated effect of early treatment on the subsequent course of bipolar disorder

Behavioral Kindling and Sensitization

Contemporary interest in the biology of recurrence of the major depressive disorders also is being driven by accumulating information regarding kindling and sensitization. Kraepelin (1) observed--and we and others have confirmed (Figure 3)--that the initial episodes of the more recurrent, "endogenous" cyclic illnesses often appear to be precipitated by environmental stress; typically these precipitants involve the stresses associated with late adolescent developmental issues. Once the first few episodes have been activated, later ones increasingly become more endogenous, occurring in the absence of environmental input. Recent research suggests that this pattern of activation may reflect a particular neurobiological process.

"Electrophysiological kindling" refers to increased behavioral and electrophysiological responsivity, either to repeated low-level electrical stimulation of the brain or to agents such as lidocaine or cocaine (in high doses) exerting local anesthetic effect. In animal studies examining kindling of the amygdala, for example, repeated once-daily stimulation for one second initially produces no observable behavioral or electrophysiological effects. However, upon repetition, after-discharges increase in frequency, duration, and complexity of waveform; eventually the animal develops a full-blown motor seizure in response to a stimulus that was previously below the threshold.

If the stimulation is repeated frequently enough, the animal will eventually develop a spontaneous seizure disorder, in which seizures occur without any exogenous stimulation, presumably because of enduring changes in brain chemistry associated with protein phosphorylation. Post et al. (37), drew an analogy between the process of central nervous system kindling and the unfolding of rapidly cycling affective illness, in which initial activation gives way, over time, to increasingly "endogenous" recurrences of the illness. Having first demonstrated that kindling in animals is blocked by carbamazepine, an anticonvulsant drug, they subsequently showed the medication to be particularly effective in reducing cycle frequency in lithium-resistant, rapidly cycling bipolar patients.

In their reviews of the carbamazepine literature, Post and Uhde (38) and Stromgren and Boller (39) (Table 5) noted that among some 300 patients (most lithium refractory), the response rate was about 65 percent (combining open and double-blind studies). Prior to the introduction of this treatment, patients were likely to have spent as much as two-thirds of their lives in either a depressed or manic state. Carbamazepine responders, by way of contrast, are, on average, symptom free approximately 85 percent of the time.

Recently, other anticonvulsants have been examined as potential prophylactic agents in manic-depressive illness. To date, the prophylactic effect of valproate has been evaluated in more than 200 bipolar patients, half of whom have been judged as responders. Studies conducted in Munich (40), moreover, suggest that carbamazepine-resistant patients may be responsive to valproic acid. The situation may be akin to that which is common in using antidepressants; i.e., different groups of patients may respond to different anticonvulsants depending, perhaps, on the nature, location, or type of seizure.

"Sensitization" describes a kindling-like phenomenon which can be produced through the use of psychomotor stimulants. Animal and clinical studies have shown that repeated, intermittent use of a drug such as cocaine--at dosages that initially had little or no effect--results in progressively more pronounced behavioral responses. Since the environmental context in which the animal originally received the drug appears to be important to its later increases in responsivity (that is, in time, the response can be elicited simply by placing the subject in the setting where the drug previously had been administered) a conditioning component may be involved. For the clinician, the phenomenon of sensitization is especially important because cocaine is among the drugs most frequently abused by affectively ill patients whose vulnerability to kindling phenomena may already be heightened. Behavioral sensitization appears to involve a dopamine substrate but can also be modified by

TABLE 5. Carbamazepine Prophylaxis in Manic-Depressive Illness

Study	Patients N	Diagnosis	Design	mg / day CBZ (blood level)	Other Drugs	Duration	Results
Controlled Studies							
Ballenger & Post, 1978b	10 CBZ	6 BP 2 UP 2 SA	CBZ vs PBO double-blind controlled on - off	200-1600	Acute treatments added when necessary in 3 patients	Varied	7/10 Improved
Okuma et al., 1981	12 CBZ 10 PBO	MDI	CBZ vs PBO double-blind	400-600 .(5.6 ± 2.0μg/ml)	Acute treatments added during episode breakthroughs	12 mos	6/10 Improved on CBZ
Placidi et al., 1986	29 CBZ 27 LI	20 CAD 9 ADSF 19 CAD 8 ADSF	CBZ vs LI random assignment	400 CBZ 300 LI (7-12 mg/L CBZ) (0.6-1.0 mEq/L LI)	Acute treatments added during episode breakthroughs	2-36 mos	At least 2/3 from each group were very much to moderately improved within 3 mo. Diagnostic groups not separated
Watkins et al., 1987	19 CBZ 18 LI	20 BP 17 UP	CBZ vs LI double-blind random assignment	5-12 mg/L CBZ 0.4-0.9 mEq/L LI	Acute treatments added for episode breakthroughs (63% of CBZ patients, 61% of LI patients)	16 mos (CBZ) 20 mos (LI)	Approximately 75% significantly improved on each; but LI associated with a significantly longer remission (16 mo vs 9.4 mo; $p < 0.001$)
Lusznat et al., 1988	20 CBZ 20 LI	Mania or hypomania	12 month follow-up after double blind random assignment	200 CBZ 400 LI (0.6-1.2 mg/ml CBZ) (0.6-1.4 mmol/ml LI)	Acute treatements (antidepressants or neuroleptics) added for episode breakthroughs		9/20 CBZ patients vs 5/20 LI patients were "satisfactory responders"

Summary of open and controlled studies

- •Most were LI resistant prior to CBZ administration
- •CBZ appears effective in both rapid cyclers and nonrapid cyclers
- •Some patients have a better reponse to the combination of CBZ and LI than either drug alone

Overall improvement rate: 271/417 (65%)

CBZ = carbamazepine, PBO = placebo, LI = lithium, CAD = "classic" affective disorder, ADSF = affective disorder with schizophrenic features, SA = schizoaffective

Post and Uhde, 1988, Strömgren and Boller, 1985, and Prien and Gelenberg, 1989, revised and updated neuropeptides, including sex hormones, enkephalins, and vasopressin.

The clinical relevance of the kindling and sensitization models to early intervention and prevention of fundamentally recurrent disorders such as major depression and mania seems to have been anticipated by Benjamin Rush, who nearly two centuries ago observed that,

> "In all forms and combinations of madness that have been described, the duration of the disease, after it is completely formed, seems to be as much fixed by nature as the duration of any autumnal fever. It may be weakened, and life may be preserved during its continuance, but, unless it be overcome in its first stage, it generally runs its course, in spite of all the power of medicine." (41)

If, as Kraepelin proposed, stress activates the illness early on, pharmacologically blocking or attenuating the effects of that stress may effectively prevent the onset of the chronic disease.

While the possibility is intriguing, testing such a primary prevention strategy puts considerable premium on the development of genetic markers for the major depressive disorders. With such markers, it will be possible to prevent potentially damaging stresses early in the vulnerable individual's life.

Biological Rhythms

A third approach to exploring the biology of recurrence involves the study of biological rhythms. The principal rhythms of the body, "diurnal" or "circadian" rhythms, are controlled by a biological clock that regulates human systems in relation to the 24-hour day. On the other hand, longer term rhythms are called "infradian." Indeed, one might posit that manic-depressive illness is an expression of an infradian rhythm. Halberg (42) and Kripke (43) have hypothesized that dysynchrony among circadian rhythms can generate occasional infradian rhythms by a so-called "beat phenomenon" generated by two or more peaks coinciding as different rhythms oscillate out of synchrony with one another; that is, as rhythms go in and out of phase with each other. To that point, considerable evidence points to disturbances of circadian rhythms in patients with manic-depressive illness. Thus, interest in the illness as an infradian rhythm requires attention to circadian abnormalities.

The principal infradian rhythm observed in nature is seasonal, and the classical literature, reviewed by Wehr and Rosenthal (44), refers often to the seasonality of major depressive illness. Annual rhythms, moreover, may represent a special case of the imposition of an environmental influence on the illness, providing a seasonal timing of episodes.

Circadian Rhythms

The body appears to be maintained by two primary oscillators: a "strong" oscillator which is generally believed to control such functions as temperature, REM sleep propensity, cortisol secretion (and probably other biochemical rhythms), and cognitive and psychomotor performance, and a secondary "weak" oscillator which, under normal conditions, controls the activity-rest, sleep-wakefulness cycle and a variety of sleep-related neuroendocrine activity. The strong oscillator, which is almost impervious to environmental influence, in effect drives the weak oscillator.

Wehr and Goodwin (45) reviewed all studies in which the circadian pattern of a biological or physiological variable in depressed patients was considered. They concluded that in the majority of studies, compared with control subjects, the strong oscillator's phase position among the depressed patients was variably advanced, generally occurring 1 to 4 hours earlier. A major indicator of the strong oscillator is core body temperature: normally, temperature falls through the evening and night, reaching a low point in the last third of the night, and then begins to rise as dawn and wakefulness approach. In many patients with major depression, particularly those with "endogenomorphic symptoms," the temperature reaches its low point about three to four hours earlier; as a result, these patients appear to "start their day" in the middle of the night.

The putative phase advance of the strong oscillator can be manipulated by modification of the sleep cycle such as partial sleep deprivation. In partial sleep deprivation, the patient may be awakened in the middle of the night and required to remain awake through that entire day; in effect, such a procedure serves to temporarily re-establish the normal relationship between the sleep-wakefulness cycle and the strong oscillator. An extension of this approach entails advancing the entire sleep period. Going to sleep earlier than normal and waking up early offers a way of restoring a normal relationship between sleep and the oscillator without the disadvantages of actual loss of sleep.

A review of the world's literature on sleep deprivation studies involving nearly 1,500 patients reveals an overall improvement rate of about 60 percent (Table 6). This rate--which remains constant regardless of whether sleep deprivation is partial or total--is roughly that found with tricyclics in controlled studies. In a direct comparison of sleep deprivation during the first half versus the second half of the night, Wehr et al. (46) have shown that the antidepressant effect is confined to the latter, suggesting that the therapeutic effect depends on being awake in the second half of the night, rather than on the loss of sleep *per se*.

Although the effect of sleep deprivation is rapid and dramatic, it is generally not sustained beyond the first or second day. In phase advance, where the patient can continue the schedule because sleep is adequate, remissions may persist for 10 to 14 days before the clock apparently adjusts (46, 47).

In bipolar patients, however, sleep deprivation is not always benign; like other antidepressant treatments, it can precipitate hypomania or mania. Wehr et al. (48) deprived a group of depressed, rapid cycling, manic-depressive patients a full night of sleep, and observed that about half went into manias (several requiring treatment) that persisted for days or weeks; in some cases, patients switched back into depression after recovery sleep.

TABLE 6
Antidepressant Effects of Sleep Deprivation

Technique	Studies N	Patients N	Response[a] %
Total SD	60	1,181	57[b]
Partial SD	10	182	64
Selective REM Deprivation	3	57	56
Totals	73	1,420	59

SD = sleep deprivation
[a]Average response rate (weighted)
[b]BP = 74%, UP = 52%

Adapted from Wehr et al., unpublished

Wehr (49) has theorized that the relationship between various stressors and the onset of mania may be operating through a final common pathway of sleep reduction. He cites sleep reductions that occur, for example, as a function of travel, shift work, and medical emergencies, as well as emotional reactions and the use, abuse, or withdrawal from certain drugs. From a clinical perspective, these effects clearly suggest the need to protect the regularity of sleep for bipolar patients, including the judicious use of short-term sedatives/hypnotics.

Annual Rhythms/Seasonality

The association of seasonal rhythms and manic-depressive illness did not go unnoticed by Kraepelin, who wrote, "repeatedly I saw in these cases moodiness set in autumn and pass over in spring, 'when the sap shoots in the trees,' to excitement corresponding in a certain sense to emotional changes which come over even healthy individuals after changes of the seasons," (1, p. 139). Wehr and Rosenthal (44) have suggested several reasons why these original observations have been largely forgotten: a decline in the ancient humoral theories that were tied into the seasonality; a tendency of the internal focus of psychoanalytic theory and biochemical theories to diminish attention to the impact of environmental influences on patients; and insulation from natural seasonal changes by reliance on modern techniques of air conditioning and heating; a cultural shift from a cyclical to a linear perception of time; and the masking of seasonal influences by treatments.

As noted previously (Figure 1), the average cycle lengths drawn from several longitudinal studies tend to approximate multiples of twelve months, initially on a multi-year pattern (i.e., with free-intervals of several years occurring between initial episodes of illness) before settling into an average recurrence pattern that appears to be annual. Analysis of the frequency distribution of individual cycle lengths for the patients studied by Zis, Grof, and Goodwin (50) suggests that this annual signal is due to a subgroup with exclusively annual rhythms.

Current hypotheses linking recurrences of affective disorders, and related phenomena such as suicide, to seasonality have focused on two related but somewhat different explanations: recurrence as a function of extremes in the length of the photoperiod (summer and winter) or extremes in the rate of change in the ratio of light and dark (spring and fall equinoxes). The seasonal extreme hypothesis would account for winter depression and the summer peak for manias and hypomanias.

Criteria for seasonal affective disorders ("winter depressions") described by Rosenthal and colleagues (51) include recurrent fall or winter major depressions for at least two winters with regular remission in the spring. A variable portion of those with regular winter depressions will become hypomanic in the spring or summer; averaging all of the studies together, slightly more than half of the patients with winter depression have hypomania in the spring/summer; that is, they are bipolar II. On the other hand, the rate of change hypothesis could account for the spring and fall peaks for "typical" depression and suicide.

Just as rapidly cycling patients are informative about patterns of recurrence in bipolar illness, seasonal patients have served as an important source of information regarding the nature of recurrent affective disorder generally. While about one-half of patients with seasonal affective disorder report a family history of affective disorder, only about 15 percent report a family history of seasonal affective disorder (52), a pattern that suggests that seasonality, if not seasonal affective disorders, may be genotypically independent.

Studies are now underway designed to obtain precise data from patients' families and to clarify questions regarding the genetic commonalities and differences.

Goodwin and Jamison (53) have hypothesized that, in part, the vulnerability to manic-depressive illness involves increased sensitivity to light. Thus, the normal influence of seasonal variation in light--its influence on mood, sleep and energy--is amplified, producing affective episodes. Another way to express this hypothesis is that given the existence of a normal energy variation associated with the seasons (people tend to be up in the summer and down in winter) it is not unlikely that patients who have a certain form of bipolar illness are more vulnerable to summer light effects. When one considers total seasonal energy output, an energy conservation model would predict mania or hypomania in the summer followed by a compensatory depression in the winter.

Early research addressing the question of light sensitivity arguably has yielded one of the few state independent markers for bipolar illness. Lewy et al. (54, 55) have shown that, compared to normal controls, manic-depressive patients are supersensitive to light, as reflected by a lower threshold required to reduce nighttime plasma melatonin levels. Nurnberger et al. (56) studying euthymic bipolar patients off medications, also found that the patients had a greater suppression in melatonin with light compared with controls. In the same study, these investigators examined children of manic-depressive parents. These children, at high risk for the illness, have a high rate of melatonin suppression by light: 57% met criteria, compared to the control rate of 15%. The sensitivity, moreover, demonstrated a clear genetic progression; among children with one parent ill, the suppression rate was 33%; with two parents ill, 57%. In patients with affective disorder, the rate was 91% (55).

Questions of seasonality and major depressive disorder may be explained by means of a two-season model or a four-season model. The two season model focuses on winter and summer, specifically the impact of seasonal extremes, as addressed by Wehr. An alternate model directs attention to the rate of change in the photoperiod, in order to explain spring and fall peaks. Different types of depression may be involved in the spring onsets as opposed to the winter onsets. The latter appear to be differentiated by hypersomnia, hyperphagia, anergia, carbohydrate craving, and weight gain--symptoms considered atypical in unipolar depression but common in bipolar patients. On the other hand, the pattern of major depressions with an onset peak in the spring (or early fall) tend to have typical "endogenous" symptoms, including insomnia, anorexia, weight loss, and agitation.

Finally, one might construct an hypothesis that the genetic defect in manic-depressive illness involves the circadian pacemaker and/or systems which modulate it, including light sensitivity. Many symptoms show diurnal variation. Circadian abnormalities can produce long-term rhythmic or periodic disturbances, perhaps including mood cycles. Indeed, most, if not all, of the state dependent biological changes that have been reported in the last 20 years might simply be reflections of disturbed circadian rhythms. Circadian systems serve a major regulatory role in the central nervous system and the reported biological changes in affective illness are perhaps best described as reflecting dysregulation, which is increasingly recognized as a more appropriate concept than a simple excess or deficiency of a particular substance. Also, the major state independent finding in bipolar illness--i.e., sensitivity to light--involves the circadian system. Thus, a genetic defect in regulatory systems resulting in a defective circadian oscillator could lead to a CNS which is poorly buffered from normal environmental (perhaps seasonal) perturbations--that is, changes in the length of the photoperiod or its rate of change. This vulnerability may increase with each successive episode to a point where the illness recurs annually or seasonally.

SUMMARY

Overdue acknowledgement in the U.S. that the affective disorders are fundamentally recurrent has stimulated a new focus on the biology of recurrence. Information obtained through research on the effects of drugs on cycle length, on kindling and sensitization, and on biological rhythms and seasonality, independently and cumulatively have important implications for clinical management of the disorders. In addition to the obvious pharmacological implications, new research suggests the importance of: early, aggressive treatment; a bias towards prophylaxis; enhancement of circadian integrity through regular schedules of sleep, meals, and exercise, and attentiveness to disruptions of this schedule which may be occasioned by jet lag, stress, or event-related insomnia; use of sleep-inducing hypnotic drugs when sleep is likely to be disrupted, particularly in bipolar patients; and avoidance of alcohol and other drugs that disrupt biological rhythms and have the potential of kindling the central nervous system.

REFERENCES

1. Kraepelin E: Manic-Depressive Insanity and Paranoia. Translated by RM Barclay. Edited by GM Robertson. Edinburgh, ENS Livingstone. Reprinted New York, Arno Press, 1976
2. Leonhard K, Berman R (trans), Robins E (ed): Aufteilung der Endogenen Psychosen [The Classification of Endogenous Psychoses], 5th ed. New York, Irvington Publishers, Inc, 1979
3. Angst J: Zur Atiologie und Nosologie endogener depressiver Psychosen. Berlin: Springer, 1966
4. Perris C: A study of bipolar (manic-depressive) and unipolar recurrent depressive psychoses. Acta Psychiatr Scand 42(suppl): 194, 1966
5. American Psychiatric Association. Diagnostic and Statistical Manual of Mental Disorders. 3rd ed. Washington, DC: The Association, 1980
6. American Psychiatric Association. Diagnostic and Statistical Manual of Mental Disorders. 3rd ed.-revised. Washington, DC: The Association, 1987
7. Mandell AJ: From molecular biological simplification to more realistic central nervous system dynamics: An overview. In: R Michels, JO Cavenar Jr, HKH Brodie, AM Cooper, SB Guze, LL Judd, GL Klerman, AJ Solnit, eds: Psychiatry. Vol 3. Chapter 72. London: JB Lippincott, 1985. pp. XXXX
8. Post RM, Jimerson DC, Ballenger JC, Lake CR, Uhde TW, Goodwin FK: Cerebrospinal fluid norepinephrine and its metabolites in manic-depressive illness. In: RM Post, JC Ballenger, eds: Neurobiology of Mood Disorders. Baltimore: Williams & Wilkins, 1984. pp 539-553
9. Keller MB, Klerman GL, Lavori PW, Coryell W, Endicott J, Taylor J: Long-term outcome of episodes of major depression. JAMA 252:788-792, 1984
10. Krauthammer C, Klerman GL: The epidemiology of mania. In Manic Illness. Shopsin B (ed), Raven Press, New York, pp 11-28, 1979
11. Zis AP, Goodwin FK: Major affective disorder as a recurrent illness: A critical review. Arch Gen Psychiatry 36:835-839, 1979
12. Keller MB, Lavori PW, Endicott J, Coryell W, Klerman GK: "Double depression": two-year follow-up. Am J Psychiatry 140:689-694, 1983
13. Tsuang MT, Lyons MJ, Faraone SV: Problems of diagnoses in family studies. J Psychiat Res 21:391-399, 1987
14. Gershon ES, Guroff JJ: Information from relatives: Diagnosis of affective disorders. Arch Gen Psychiatry 41:173-180, 1984
15. Angst J: The course of affective disorders: II. Typology of bipolar manic-depressive illness. Arch Psychiat Nervenkr 226:65-73, 1978

16. Egeland JA, Hostetter AM: Amish Study, I: Affective disorders among the Amish, 1976-1980. Am J Psychiatry 140:56-61, 1983
17. Coryell W, Keller M, Endicott J, Andreasen N, Clayton P, Hirschfeld R: Bipolar-II illness: Course and outcome over a five-year period. Psychol Med 19:129-141, 1989
18. Grof P, Angst J, Karasek M, Keitner G: Patient selection for long-term lithium treatment in clinical practice. Arch Gen Psychiatry 36:894-897, 1979
19. Crane GE: The psychiatric side effects of iproniazid. Am J Psychiatry 112:494-501, 1956
20. Angst J: Switch from depression to mania: A record study over decades between 1920 and 1982. Psychopathology 18:140-154, 1985
21. Dunner DL, Patrick V, Fieve RR: Rapid cycling manic depressive patients. Compr Psychiatry 18:561-566, 1977
22. Kukopulos A, Caliari B, Tundo A, Minnai G, Floris G, Reginaldi D, Tondo L: Rapid cyclers, temperament, and antidepressants. Compr Psychiatry 24:249-258, 1983
23. Kukopulos A, Reginaldi D, Laddomada P, Floris G, Serra G, Tondo L: Course of the manic-depressive cycle and changes caused by treatments. Pharmakopsychiatr Neuropsychopharmakol 13:156-167, 1980
24. Wehr TA, Goodwin FK: Rapid cycling in manic-depressives induced by tricyclic antidepressants. Arch Gen Psychiatry 36:555-559, 1979
25. Wehr TA, Sack DA, Rosenthal NE, Cowdry RW: Rapid cycling affective disorder: Contributing factors and treatment responses in 51 patients. Am J Psychiatry 145:179-184, 1988
26. Quitkin FM, Kane J, Rifkin A, Ramos-Lorenzi JR, Nayak DV: Prophylactic lithium carbonate with and without imipramine for bipolar-I patients: A double-blind study. Arch Gen Psychiatry 38:902-907, 1981
27. Schou M: Lithium as a prophylactic agent in unipolar affective illness: Comparison with cyclic antidepressants. Arch Gen Psychiatry 36:849-851, 1979
28. Akimoto H, Nakakuki M, Honda Y, Takahashi Y, Toyoda J, Sasaki K, Machiyama Y: Clinical evaluation of the effect of central stimulants, MAO inhibitors, and imipramine in the treatment of affective disorders. In: Proceedings of World Congress of Psychiatry, 3rd, 1961. Toronto: University of Toronto Press, 1962-1963. pp 958-963
29. Berridge MJ: Inositol trisphosphate, calcium, lithium, and cell signaling. JAMA 262:1834-1841, 1989
30. Lloyd KG, Zivkovic B, Scatton B, Morselli PL, Bartholini G: The GABAergic hypothesis of depression. Prog Neuropsychopharmacol Biol Psychiatry 13:341-351,1989
31. Benfield P, Heel RC, Lewis SP: Fluoxetine: A review of ite pharmacodynamic and pharmacokinetic properties, and therapeutic efficacy in depressive illness. Drugs 32:481-508, 1986
32. Gjessing RR: Contributions to the Somatology of Periodic Catatonia.

Edited by LR Gjessing, FA Jenner. Oxford: Pergamon Press, 1976
33. Stancer HC, Furlong FW, Godse DD: A longitudinal investigation of lithium as a prophylactic agent for recurrent depressions. Can Med Assoc J 15:29-40, 1970
34. Cowdry RW, Wehr TA, Zis AP, Goodwin FK: Thyroid abnormalities associated with rapid-cycling bipolar illness. Arch Gen Psychiatry 40:414-420, 1983
35. Bauer MS, Whybrow PC: Rapid cycling bipolar affective disorder: Thyroid function and response to adjuvant treatment with high-dose thyroxine. Abstract of paper presented at the 43rd annual meeting of the Society for Biological Psychiatry, May, 1988
36. Hatterer JA, Kocsis JH, Stokes PE: Thyroid function in patients maintained on lithium. Psychiatry Res 26:249-258, 1989
37. Post RM, Rubinow DR, Ballenger JC: Conditioning, sensitization, and kindling: Implications for the course of affective illness. In: RM Post, JC Ballenger, eds: The Neurobiology of Mood Disorders. Williams & Wilkins, 1984. pp 432-466
38. Post RM, Uhde TW: Carbamazepine as a treatment for refractory depressive illness and rapidly cycling manicdepressive illness. In: J Zohar, RH Belmaker, eds: Special Treatments for Resistent Depression. New York: Spectrum Press, 1985. 281-288
39. Stromgren LS, Boller S: Carbamazepine in treatment and prophylaxis of manic-depressive disorder. Psychiatry Dev 4:349-367, 1985
40. Emrich HM, Dose M, Gunther R, Von Zerssen D: The use of valproate and oxcarbamazepine in affective disorders. In: P Pichot, P Berner, R Wolf, K Thau, eds: Psychiatry: The State of the Art. New York: Plenum Press, 1985. pp 455-458
41. Rush B: Medical Inquiries and Observations Upon the Diseases of the Mind. Philadelphia: Kimber and Richardson, 1812
42. Halberg G: Physiologic considerations underlying rhythmometry, with special reference to emotional illness. In: J DeAjuriaguerra, ed: Cycles Biologiques et Psychiatrie. Symposium Bel-Air III. Geneva, Masson et Cie, 1968. pp 73-126
43. Kripke DF, Mullaney DJ, Atkinson M, Wolf S: Circadian rhythm disorders in manic-depressives. Biol Psychiatry 13:335-351, 1978
44. Wehr TA, Rosenthal NE: Seasonality and affective illness. Am J Psychiatry 146:829-839, 1989
45. Wehr TA, Goodwin FK: Biological rhythms and psychiatry. In: S Arieti, HKH Brodie, eds: American Handbook of Psychiatry: Vol. 7, Advance and New Directions. 2nd ed. New York: Basic Books, 1981. pp 46-74
46. Wehr TA, Wirz-Justice A, Duncan W, et al: Phase advance of the circadian sleep-wake cycle as an antidepressant. Science 206:710-713, 1979
47. Sack DA, Nurnberger J, Rosenthal NE, Ashburn E, Wehr TA: The poten-

tiation of antidepressant medications by phase advance of the sleep-wake cycle. Am J Psychiatry 142:606-608, 1985

48. Wehr TA, Goodwin FK, Wirz-Justice A, Breitmeier J, Craig C: 48-hour sleep-wake cycles in manic-depressive illness: Naturalistic observations and sleep-deprivation experiments. Arch Gen Psychiatry 39:559-565, 1982
49. Wehr TA, Sack DA, Rosenthal NE: Sleep reduction as a final common pathway in the genesis of mania. Am J Psychiatry 144:201-204, 1987
50. Zis AP, Grof P, Goodwin FK: The natural course of affective disorders: Implications for lithium prophylaxis. In: TB Cooper, S Gershon, NS Kline, M Schou, eds: Lithium: Controversies and Unresolved Issues. Amsterdam: Exerpta Medica, 1979. pp 381-398
51. Rosenthal NE, Sack DA, Gillin JC, Lewy AJ, Goodwin FK, Davenport Y, Mueller PS, Newsome DA, Wehr TA: Seasonal affective disorder: A description of the syndrome and preliminary findings with light therapy. Arch Gen Psychiatry 41:72-80, 1984
52. Hellekson C: Phenomenology of seasonal affective disorder: an Alaskan perspective. In: NE Rosenthal, MC Blehar, eds: Seasonal Affective Disorders and Phototherapy. New York: The Guilford Press, 1989. pp. 33-45
53. Goodwin FK and Jamison KR: Pathophysiology: critical evaluation, integration, and future directions. In: FK Goodwin and KR Jamison: Manic-Depressive Illness. New York, Oxford University Press (in press, 1990)
54. Lewy AJ, Wehr TA, Goodwin FK, Newsome DA, Rosenthal NE: Manic-depressive patients may be supersensitive to light. Letter. Lancet 1:383-384, 1981
55. Lewy AJ, Nurnberger JI, Wehr TA, Pack D, Becker LE, Powell R-L, Newsome DA: Supersensitivity to light: Possible trait marker for manic-depressive illness. Am J Psychiatry 142:725-727, 1985
56. Nurnberger JI Jr, Berrettini W, Tamarkin L, Hamovit J, Norton J, Gershon ES: Supersensitivity to melatonin suppression by light in young people at high risk for affective disorder: A preliminary report. Neuropsychopharm 1:217-223, 1988

chapter 11

Perspectives In The Study Of Alzheimer's Disease

Martin Roth, M.D., Sc.D., F.R.C.P., F.R.C. Psych. (U.K.)

INTRODUCTION

At the beginning of this century life expectancy at birth in the affluent countries was in the mid-forties. At the present time it is in the seventies and, as mortality rates are declining more rapidly for those over the age of 70 years, the older segment of the population, those over the age of 80 in particular, are growing disproportionately. In consequence, prevalence of chronic diseases that incapacitate aged people and render them dependent on their families and on health and welfare services is increasing at an accelerating rate. It is the degenerative disorders of the brain that constitute the most pressing problem for they destroy the mental faculties and deprive old and young persons alike of their personal identity, reducing them in the end to a vegetative life. Families do their best to cope, but in the advanced stages of Alzheimer's disease (AD) institutional care often becomes unavoidable and pressures on health and social services are straining at the seams.

AD is the most common and the most serious of the group of disorders as it is the sole cause of two-thirds of the dementias that affect about 5-7% of those aged 65 and over and between 15 and 20% of those over 80. Each case presents different challenges for the psychiatrists, family doctors, and social workers for no two cases are quite alike. This paper will be mainly confined to some of the developments in clinical and neurobiological research into AD in recent years. They offer hope that we may in the near future acquire deeper understanding of the condition and possibly learn methods of treatment that will prove effective in alleviating or arresting it in its early stages of development.

THE STRUCTURAL CHANGES

It seems logical to commence with the structural changes. They

Published 1990 by Elsevier Science Publishing Co., Inc.
Psychiatry: Past Reflections–Future Visions
B.T. Taylor and I.J. Taylor, Editors

were the starting points of Alzheimer's discovery but have been demoted by some investigators who regard them as being probably secondary to neurotransmitter deficits or to the changes in brain metabolism which have been described in AD (1).

In 1977, a special committee was appointed by the Medical Research Council of Great Britain to report on the state of knowledge regarding the origins. They posed a number of questions regarding the nature and significance of the structural changes. The first question inquired whether nerve cell loss in Alzheimer's disease exceeded that in aged matched controls. The second question concerned the relationship between neuronal loss on the one hand and plaques and tangles on the other. Were the latter mere epiphenomena; non-specific and unimportant debris that marked the sites of neuronal destruction? The third question inquired: "to what degree is the affliction diffused throughout the brain?" Were the lesions consistently confined to certain cortical areas leaving others intact? Was it possible to identify the functional characteristics of the subsystems affected by lesions?

Recent developments have given clear answers to some of these questions. It has been established that neuronal counts show a significant fallout predominantly in the fronto-temporal cortex when compared with mentally well preserved controls. That outfall occurs has been called into question in recent years by Terry et al. (2) but conceded on the strength of later findings by the same group of workers (3). A recent study found that the loss extends from 23-43% in different critical areas (4). The reduction is confined to the large pyramidal cells with their long axonal paths and large energy expenditure. As there is no corresponding loss of smaller cell groups there must be a true fallout of neurones.

A positive answer has also been given to the second question; there is an inverse and significant correlation between plaque and tangle formation on the one hand and neuronal loss in the homologous part of the opposite cerebral hemisphere on the other. It is noteworthy that the correlations are in the predicted direction: the fewer the number of neurones estimated the larger the plaque and tangle counts (4). Positive correlations would have been devoid of meaning.

The answer that has been given to the third question is that, while plaques and tangles are widely distributed over the cortex, neuronal loss is confined to certain cortical regions: the superior, middle and inferior frontal gyri, the cingulate gyrus and superior and middle temporal gyri. Although neuronal counts are also decreased in parietal and occipital gyri, they do not differ significantly from counts in controls (4).

The findings in the course of a number of PET scan studies using 18-F-deoxyglucose have revealed reduced glucose utilization in the temporal and parietal areas (5,6). These findings are in conflict with post-mortem estimates of cortical cellular density in two respects. Cellular fallout in the parietal region has not been found at significant levels in some studies (4). And sparing of the frontal lobes in PET studies clashes with other evidence that there is neuronal loss in this region. Neurotransmitter deficits in respect of noradrenaline,GABA and somatostatin which are localized to the frontal and temporal cortex (also in cingulate cortex in the case of Noradrenaline) but have not been found in parietal or occipital cortex (7).

The focal abnormalities recorded with the aid of PET scans may result from metabolic disturbance alone. However, the absence of neuronal fallout does not necessarily signify that parietal and occipital lobes are functionally intact. They are the site of tangle and plaque formation, although this is less intense than in fronto-temporal cortex. The significance of PET findings in Alzheimer's would be clarified if the results of scans *in vivo* could be compared with morphological studies post-mortem. This might shed new light on certain paradoxical findings in relation to the neurobiology of Alzheimer's disease (8).

INTERCORRELATIONS BETWEEN IN VIVO AND POST-MORTEM FINDINGS

In a recent study by Mountjoy et al. (9) of the intercorrelations between the scores on measures of dementia recorded during life, measurements of structural features and neurochemical deficits in Alzheimer's disease were systematically investigated in 102 patients and control subjects. Pearson correlations between these variables estimated in nine cortical areas showed a high correlation in all nine areas between dementia score, plaque counts and neurofibrillary tangles: in most areas tangles showed a higher correlation with dementia scores than plaques. Only in the cingulate cortex was there a highly significant correlation with neuronal counts. Measurements of ChAT activities in sixteen areas of cortex were all correlated highly significantly (p 0.001) with dementia score. But this showed no significant association with ChAT activity in the cerebellar cortex. An examination of GABA activity in the same cortical areas revealed only a single barely significant correlation in Brodmann area 9.

A detailed investigation of Brodmann areas 10, 24 and 21 and of hippocampus showed plaque counts and tangle estimates to be significantly correlated with the dementia score in all sites, the correlations being in the predicted direction, namely positive; in other words, the greater the intensity of Alzheimer changes the more severe the dementia. ChAT activity was also significantly correlated with dementia score in each of these areas, but GABA was not. Noradrenaline (NA) was significantly correlated with dementia score only in Brodmann area 24, the level of significance being similar to that for ChAT. In Brodmann area

21 somatostatin and ChAT were equally well correlated with dementia score. But the correlation with dopamine was positive; (the higher the dopamine measurement, the more demented the subject) and therefore difficult to interpret.

The most striking finding was the high correlation between ChAT activity and dementia score in all areas of cerebral cortex investigated. But somatostatin in the temporal lobe and Noradrenaline in the cingulate gyrus proved also to have significant correlations with level of dementia measured by the Blessed-Roth Scale (10).

In summary, a number of the neurochemical deficits found in AD show significant correlations with measures of dementia undertaken during life. And with the conspicuous exception of dopamine, all the correlations are in the predicted direction and therefore interpretable. In the light of these findings the structural and neurochemical changes are likely to be different expressions of a unitary aetiological process underlying the dementia observed during life. The nature of this process is unclear at the present time, but an increasingly coherent picture is appearing from the body of data reviewed in this section and certain other lines of evidence that will be briefly reviewed.

THRESHOLD EFFECTS IN ALZHEIMER'S DISEASE

Theories of causation in Alzheimer's disease have to take account of the presence of threshold effects in relation to the structural changes (10,11,12) and therefore probably in the other neurobiological phenomena correlated with them.

There is no change in the cerebral cortex of patients with Alzheimer's disease that is not found in less marked degree in the brain of well-preserved elderly subjects. But the severity of the changes in the post-mortem brain in terms of intensity of plaque and tangle formation is almost invariably in excess of a certain threshold level in those who develop the disease (10). If a method of containing plaque and tangle formation (the latter in particular) below threshold levels were to be discovered, a means of averting or controlling the development of AD would have become available. As neuronal outfall shows consistent negative correlations with these Alzheimer changes in different cortical regions, there is presumably a threshold level also in respect of neuronal outfall. But this is not for the present definable in quantitative terms. In addition to older observations the threshold hypothesis is supported by other lines of evidence.

a) Sub-threshold levels of Alzheimer pathological change have been found with concomitant sub-threshold amounts of infarction in some patients with indubitable dementia during life (12). The two types of change had probably been summated giving rise to a total amount of cerebral damage which exceeded the threshold limit beyond which progressive mental deterioration is initiated.

b) In the case of "dementia pugilistica" the commencement of dementia may not occur until a number of years have elapsed between the cessation of boxing and the commencement of intellectual and personality deterioration. This suggests a "threshold" effect arising from the aggregation of damage due to trauma with the age-related decline in number of cerebral neurons.

c) A threshold phenomenon similar to that in Alzheimer's disease appears to operate in the evolution of Parkinson's disease. No disability is manifest clinically until there has been an outfall of 80-85% of the neuronal population of the substantia nigra and the dopamine of the striatum has been depleted by 50% or more. During the pre-clinical stage two compensatory mechanisms operate. There is increased turnover and release of dopamine as reflected in the increased concentration of homovanilic acid in relation to dopamine in the striatum. The second compensatory mechanism comprises an increase in the sensitivity of dopaminergic post-synaptic receptors. In the course of some decades this compensation for the cellular loss in the substantia nigra fails. The symptoms of Parkinsonism then make their appearance.

There is for the present no firm evidence of compensation of this character in the case of Alzheimer's disease. The variation in respect of cerebral neurotransmitter in elderly subjects and the extent to which it parallels the variance in Alzheimer structural changes and neuronal counts merits investigation. Advances in imaging techniques may make it possible to visualize tangles of plaques and so provide quantifiable markers of the pre-symptomatic stage of Alzheimer's disease and the extent to which the pathological changes have advanced towards threshold levels.

THE SIGNIFICANCE OF LESIONS IN SUBCORTICAL NUCLEI

Until a few years ago it appeared that lesions discovered in a number of subcortical nuclei in patients with Alzheimer's disease might prove important in its causation. There are very few cholinergic, noradrenergic or serotonergic indigenous neurons in the cerebral cortex. The input of these transmitters is provided by projections from the nucleus basalis of Meynert (and the septal nuclei and nearby structures), the nucleus locus ceruleus, and the raphe nuclei, respectively. An outfall of pyramidal cells from the nucleus of Meynert was originally reported by Pilleri (13) and later by Whitehouse et al. (14). Massive cell loss from the nucleus ceruleus has been established with the aid of total counts of its neuronal population by Bondareff et al. (15) and of neurofibrillary tangles by Curcio and Kemper (16). Loss of cells from these subcortical nuclei and the consequent severance of their cortical projection seemed a possible line of explanation for a range of neurotransmitter deficits for plaque and tangle formation and possibly for cortical neuronal outfall and dementia of AD.

Several lines of evidence are incompatible with such theories. Less than 5% of cortical synapses are mediated by cholinergic and aminergic and serotoninergic transmitters taken together. Interruption of these projections cannot therefore account for extensive plaque and tangle formation or neuronal loss of AD. Interruption of these projections does not generate any Alzheimer changes in the cortex. In Parkinson's disease an even more extensive outfall of cells from the Meynert and locus ceruleus nuclei is found but without plaque and tangle formation in the cortex and often with no evidence of associated dementia. Finally, lesions in subcortical nuclei are neither sufficient nor necessary causes; loss of cells from subcortical nuclei is often absent from cases of late onset or Type I Alzheimer's and is particularly characteristic of cases of early onset (Type II). Yet in the late onset cases of AD the characteristic structural changes of this condition are present in the cerebral cortex. What then are the minimal pathological and neurochemical lesions associated with a disorder that satisfies the diagnostic criteria of Alzheimer's disease?

CLINICAL COMPARISON OF EARLY AND LATE ONSET CASES

There is a dearth of information regarding the clinical features that could serve to differentiate with confidence Type I and Type II forms of Alzheimer's disease. In a recent investigation of 35 early onset and 86 late onset cases, females were predominant in the latter, but sex distribution was equal in the pre-senile subjects. Echolalia was more common in the earlier than late onset cases but increase in muscle tone usually on the left side and abnormal gait were more prevalent in the late onset group. No significant difference in respect of parietal lobe clinical features was found but the findings of Lauter (17) suggest that such deficits tend to become less common and less conspicuous as age of onset increases. Criteria for the clinical differentiation of Type I and Type II cases have been discussed elsewhere (8).

DIFFERENTIATION OF TYPES I AND II ON THE BASIS OF STRUCTURAL CHANGES

Senile plaques are present in cerebral cortex in both Type I and Type II Alzheimer's disease but also in well preserved elderly control subjects (Table 1). However, in the latter subthreshold values are registered for plaques in the majority of cases (8,10). Neurofibrillary tangles are present in the cortex of both Type I and Type II cases, but in elderly controls they are confined to the hippocampus with a few stray cortical tangles in a minority. Hence when the cerebral cortex shows abundant tangle formation in many areas, the finding has an almost indubitable significance. AD will have almost invariably been manifest in the patient during life.

As far as fallout of neurons is concerned, inquiries with image-analysing equipment have shown reductions both in the Type I and Type II syndromes. But only Type II cases have been found to have suffered fallout significantly in excess of controls (4). The reduction in number of neurons predominates in the large pyramidal cells of the temporal, frontal and cingulate tyri. The cells affected by tangle formation in Type I cases may be functionally impaired. But with due reservation for possible limitations in the accuracy of existing techniques of neuron counting, two statements can be made. The first is that outfall of neurons beyond age-specific levels does not constitute one of the essential conditions for the emergence of dementia, for it is not found in one version of Alzheimer's disease. The second is that the neurofibrillary tangle, found both in cortex and subcortical nuclei, emerges as the most specific structural change differentiating brains of normal aged subjects from patients with AD.

CONTINUITIES AND DISCONTINUITIES BETWEEN WELL PRESERVED AGED AND ALZHEIMER'S DISEASE

Data which have been published elsewhere (7,18,8) show that there are continuities between normal cerebral aging and AD in respect of certain variables and discontinuities in respect of others. A significant decline in concentration of noradrenaline in several cortical areas of early onset cases (Type II) has no counterpart in the cerebrum of well preserved aged people; there is no significant difference in this respect between the brains of patients with AD of late onset and controls. The same statement can be made in respect of GABA. The Type II syndrome departs from the neurobiological changes that characterize normal aging in respect of the deficits in levels of noradrenaline and somatostatin. It differs both from the Type I syndrome and normal aging in respect of the marked decline of GABA levels in frontal and temporal cortex. It shares one qualitative difference from normal cerebral aging with the late onset syndrome: the appearance of extensive neurofibrillary tangle formation in the cerebral cortex.

TABLE 1

STRUCTURAL DIFFERENCES BETWEEN WELL PRESERVED AGED SUBJECTS AND PATIENTS WITH ALZHEIMER'S DISEASE OF EARLY ONSET AND LATE ONSET

VARIABLE	WELL PRESERVED AGED	ALZHEIMER'S DISEASE OF LATE ONSET	ALZHEIMER'S DIS. OF EARLY ONSET
Senile plaques in cortex	+ (aub-threshold)	++ (post-threshold)	+++ (post-threshold)
Neurofibrillary tangles in hippocampus	+	++	+++
NF tangles in cerebral cortex	-	++	+++
Outfall of neurones	Age related decline	No significant difference from controls	Significant difference from controls in frontal and temporal lobes

- = Change minimal or absent

\+ = Limited increase in pathological change

++ = Moderate increase in pathological change

+++ = Intense plaque or tangle formation in association neucortical areas

However, there is a measure of continuity in respect of the age related decrease in ChAT activity which already proves to be inversely correlated with plaque counts in the normal aged, a trend which exhibits a progressive increase as the comparison is extended to late onset cases and thence to early onset Alzheimer's disease. There is probably a similar continuity in respect of the transmitter 5HT since receptors have been shown to decrease in number in the cerebral cortex of normal controls. In AD, presynapitc 5HT markers are affected with greater severity in early than in late onset forms.

When these data are considered in conjunction with those displayed in Table 1, which shows the structural differences between brains of well preserved elderly subjects and those with the two forms of AD, the minimal conditions for developing the most benign form of the disorder can be tentatively defined. There is a quantitative increase in plaque formation which moves from sub-threshold to post-threshold levels. The rise in the number of hippocampal tangles can also be interpreted as a quantitative change. In contrast, the intensive proliferation of neurofibrillary tangles (NFT) in the cerebral cortex has the characteristics of a qualitative shift in that the normal cerebral cortex of the elderly contains only an occasional or no NFT. The absence of significant neuronal outfall in the late onset form cannot be due to the prior fallout of tangle bearing cells. Tangle formation is even more intensive in the early onset cases, but cell counts in columns in the same regions of the contralateral cortex show a 25-40% decrease in the larger pyramidal cells of the frontal and temporal cortex.

As the decline in ChAT activity and that in respect of 5HT markers are circumscribed and can be interpreted as an accentuation of normal aging, and since the decline of somatostatin is localized to the temporal lobes, the NF tangle which is also found in abundance in subcortical nuclei emerges as the most qualitatively distinct feature of the "minimal" or late onset form of AD. It dominates the transition from normal cerebral aging to the most benign or Type I form of AD. The structural and neurochemical characteristics of NF may therefore carry important clues regarding the nature of the basic changes underlying the cerebral degeneration and dementia of AD.

STRUCTURAL AND NEUROCHEMICAL THEORIES FOR CAUSATION OF ALZHEIMER'S DISEASE

It will be apparent from the foregoing discussion that neurochemical and structural theories are in rivalry with one another in relation to the causation of AD. It is possible that they will prove to be complementary rather than mutually exclusive. The cholinergic theory has dominated thinking about etiology and possible treatment of this disorder during the past ten years. It is, therefore, necessary to consider whether it could be the primary factor antecedent of structural change. This question is all the more pertinent in the light of the fact that in the late onset form (Type I) a significant outfall of neurones in excess of that in well preserved controls is not in evidence.

THE RELEVANT LINES OF EVIDENCE FOR A NEUROCHEMICAL ETIOLOGY ARE AS FOLLOWS:

(a) The cholinergic deficit is not only the most extensive of the neurochemical lesions in AD. From its correlation with indices of structural change it would appear to be more intimately linked with the process of cerebral degeneration than any of the other neurochemical deficits found in Alzheimer's disease and this receives further support from its correlations with measures of dementia also unmatched by any other transmitter.

(b) However, attempts to boost cholinergic function in the cerebrum by pharmacological means have proved disappointing. The proportion of synapses mediated by cholinergic transmitters does not amount to more than 1% in the human cerebral cortex. The cholinergic hypothesis cannot therefore account for either the extensive distribution of neurofibrillary tangles and plaques or the neuronal fallout over extensive areas of cerebral cortex.

(c) There is no evidence to suggest that interruption of the cholinergic projection gives rise to plaques and/or tangles (19).

(d) The psychological effects of scopolamine and their reversal by physostigmine have been drawn upon in support of the cholinergic hypothesis. The administration of scopolamine gives rise to a recent memory deficit. It bears very little resemblance to the profile of cognitive deficits of AD. Moreover, from an early stage AD entails abnormalities in mental functioning wider than defects of memory and learning.

(e) Heavy outfall of neurons from the cells of origin of the cholinergic projection in the nucleus of Meynert (as also the nucleus locus ceruleus) are common in Parkinson's disease but dementia is found in only a minority of cases.

THE EVIDENCE THAT FAVORS A PRIMARILY STRUCTURAL CAUSATION IN ALZHEIMER'S DISEASE IS AS FOLLOWS:

1) It is the neurofibrillary tangle that, with some exceptions,

exhibits the highest correlations with the indices of neurochemical deficit and with ChAT activity in particular. Tangle formation is the structural alteration most consistently found in the subcortical nuclei. Of all structural changes it is also the intensity of tangle formation which shows the highest correlations with measures of dementia recorded during life (9).

2) Tangle counts are also highly correlated with neuronal counts in a manner that accords with hypotheses about the aetiological role of the tangle; thc lower the counts of neurons, the higher the intensity of tangle formation in homologous regions of contralateral cortex. This also holds for plaques, but the phf that fill the neurites in the plaque periphery are identical with those in NFT. The destruction of neurons is almost certainly the ultimate cause of the downward course followed by Alzheimer's disease. In addition to the association with tangles, neuronal counts prove to have significant correlations with ChAT activity.

3) The neuritic components of plaques are made up of swollen dystrophic terminals although, as the observations of Probst (20) have demonstrated, they contain a mixture of degenerative and regenerative neuritic changes: the latter refers to the apparent sprouting of some axonal processes entering plaques. Neurofibrillary tangles are highly resistant to solvents and the paired helical filaments of which they are constituted develop inside the perikaryon. In the mentally intact aged they are almost entirely confined to the hippocampus. In AD they are diffusely distributed in the cerebral cortex from an early stage in the development of the disease. Tangles are located within neurons often filling them in their entirety until they are released on rupture of the cell membrane into the neuropil as "ghost tangles." They are likely to be closer than plaques to the process of neuronal destruction and outfall.

INQUIRIES INTO THE STRUCTURE AND COMPOSITION OF THE PAIRED HELICAL FILAMENT (PHF)

A great deal of scientific effort has, therefore, been directed towards the characterization of the protein of which PHF are constituted. Wischik, Crowther and their colleagues studied the sub-unit organization of the paired helical filaments (PHF) which constitute the main part of Alzheimer tangle (21,22,23).

Investigation with the aid of visual diffraction and computerized image reconstruction has shown PHF to consist of a double helical stack of transversely oriented subunits giving the overall shape of a ribbon twisted into a left-handed double helix (21,22,23). In structure it resembles filaments which might arise by *de novo* polymerisation--in this case perhaps by assembly of an aberrant protein which accumulates in great abundance in affected neurons. It is the aggregation of this highly insoluble polymer within the perikaryon that gives rise to the tangle with damaging effects upon neuronal function as reflected in the high inverse correlations between tangle estimates and measures of dementia.

Recent investigations have shed fresh light on the molecular composition of the paired helical filament. Wischik et al. (24) used the proteolytic enzyme pronase to remove the outer fuzzy coat of the central core of the paired helical filament (PHF). They were then able to solubilize two peptides from this inner core. This enabled Goedert et al. (25) to isolate a complementary DNA which proved to be the parent molecule of the two PHF core peptides. The sequence of this precursor molecule revealed it to be the human equivalent of Tau protein. The two peptides (9.5kD and 12kD) were found to be derived from the central region of the amino acid sequence of Tau. The remaining parts of the Tau molecule, the C and N terminals, were situated in the fuzzy coat of PHF which had served to conceal the epitope of the central part of Tau molecule in the inner core.

The molecular mass of the subunit of the paired helical filament (PHF) is 120kD. After pronase treatment which removes C and N terminals of the Tau molecule, which probably constitutes the whole of the "fuzzy coat" of PHF, the molecular mass is 100kD (24). It seems probable that one molecule of Tau is bound per subunit of the paired helical filament. As the peptide fragments that remain within the core of the paired helical filament after pronase treatment have a molecular mass of 9.5 and 12kD (26). Tau protein must make up about a quarter of each subunit of the PHF. A substantial proportion of the total cellular pool of Tau protein must therefore be segregated in Alzheimer's disease within nerve cells containing PHF. This protein is concerned with the building and maintenance of the microtubular part of the cytoskeleton. It has been observed that in the presence of tangle formation and also in cells without visible tangles there is deformation and disappearance of microtubules and neurofilaments (27). The immobilization of Tau protein within tangle bearing cells would be expected to cause progressive impedance of axonal transport. This would ultimately cause destruction of the neurons in which they develop. A recent study has shed further light on the steps in the process that leads ultimately to the destruction of neurones by proliferation of tangles (NFT). In the final stage the cell membrane is ruptured and NFTs are shed in the form of degraded extra cellular tangles into the micropil (28).

Discovery of the composition of that part of the paired helical filament (about 70-75% which remain for the present unidentified) might therefore shed further light on the manner in which the destruction of neurons, the central feature of the Alzheimer form of cerebral degeneration, is brought about.

CONCLUSIONS

This paper has been necessarily confined to one line of research into the condition. It is possible that inquiries that have pursued other paths (29,30,31) will arrive sooner at the root causes of this condition than studies that have focused on the neuro-fibrillary tangle. This structure is, however, the only intracellular degenerative change in AD. It is more highly correlated with cognitive deficits and wider measures of dementia during life than any other change, than any other structural or neurochemical change in the cerebrum (32). The paired helical filaments of which tangles are constituted are also to be found in abundance in the neuritic components of the senile plaque the other most prominent feature of the pathology of AD (33,34).

The view that the beta amyloid protein is a major etiological factor in the genesis of AD is called into question by the findings that there is no correlation between the distribution of beta amyloid protein precursor in mRNA and the pathology of AD (36), and that overproduction of beta amyloid protein precursor in RNA is unlikely to be responsible for amyloid beta protein deposition in AD. Further, there is no firm evidence that deposition of amyloid is correlated with cognitive impairment and considerable evidence against any association between them (35).

The neurofibrillary tangle and its main constituent PHF is of central importance in that proliferation of tangles in the cerebral cortex is the most conspicuous change that differentiates Alzheimer's disease from the phenomena of normal cerebral aging. The 25-40% outfall of pyramidal neurons in the frontotemporal and other cortical regions is therefore likely to be due in a large part to the accumulation of tangles and the dystrophic neurities in the corona of plaques which contain PHF identical with those in the tangles and the changes in cerebral metabolism closely associated with these structural components of the degenerative process in AD. Recent investigations have shown that the Tau protein constitutes about 25% of each subunit of the paired helical filament (26) and more recent studies have begun to shed light on the process, mediated by tangles, that culminates the destruction of neurons in Alzheimer's disease (28).

Future inquiries should help to decide between such rival theories of causation or achieve a synthesis that shows them to be complementary. Such an achievement would bring hope of relief nearer for the worst affliction of later life.

REFERENCES

1. Hoyer S, Frolich L, Lauterback M, van den Bosch de Aguilar P: Animal models in dementia research: metabolic changes after intracerebroventricular injections of bromopyruvate, AF64A and Alzheimer brain Homogenates In Modern Trends in Aging Research, Courtois Y, Faucheux B, Forette B, Knook DL, Treton JA: (eds) 541-550 John Libbey & Company Ltd. London, Montrouge, 1986
2. Terry RD, Fitzgerald C, Peck A, Millner J, Farmer P: Cortical cell counts in senile dementia. J. Neuropathol Exp Neurol 36:633, 1977
3. Terry RD, Peck A, DeTersa R, Schecter R, Horoupian DS: Some morphometric aspects of the brain in senile dementia of the Alzheimer type. Ann. Neurol. 10:184-192, 1981
4. Mountjoy CQ, Roth M, Evans NJR, Evans HM: Cortical neuronal counts in normal elderly controls and demented patients. Neurobiol. Aging 4:1-11, 1983
5. Deleon MJ, George AE, Ferris SH, et al: Positron emission tomography assessments of the aging human brain. J. Comput Assist Tomogr. 8:88-94, 1984
6. Chase TN, et al: Regional cortical dysfunction in Alzherimer's disease as determined by positron emission tomography. Ann. Neurol. 15 (Suppl.) S170-S174, 1984
7. Rossor MN, Iversen LL, Reynolds GP, Mountjoy CQ, Roth, M: Neurochemical characteristics of early and late onset types of Alzheimer's disease. Br. Med. J. 288:361-364, 1984
8. Roth M: The association of clinical and neurological findings and its bearing on the classification and etiology of Alzheimer's disease. Br. Med. Bull. 42:42-50, 1986
9. Mountjoy CQ, Rossor MN, Iversen LL, Roth M: Correlation of cortical cholinergic and GABA deficits with quantitative neuropathological findings in senile dementia. Brain 107:507-518, 1984
10. Blessed G, Tomlinson BE, Roth M: The association between quantitative measures of dementia and of senile change in the cerebral grey matter of elderly subjects. Br. J. Psychiatry 114:797-811, 1968
11. Roth M, Tomlinson B, Blessed G: The relationship between quantitative measures of dementia and the degenerative changes in the cerebral grey matter of elderly subjects. (Abridged). Proceedings of the Royal Society of Medicine, 60, 254-258, 1967
12. Roth M: Classification and etiology in mental disorders of old age; some recent developments. In: Recent Developments in Psychogeriatrics, Kay DWK, Walk A (eds) Ashford: Hedley Bros. 1-18, 1971
13. Pilleri G: Kluver-Bucy syndrome in man. A clinicoanatomical contribution to the function of the medial temporal lobe structures. Psychiatrie Neurol. 152:65-103, 1966
14. Whitehouse PJ, Price DL, Struble RG, Clark AW, Coyle JT, DeLong

MR: Alzheimer's disease and senile dementia: loss of neurons in the basal forebrain. Science 215:1237-1239, 1982
15. Bondareff W, Mountjoy CQ, Roth M: Loss of neurons of origin of the adrenergic projection to cerebral cortex (nucleus locus ceruleus) in senile dementia. Neurol. 32:164-168, 1982
16. Curcio CA, Kemper T: Nucleus raphe dorsalis in dementia of the Alzheimer type: neurofibrillary changes and neuronal packing density. J. Neuropath. Exp. Neurol 43:359-368, 1964
17. Lauter H, Meyer JE: Clinical and nosological concepts of senile dementia. In: Senile Dementia: Clinical and Therapeutic Aspects. Muller CH, Ciompi, L. Hubner (eds) Bern, 1968
18. Rossor MN, Iversen LL: Non-cholinergic neurotransmitter abnormalities in Alzheimer's disease. BMB 42 No. 1:70-74, 1986
19. Price DL, Whitehouse PJ, Struble RG, Price DL, Cash LC, Hedreen JC, Kitt CA: Basal forebrain cholinergic neurons and neuritic plaques in primate brain. In: Katzman R (ed) op. cit. 65-77, 1983
20. Probst A: Neuritic changes in Alzheimer's disease and established in neuritic plaques as shown by Golgi impregnation and method. A review. In: Pilleri G, Tagliavini F (eds) Brain Path. vol I, 1984
21. Wischik CM, Crowther RA, Stewart M, Roth M: Subunit structure of paired helical filaments in Alzheimer's disease. J. Cell. Biol. 100: 1905-1912, 1985
22. Crowther RA, Wischik CM, Stewart M: Analysis of the structure of paired helical filaments. Proc EMSA 43:734-737, 1985
23. Wischik CM, Crowther RA: Subunit structure of the Alzheimer tangle. Br. Med. Bull. 42:51-56, 1986
24. Wischik CM, Novak M, Edwards PC, Klug A, Tichelaar, Crowther RA: Structural characterization of the core of the paired helical filament of Alzheimer disease. Proc. Natl. Acad. Sci. 85:4884-4888, 1988a
25. Goedert M, Wischik CM, Crowther RA, Walker JE, Klug A: Cloning and sequencing of the cDNA encoding a core protein of the paired helical filament of Alzheimer Disease: Identification as the microtubule-associated protein tau. Proc. Natl. Acad. Sci9. 85:4051, 1988
26. Wischik CM, Novak M, Thogersen HC, Edwards PC, Runswick MJ, Jales R, Walker JE, Milstein C, Roth M, Klug A: Isolation of a fragment of tau derived from the core of the paired helical filament of Alzheimer disease. Proc. Natl. Acad. Sci. 85:4506-4510, 1988b
27. Gray EG et al.: Neuropath Appl. Neurobiol. 13:91-110, 1987
28. Bondareff W, Wischik CM, Novak M, Amos WB, Klug A, Roth M: Molecular Analysis of Neurofibrillary degeneration in Alzheimer's disease: An Immunohiustochemical Study. In Press, American Journal of Pathology, 1990
29. Beyreuther K, Weidemann A, Salbaum JM, Dyrks T, Multhaup G,

Fischer P, Hilbnich C, Konig G, Beer J, Bunke D, Monning U, Simms G, Martins R, Rumble B, Masters CL: Alzheimer's disease A4 protein and the PAD gene product. In Current Communications in Molecular Biology. The Molecular Biology of Alzheimer's disease. 71-79. Cold Spring Harbor Laboratory, New York, 1988

30. Masters CL, Martins R, Simms G, Rumble B, Fuller S, Hutchinson L, Beer J, Hilbich C, Dyrks T, Fischer P, Weidemann A, Monning U, Multhaup G, Cramer M, Salbaum, JM, Wehr S, Beyreuther K: The molecular basis of cerebral amyloidosis in Alzheimer's disease and the unconventional virus disease. In: Pouplard-Barthelaix, Emile J, Christen Y (eds). Immunology and Alzheimer's disease. Springer, Berlin Heidelberg New York Toky, 1988
31. Mountjoy CQ, Rossor MN, Evans NJR, Reynolds GP, Evans H, Roth M, Iversen LL, Emson P: Biochemical and neuropathological changes in the brain and their correlation to the severity of dementia in Alzheimer's disease In: Biological Psychiatry 1985; Shagass C, et al. (eds.) Elsevier Science Publishing Co. Inc. 1415-1417, 1986
32. Masters CL, Multhaup G, Sims G, Poltgeisser J: Neuronal origin of a cerebral amyloid: neurofibrillary tangles of Alzheimer's disease contain the same protein as the amyloid plaque cores and blood vessels. Proc. Natl. Acad. Sci. USA, 1985
33. Metuzals J, Montpetit V, Clapin DF: Organization of the neurofilamentous network. Cel. Tiss. Res. 214:455-482, 1981
34. Perry G, Rizzuto N, Autilio-Gambetti L, Gambetti P: Paired helical filaments from Alzheimer's disease patients contain cytoskeletal components. Proc. Natl. Acad. Sci. USA 82:3916-3920, 1985
35. Dickson C et al: Neurobiology of Aging, 1988. Glenner GG, Wong CW: Alzheimer's disease: initial report of the purification and characterization of a novel amyloid protein. Biochem. Biophys. Res. Comm. 120:885-890, 1984
36. Goedert M: Neuronal localization of amyloid data protein precursor mRNA in normal human brain and in alzheimer's disease. The EMBO Journal, Vol. 6, #12, pp. 3627-3632, December 1, 1987

chapter 12

Quo Vadis? The Future Of Psychopharmacotherapy

Frank J. Ayd, Jr., M.D., L.F.A.P.A.

Almost forty years have passed since modern psychopharmacotherapy was inaugurated by the discovery of the psychotropic effects of the first neuroleptic, chlorpromazine. In this short period of time, molecular manipulators have synthesized and pharmacologists and toxicologists have screened hundreds of putative psychoactive compounds. Consequently, today a psychopharmacotherapist may prescribe:

1. Neuroleptics;
2. Antidepressants;
3. Anxiolytics;
4. Sedatives and hypnotics;
5. Mood stabilizers; and
6. Miscellaneous.

Each of these groups of psychotropics consists of one or more subgroups. Neuroleptics include:

1. Phenothiazines;
2. Butyrophenones;
3. Thioxanthenes;
4. Dihydroindolones;
5. Dibenzoxazepines;
6. Diphenylbutylpiperidines;
7. Benzamides; and
8. Miscellaneous.

All these neuroleptics share one common property, aside from therapeutic efficacy. Namely, the capacity to evoke diverse signs and

Psychiatry: Past Reflections–Future Visions
B.T. Taylor and I.J. Taylor, Editors

symptoms of extrapyramidal reactions. For this reason, these EPS-inducing neuroleptics are classified typical neuroleptics to distinguish them from a subsequently developed group of atypical neuroleptics, so characterized because they seldom, if ever, evoke an extrapyramidal reaction.

ATYPICAL NEUROLEPTICS

There is intense clinical and research interest in atypical neuroleptics. There are two important reasons for this, one old, and the other of recent origin. Neuroleptic-induced extrapyramidal reactions have always been problems for patients and their therapists. Early onset extrapyramidal reactions, such as akinesia, akathisia, and parkinsonism, are distressing to patients, and are often responsible for noncompliance and loss of therapeutic benefits. Late onset extrapyramidal reactions, particularly tardive dyskinesia and other tardive extrapyramidal syndromes, have become the basis of an escalating number of malpractice suits. Thus, for therapeutic and medical-legal reasons, there is a concerted effort to develop atypical neuroleptics which would be as effective as typical neuroleptics, without causing extrapyramidal symptoms. Some atypical neuroleptics, clozapine, for example, have been marketed in various countries. Their limited efficacy and nonneurological side effects have detracted from their usefulness. Hence it can be predicted with reasonable certitude that in the immediate future there will be an unrelenting search for new atypical neuroleptics that will seldom, if ever, evoke an extrapyramidal reaction, will be more efficacious than clozapine, and, most important, will not cause toxic effects such as agranulocytosis, disturbances in temperature regulation, seizures, hypersalivation, or excessive weight gain.

Until effective and safe atypical neuroleptics become available, therapists will continue to do what they have been doing recently. They will prescribe low dose neuroleptic therapy for acute and chronic patients, especially for maintenance therapy. They will administer neuroleptics intravenously more frequently than they have in the past. They will use various neuroleptic-sparing therapeutic regimens, such as prescribing concomitantly neuroleptics and benzodiazepines, or neuroleptics and lithium. Furthermore, they will administer progressively lower depot neuroleptic doses and at the same time progressively lengthen the interval between injections. They also will use drug holidays or targeted or intermittent neuroleptic therapy more often, especially for maintenance therapy.

The object of all these regimens is to provide patients with therapeutic benefits of typical neuroleptics with minimal incidence of mild to moderate adverse reactions, particularly extrapyramidal reactions and especially tardive dyskinesia and other tardive extrapyramidal syndromes. This is possible because low-neuroleptic doses for the shortest possible period are less likely to cause adverse neurological responses. Thus, until new typical or atypical neuroleptics become available, therapists will increasingly use neuroleptics in ways designed to maximize their positive effects and minimize their negative effects.

All typical and atypical neuroleptics to date have relieved positive schizophrenic symptoms but have had little impact on negative schizophrenic symptoms. For this reason, there has been and there will be efforts to develop compounds that will alleviate both positive and negative symptoms in schizophrenics. There are some new compounds, remoxipride, resperidone, and ritanserin, for example, that seem to alleviate positive and negative symptoms while showing a lower potential to evoke extrapyramidal reactions. There are good reasons to believe that these new psychotropics will be widely used and that there will be a number of similar antipsychotics developed and marketed in the future.

In the past thirty years, there has been a steady increase in the number and types of antidepressants, ranging from the tricyclics to other cyclic and noncyclic monoamine oxidase inhibitors (MAO) compounds. In addition, the MAOs now consist of type A inhibitors, which interact with tyramine, type B, which do not interact with tyramine, and a mixed type A-B. Since type B inhibitors abolish the need for the dietary restrictions that plague the use of type A inhibitors, there is considerable interest in the type B inhibitors for clinical and medical-legal reasons. If type B inhibitors are as effective as other MAOs and non-MAOs, there is no doubt that some clinicians will prescribe these substances with increasing frequency, especially for the elderly. In addition, if there is minimal or no risk of adverse interactions with tyramine and other substances, sympathomimetics, for example, so that the risk of severe hypertensive crises is minimal, medical-legal restraints on their use will be practically non-existent, and physicians will be inclined to prescribe them.

Interest in the MAOs and an increase in their use has been spurred by controlled studies documenting their antidepressant efficacy and by the recent demonstration of their efficacy in the treatment of eating disorders, particularly bulimia, in the treatment of panic disorder, with or without agoraphobia, and in the treatment of mixed anxiety and depressive disorders.

Despite the developments related to the MAOs and their therapeutic applications, it is my conviction that there will not be a substantive increase in MAO prescription. There are two valid reasons for this belief. First, controlled comparative studies have not been done that confirm that all types of MAOs are as effective and as safe as other antidepressants, especially some of the newer antidepressants. Second, the negative perceptions about the dangers and limited efficacy of MAOs are so deeply ingrained that only a minority of physicians will be inclined to prescribe them, except for patients with treatment-resistant depressions.

There is data indicating that MAOs may benefit some depressed patients refractory to cyclic and other non-MAO antidepressants. There also is data that co-prescription of an MAO with a tricyclic and other non-MAO antidepressants can result in the augmentation of the antidepressant effects of the non-MAOs. Also, combined MAO-lithium therapy for some refractory patients may be more effective than either drug alone. Hence, there may be increasing use of MAOs combined with other drugs for treatment-refractory depressives.

Returning to the non-MAO antidepressants, there is no doubt that there will be a continuation of the current endeavor to develop newer ones that retain the efficacy of their predecessors, are safer when taken in overdose, and lack or have much less sedative, anticholinergic, cardiovascular and other potentially troublesome and serious pharmacological effects. At the August 1988 Collegium of Internationale Neuro-psychopharmacologicum (CINP) meeting, there were presentations on more than twenty putative new antidepressants, many of them being serotonin re-uptake inhibitors. There is a great deal of interest in these serotonin re-uptake inhibitors. However, before more of these drugs are synthesized and made available for clinical trial, a cautionary note is in order.

The development of serotonin re-uptake inhibitors has indeed provided a series of potential antidepressant drugs, which, early in their clinical evaluation, appeared to offer many significant advantages over the tricyclic antidepressants: less cardiotoxicity, fewer anticholinergic side effects, and a claim, for some, of more rapid onset of action. While these are welcome gains, they may be offset by a pattern of side effects peculiar to these agents, mainly, gastrointestinal upsets, insomnia, and akathisia-like symptoms. The initial enthusiasm for serotonin re-uptake inhibitors has been tempered somewhat by the unfortunate side effects of zimiledine. The paucity of studies of intermediate and long-term administration of the new serotonin re-uptake inhibitors should make us cautious about uncritically proclaiming the virtues of these new antidepressants in the treatment of depressive illness.

ANXIOLYTICS

Whether or not there will be more benzodiazepines marketed as anxiolytics is difficult to forecast. New benzodiazepine anxiolytics will have to compete with more generic benzodiazepines, as well as proprietary benzodiazepines, which some physicians will always prescribe in preference to a generic or a newly-introduced anxiolytic. The growing professional and public awareness of the risk of dependence on therapeutic doses of all benzodiazepines is responsible for a gradual decline in prescription of benzodiazepines. Additionally, the growing professional awareness of the deleterious physical and cognitive effects of benzodiazepine usage also is effecting the prescription of at least some benzodiazepines.

Because of concern about overuse, abuse, and withdrawal reactions, there are in many western countries escalating anti-benzodiazepine movements with demands that some be taken off the market and that the prescription of the remainder be restrained. Already, this is happening in England.

Just as many doctors voluntarily stopped prescribing barbiturates and meprobamate because of their abuse and other liabilities, more and more doctors are voluntarily limiting their prescription of benzodiazepines. Thus, these trends may be the beginning of the ultimate replacement of benzodiazepines by new anxiolytics.

Finally, the slow but steady increase in litigation based on instances of benzodiazepine dependence and withdrawal is prompting some doctors to look for alternatives to benzodiazepines, which will be effective anxiolytics without posing risk of dependency and withdrawal. At the moment, buspirone is the only marketed non-benzodiazepine that is an effective anxiolytic that has a very low or nonexistent dependency and withdrawal risk, has no adverse cognitive or psychomotor interaction with alcohol, has little or no abuse potential, even in alcoholics, and is relatively nontoxic when taken in overdose. It is not surprising, therefore, that relatives of buspirone are now in clinical trials. Of these, gepirone, which is similar to buspirone except that it does not bind to dopamine receptors, has been studied most. Clinical trials of ipsapirone, another anxiolytic related to buspirone, are currently underway.

It is reasonable to predict that demand for effective anxiolytics with little or no abuse potential, little or no risk of dependency or withdrawal reactions, and with the asset of being relatively safe in overdose, will stimulate, as it already has, a search for such drugs. This has resulted in studies of alpidem as another alternative to the benzodiazepines with fewer sedative and addictive properties. Also under study is suriclone, another non-benzodiazepine anxiolytic unrelated to buspirone. Furthermore, there is some evidence that benzodiazepine partial agonists may be effective anxiolytics. This has prompted research for other partial agonists that also may be anxiolytic.

Will the benzodiazepines be replaced by new anxiolytics? The answer, in my judgement, is yes. It is conceivable that as bromides were replaced by barbiturates, and barbiturates and meprobamate were replaced by benzodiazepines, the benzodiazepines will slowly be replaced by a new group of anxiolytics.

HYPNOTICS

For several decades, benzodiazepine hypnotics have been the most commonly prescribed hypnotics in medical history. Professional and public awareness of the incidence of dependency and withdrawal reactions, as well as continuation of drug effects into the waking hours, have stimulated a search for alternative nonbenzodiazepine hypnotics.

In the United States, the triazolobenzodiazepine triazolam is the number one benzodiazepine hypnotic. Associated with its very extensive usage has been the growing realization that triazolam has other disadvantages, such as: seizures in some patients, disinhibition in others, and amnesia in still others. These liabilities, coupled with a marked increase in serious suicide attempts and successful suicides with triazolam alone or with other drugs, plus its high risk of dependency and severe withdrawal reactions in long-term users, are responsible for a growing clamor that triazolam be removed from the market, or stringent restrictions be placed on its prescription.

Ritanserin and zopiclone are new products which, at the moment, seem to be effective non-benzodiazepine hypnotics. Only time will tell if these and other non-benzodiazepine hypnotics have fewer of the disadvantages of the benzodiazepine hypnotics. If this proves to be true, then it is reasonable to forecast the replacement of benzodiazepine hypnotics by newer non-benzodiazepine hypnotics because these have less pronounced hangover effects, less risk of dependency and withdrawal and less of the untoward effects of the benzodiazepine hypnotics.

ALTERNATIVES FOR LITHIUM

In the past quarter century there has been a search for drugs that could be alternatives for lithium in treating effectively and safely patients who:

(a) may not be lithium candidates because of age, e.g. the elderly;
(b) may not be lithium candidates because of pregnancy, or renal or cardiac disorders;
(c) are unresponsive to lithium; or
(d) react adversely to lithium.

The first alternative to lithium was suggested by Okuma who, in 1973 and several times thereafter, reported that the anticonvulsant carbamazepine has both therapeutic and prophylactic efficacy in bipolar affective disorders. Okuma's pioneering work with carbamazepine sparked research on carbamazepine in Europe and the United States, especially at the National Institute of Mental Health by Robert Post. Consequently, there has been a steady increase in reports around the world attesting to the efficacy of carbamazepine, primarily as an antimanic agent and less so as an antidepressant.

The data on carbamazepine's efficacy as a mood stabilizer in bipolar patients stimulated many investigators to evaluate the efficacy and safety of other anticonvulsants for acute and prophylactic therapies of affective disorders. These include oxcarbamazepine, dipropy lactamide, sodium valproate, and clonazepam. The data accumulated thus far on these anticonvulsants, with the exception of carbamazepine and clonazepam, must be viewed as preliminary. For this reason no anticonvulsant, not even carbamazepine, has been approved by the Food and Drug Administration for the treatment of affective disorders. Nevertheless, it is now evident that there are a number of anticonvulsants that may be suitable alternatives for lithium. These drugs have acute antimanic and prophylactic effects, often with fewer side effects than lithium and without as much monitoring required. They offer hope for rapid cyclers and for the 25% of partial lithium responders and the 25% of lithium nonresponders. They also offer hope for a subgroup of depressives who, if responsive, will experience an antidepressant effect at about the same time as with a tricyclic or other antidepressants, that is, within two to three weeks. Finally, studies of the mechanism of action of these anticonvulsants alone and with other drugs may lead to new and better understanding of the basic mechanisms of affective dysregulation.

CALCIUM CHANNEL BLOCKERS

If I failed to mention the calcium channel blocking agents, this discourse on my thoughts about the future of psychopharmacotherapy would be incomplete. At the moment three calcium channel blockers--verapamil, nifedipine, and diltiazem--are approved in the United States for the treatment of certain cardiac disorders. Under study, also for cardiovascular indications, are nitrendipine, nimodipine, and flunarizine.

Interest in the calcium channel blockers as an alternate to lithium for the treatment of mania was stimulated because lithium has calcium antagonist properties, and because lithium is similar to calcium channel blockers such as verapamil in its effects on a number of organ systems. In addition, as Dubovsky and others have pointed out, other drugs used to treat affective disorders such as antidepressants, neuroleptics, and carbamazepine, inhibit calcium and have calcium channel blocking properties, but it is not clear whether these are related to the therapeutic actions of these drugs.

Of all the calcium channel blockers to date, only verapamil has been administered to a small number of manic patients. The evidence accumulated so far indicates that verapamil is effective but less so than lithium in treating acutely manic patients who are also likely to respond to lithium. No formal studies of verapamil's prophylactic efficacy have been completed. However, some clinicians have gathered some data indicating that verapamil may have prophylactic efficacy for recurrent mania.

Just as carbamazepine and other anticonvulsants with antimanic effects cannot be considered first-line drug therapy for mania, this also is true for verapamil. Nevertheless, verapamil can be useful as an alternative to lithium or carbamazepine for patients intolerant of or unresponsive to them.

It should not surprise anyone that studies of verapamil and other calcium channel blockers as antidepressants, and for the management of schizophrenia, are being done. It is too early to report the efficacy of these drugs as antidepressants and antipsychotics.

There are three other conditions in which calcium channel blockers may be useful. These are tardive dyskinesia, neuroleptic malignant syndrome, and hypertensive crises induced by monoamine oxidase inbibitors. There are reports of verapamil and diltiazem decreasing signs and symptoms of tardive dyskinesia. It is not unreasonable to consider using a calcium channel blocker for tardive dyskinesia when other therapies such as discontinuing the neuroleptic are not feasible. Furthermore, the potential antimanic or antipsychotic effect of the calcium channel blocker may make it possible to lower neuroleptic dose and thus benefit the patient.

In the last decade psychiatrists have become aware of the growing incidence of the neuroleptic malignant syndrome, a condition that clinically resembles malignant hyperthermia. Lately a number of clinicians have used calcium channel blockers with varying success to treat this syndrome.

For almost three decades, psychiatrists have looked for effective therapies for the hypertensive crises that can occur in patients being treated with certain MAOIs. Now there is evidence that chewing a 10 mg tablet of nifedipine and placing it under the tongue to expedite absorption may be rapidly effective in alleviating an MAOI-induced hypertensive crisis. Verapamil, because of its coating, is more difficult to use sublingually. However, a single oral dose of 80 mg is usually sufficient. If needed, a second 80 mg dose one hour later can be given.

Although the data on the psychiatric uses of calcium channel blockers is currently limited, it can be stated that these drugs seem to have great promise in psychiatry.

CONCLUSION

No drugs have had a greater impact on medical and psychiatric practice than the modern psychopharmaceuticals. Over the last four decades, they have had a profound influence on the treatment of emotional and mental illnesses. The psychopharmaceuticals also have had a major impact on the development of clinical pharmacology.

They have been an unprecedented contributor to the emergence of biological psychiatry, to the making of many psychiatrists, medical intranauts who explore man's inner spaces by invasive and noninvasive techniques to discover the pathophysiology of psychiatric disorders and to learn the mechanism of action of the psychotropic drugs.

The history of modern psychopharmacology and psychopharmacotherapy is not a chronicle of unlimited success. There have been some truly remarkable achievements, but there also have been disappointments. However, there has been no lessening of hopes or of determination to improve psychotropic drug therapies. In my view, the future of psychopharmacotherapy is very promising, as all contributors to it build on what we have learned and research clinicians continue to improve on all available means of evaluating the therapeutic efficacy and safety of newly developed putative psychopharmaceuticals.

chapter 13

Dependence And Abuse Of Prescribed Drugs: A Look Into The Future

Malcolm H. Lader, M.D., D.P.M., D.Sc. F.R.C. Psych.

This symposium has reflected on past advances in the care of the mentally ill and has scanned far horizons for future breakthroughs. I now introduce a new perspective, a cautionary view that technological advances can lead to personal misery as well as symptomatic relief, especially if the caring professions neglect that fundamental maxim--"Primum non nocere" (First do no harm). My topic is an adverse effect of some medications which act on the brain, namely dependence and abuse. My interest in this area has led me into various aspects of clinical and laboratory research, of treatment and management, and of the provision of services. Further afield I have become embroiled in economic and political issues, the media, regulatory affairs, and reluctantly in major medico-legal confrontations. Finally, theoretical aspects of tolerance and dependence, abuse and addiction have been explored.

In this presentation, I shall try to cover as many of these areas as possible. In some areas I shall ask questions and proffer some answers; in others the questions outnumber the answers; and in yet others, my ignorance of which questions can even be addressed will become apparent. Throughout I will concentrate on the benzodiazepine tranquillizers, although from time to time other examples will be used as being more apposite or better-studied. I shall point out our errors, not in remonstration but in resigned optimism, so that by learning from history we will not repeat those mistakes quite so readily.

DEFINITIONS

Definitions of the various aspects of drug dependence and abuse have often been contentious, as attested by the changing nomenclature over the years. Reasonably precise definitions of these terms,

Psychiatry: Past Reflections–Future Visions
B.T. Taylor and I.J. Taylor, Editors

however, are needed to discuss a specific clinical problem such as benzodiazepine dependence. The following definitions and terms are those currently accepted by the World Health Organization (WHO, 1974) (1), and for our purposes it is convenient to elaborate on these and to add certain others such as tolerance and cross-dependence:

Drug

'Any substance that, when taken into the living organism, may modify one or more of its functions.'

Drug Abuse

'Persistent or sporadic excessive drug use inconsistent with or unrelated to acceptable medical practice.' This description implies a value judgement and it is, therefore, more useful to restrict medical terms to physical and psychological dependence and then to set the medical problem into the wider social context of drug abuse.

Drug Dependence

'A state, psychic and sometimes also physical, resulting from the interaction between a living organism and a drug, characterized by behavioral and other responses that always include a compulsion to take the drug on a continuous or a periodic basis in order to experience its psychic effects, and sometimes to avoid the discomfort of its absence.' Furthermore, it is useful to distinguish between psychological (habituation) and physical dependence, although the distinction may appear somewhat arbitrary.

Psychological Dependence

'A condition in which a drug produces a feeling of satisfaction and a psychic drive that require periodic or continuous administration of the drug to produce pleasure or to avoid discomfort.'

Physical Dependence

'The development of an altered physiological state which requires continued administration of a drug to prevent the appearance of a characteristic illness, the abstinence syndrome.' The withdrawal syndrome usually involves both physical and psychological manifestations, the nature of which vary with the drug on which dependence exists. Implicit in the term 'characteristic' is the concept of a specific and time-dependent syndrome occurring on discontinuation of a drug and incorporating symptoms and signs not previously present in the drug user. The type and timing of the syndrome should be highly predictable.

Cross-Dependence

'The ability of one drug to suppress the manifestations of physical dependence produced by another and to maintain the physically dependent state.'

Tolerance

'Following repeated administration, a given dose of a drug produces a decreased effect or, conversely, increasingly larger doses must be administered to obtain the effects observed with the original dose.'

The state in which tolerance to one drug has the effect of causing tolerance to another drug of the same or a different chemical type is termed cross-tolerance.

HISTORICAL BACKGROUND

Mankind has used anxiety-allaying and pain-killing agents since the dawn of history, alcohol and opium being the major examples. For at least as long, mankind has also sought to induce abnormal mental experiences by the use of chemical substances contained in plants, cannabis, "soma," and peyotl providing instances, some of which are still in use today (Lader, 1983) (2). Thus, for millenia, we have witnessed the two strands of psychotropic drug use--for relief of symptomatic distress, and for the production of gratifying experiences. But these uses are not necessarily or even largely dictated by the pharmacological properties of the active ingredients. Social factors are far more important in determining patterns of use and misuse. For example, cocaine, the active principle of the pulped leaf of the South American coca plant, Erythroxylum coca, has been used since about 2500 BC as an aid to arduous work at high altitudes, a practice which still continues. However, the Amerindians do not use it at low altitude where symptomatic fatigue is much less. Taken out of its original context, refined and transformed with sodium bicarbonate into "crack," it has become widely abused in North America, and large amounts are beginning ominously to infiltrate Western Europe. Similar examples include alcohol, opium, cannabis and tobacco, all substances which cause few if any social problems in their natural anthropological habitat but are a major destabilizing influence on alien cultures which embrace their use too readily.

What, then, of prescribed medication, essentially drugs given for symptomatic relief? They, too, carry a social dimension but, as I will show later, of a different type. Here the problem may be excessive use or, as with a succession of anxiolytics, it may also include dependence. A series of sedative/hypnotic compounds were introduced from the mid-19th century onwards. As with their predecessor, alcohol, they were found in turn to induce dependence and to be subject to abuse. They include the bromides, paraldehyde, chloral, the barbiturates and meprobamate.

In this century, the barbiturates attained enormous popularity. It became evident quite quickly, certainly by the 1920s, that barbiturates were widely misused. Patients prescribed a barbiturate for anxiety or insomnia often increased their dose beyond therapeutic limits. Such high-dose usage was also accompanied by major and occasionally life-threatening withdrawal reactions with convulsions, confusion and psychosis. As well as such misuse, abuse in the nonmedical context became increasingly evident, culminating in the scheduling of the barbiturates under the United Nations Convention on Psychotropic Substances, 1971 (United Nations, 1977) (3).

The essential point is that the medical profession was accustomed to associate dependence, physical and psychological, with escalation of dosage. In line with this, Hollister and his colleagues (1961) (4) showed that very high doses of chlordiazepoxide, the first benzodiazepine, produced severe physical dependence with fits on withdrawal. This was accepted as an almost inevitable property of an anxiolytic. It was expected that some misuse of benzodiazepines would occur, with some patients increasing their dose beyond therapeutic levels as they became tolerant.

DEPENDENCE ON BENZODIAZEPINES

It was against this background that the benzodiazepines were introduced and burgeoned in popularity, largely replacing the barbiturates and meprobamate. It was clear that the benzodiazepines were efficacious anxiolytics especially in patients with clearly-defined Anxiety Disorders (Quality Assurance Project 1985; Rickels et al. 1978) (5,6). Side effects were usually mild and/or transient or could be obviated by lowering the dose. A major advantage over the barbiturates was the safety in overdosage of the benzodiazepines. The introduction of the benzodiazepines coincided with a pandemic of suicidal attempts and many thousands of people are alive today because they overdosed with a benzodiazepine and not a barbiturate. So impressed was the British medical profession that it mounted an official campaign to phase out the barbiturates. Implicit in that initiative in the mid 1970s was acquiescence in the growth in use of the benzodiazepines.

In contrast to the many accounts testifying to the safety of the benzodiazepines was the paucity of reports on misuse with escalation of dosage. This was epitomized in John Marks's book (1978) (7) in which he concludes that the risk of dependence is very low. After reviewing the world literature he arrived at an estimate of "approximately one case per 5 million patient months 'at risk' for all recorded cases and probably less than one case per 50 million months in therapeutic use." The medical profession and the benzodiazepine manufacturers were greatly reassured. However, the reports collated by Marks almost all described patients who had escalated their dosage beyond therapeutic levels. This, indeed, was the marker by which medical concern had been raised. Only a few criticisms were raised of Marks's anodyne conclusion although it was pointed out in the Lancet (Editorial, 1979) (8) that case reports are not a satisfactory epidemiological framework. Nevertheless, the consensus 10 years ago was that benzodiazepines were rarely abused and that the risk of dependence was low.

The usage of benzodiazepines had increased rapidly during the 1970s in line with such perceptions of safety. But a few dissentient voices were raised, mainly in the U.K. Trethowan (1975) (9) referred to the "psychotropic drug juggernaut;" Tyrer (1978) (10) pointed out the lack of knowledge concerning long-term treatment; and I wrote an article entitled "Benzodiazepines--the Opium of the Masses?" (Lader, 1978) (11). These articles, together with the Lancet editorial cited earlier, hinted at the possibility that such extensive long-term usage was on the basis of dependence at therapeutic dosage but reluctantly concluded that the evidence was sparse for the existence of such dependence and its prevalence was probably low.

Two studies should have raised the alarm. The first was a complex evaluation of cross-tolerance between the benzodiazepines, barbiturates and phenytoin (Covi et al., 1969; 1973) (12,13). Inter alia, the investigators described a minor withdrawal syndrome in anxious patients discontinuing chlordiazepoxide after 20 weeks of use. None of the patients took more than the prescribed dose. The authors suggested that long-term benzodiazepine users may represent an "addictive personality," although they had no data to support this, thus starting a hare which has run tirelessly. The studies did not excite much attention because Covi, et al. stressed the minor nature of the symptoms, did not design their studies specifically to evaluate withdrawal, and presented their results in a complicated way.

Another publication, however, was more concerned. Maletzky and Klotter (1976) (14b) reviewed the literature on diazepam dependence, pointing out its inadequacies and then surveyed 50 diazepam users. They noted that these patients tended to increase their dose and had difficulty discontinuing; they experienced anxiety, tremor and insomnia. The authors argued cogently that this represents withdrawal because the initial anxiety had resolved or the benzodiazepine had been prescribed for an indication other than anxiety. Seventeen of the 24 patients who had attempted to stop complained of new symptoms. Maletzky and Klotter caution that "the retrospective, uncontrolled nature of most of the data reported herein makes this study merely suggestive" (p. III). They point out the need for a controlled systematic trial, affirmed their intention to carry out one, but unfortunately never did so.

It was left to Peter Tyrer and myself to separately carry out the first prospective studies. Tyrer, while working in my clinic, had discussed with me his misgivings about long-term benzodiazepine use. In 1981 he published a study of 40 patients, long-term diazepam or lorazepam users, whose benzodiazepine was tapered off and placebo or propranolol substituted (Tyrer et al., 1981) (14a). This study confirmed the reality of normal-dose dependence as evidenced by a physical withdrawal syndrome, showed that stopping lorazepam was attended by a more severe syndrome with a higher resumption rate than stopping diazepam, and provided an estimate of the incidence of withdrawal reactions among long-term users at about one-third.

CLINICAL STUDIES

My own studies over the past decade have been mostly laboratory-based (Petursson and Lader, 1984; Higgitt et al., 1988) (15,16). They provide an illustration of the use of a range of techniques in the investigation of a clinical problem.

Our first pilot study was purely descriptive. We tapered off medication in a small group of high-dose misusers and a small group of normal dose therapeutic users and found that withdrawal syndromes supervened in both and were similar in type and severity (Hallstrom and Lader, 1981) (17). It was also evident that quite elaborate control procedures were needed to establish beyond doubt the existence of a normal dose dependence syndrome and to overcome the scepticism of prescribers.

The methodological problems were many. Firstly, the discontinuation had to be double-blind. Not only was placebo-substitution essential but the actual time of substitution needed to be kept blind to both patients and observers. We did this by allocating patients randomly to groups who underwent placebo substitution at different times. This minimized the problem of pseudowithdrawal when patients develop anxiety symptoms as the dosage is reduced (Winokur and Rickels, 1981).

(18). A second problem concerns the provenance of the patients. If they had previously tried to withdraw and developed symptoms, they are likely to do so again. If only such patients are referred to psychiatrists or to special withdrawal clinics, then the incidence of withdrawal will be 100%, as in our extensive series. Compliance is another difficult factor, and repeated urinary screening for benzodiazepines is useful to monitor this. Finally, very few studies of long-term benzodiazepine usage have been prospective in design. We still know little of the natural history of benzodiazepine use in its main habitat, namely general practice, although one study suggests that about a fifth of people started on these drugs are still taking them 6 months later (Williams et al., 1982) (19). Carrying out such studies under the constraints of a formal clinical trial may also have ethical implications if attempts are made to continue patients long-term without attempting withdrawal.

The clinical phenomena attending benzodiazepine withdrawal have been well-documented and fall roughly into three groups (Petursson and Lader, 1984) (15). The first group comprise psychological symptoms such as anxiety and tension, agitation and restlessness, irritability, lack of energy, impaired memory and concentration, depression and depersonalization. The second encompasses bodily symptoms of anxiety and includes sleep and appetite disturbance, headache, muscle pains and twitching, nausea, tremor and sweating. The third are perceptual and general symptoms of metallic taste, hyperosmia, paresthesia, photophobia, incoordination, a sense of perpetual movement, hyperacusis, hypersensitivity to touch and pain and a "flu-like" illness. Occasional severe features include paranoid reactions, hallucinations, confusion and convulsions. Many but by no means all of these symptoms are seen in anxiety disorders but not usually so intensively or chronically. Nevertheless, it has been suggested that it is difficult if not impossible to distinguish between withdrawal and the original anxiety recurring. This is not usually so: the withdrawal syndrome is usually time-locked to discontinuation, depending on the elimination half-life of the benzodiazepine, and usually subsides over a few weeks; recurrence of anxiety is much less predictable and it usually persists. Furthermore, some patients were started on benzodiazepines for non-psychiatric reasons; e.g., muscle spasm, and first suffer psychological symptoms on withdrawal. Nevertheless, some patients undoubtedly suffer mixed syndromes with both withdrawal and recurrence anxiety.

The benzodiazepine withdrawal syndrome is not clinically unique, resembling in many respects that seen on abstinence from alcohol or a barbiturate. It is thus a variant of the sedative/hypnotic withdrawal syndrome. Also, it lies on a continuum from the much more common rebound syndrome seen after discontinuing a benzodiazepine after even short-term use. Rebound insomnia is a specific type of withdrawal sleep disturbance characterized by a worsening of sleep above pretreatment levels following abrupt discontinuation of benzodiazepine hypnotics with rapid elimination rates (Kales et al., 1983; Lader and Lawson, 1987) (20,21). A lesser form of the syndrome is seen when insomnia worsens for a night or two after discontinuation relative to the drugged period. More recently it has become apparent that an analogous anxiety syndrome occurs after the withdrawal of anxiolytics given short-term, especially when discontinued abruptly (e.g. Fontaine et al., 1984) (22). In one of our own studies, anxious patients were treated with lorazepam in an average dose of 3 mg/day for four weeks. Abrupt discontinuation was followed by marked and distressing rebound anxiety in nearly half the patients and we modified the protocol thereafter to allow gradual withdrawal over 2 weeks. Such tapering should be regarded as good clinical practice even when the benzodiazepine has been given for only a few weeks.

Another form of rebound anxiety is "interdose anxiety" (Herman et al., 1987) (23). The patient is usually being treated for panic anxiety with high doses of an intermediate-acting benzodiazepine such as alprazolam. Although the panics may remain blocked, generalized anxiety levels rise just before the next dose is due. The drug is thus eagerly anticipated ("clockwatching"), surely a form of psychological dependence.

The natural history of benzodiazepine withdrawal is not clearly understood. Although most patients experience a fairly short-term syndrome, some have protracted illnesses with severe and incapacitating symptoms (Ashton, 1984) (24). Nor is the eventual outcome clearly documented. In many series, total abstinence is only attained in 30-70% of patients. Patients with previous minimal or no psychiatric disturbance do best (Rickels et al., 1986) (25). Psychiatric clinics seem to attract particularly severe, disabled and chronic benzodiazepine users.

MANAGEMENT OF WITHDRAWAL

As the more severe symptoms of withdrawal such as psychosis and fits are most likely to follow abrupt withdrawal, tapering the dose is universally accepted as not only advisable but essential (Tyrer and Sievewright, 1984) (26). What is more contentious is the optimal rate of withdrawal (Higgitt et al., 1985; Editorial, 1987) (27,28). Four weeks is the minimum period after more than 6 months' use, and programs as long as 16 weeks have been advocated. Indeed, some self-help agencies suggest a month of tapering for every year of use. No comparative data support any suggestions. There is no evidence that very slow tapering obviates symptoms and it may merely prolong the agony. Our strategy is try fairly brisk withdrawal, say over 6-8 weeks, and only to slow down if the symptoms become intolerable.

One can usefully substitute a long-acting for a short-acting benzodiazepine, say 10 mg of diazepam for 1 mg of lorazepam and then, after stabilization, taper off the diazepam. However, because it takes 4-5 elimination half-lives for the increase in diazepam to take effect, typically as long as a week, and 4-5 half-lives for the lorazepam to restabilize at a lower level, say only 48 hours, it is sensible to add the diazepam, wait two to three days, and then to lower the lorazepam dosage.

Adjunctive therapies have been tried. A beta-adrenoceptor antagonist may lessen some symptoms but clonidine, perhaps for reasons I will outline later, is ineffective (Goodman et al., 1986) (29). Non-benzodiazepine anxiolytics such as buspirone are noncross tolerant with the benzodiazepines and do not help withdrawal (Schweizer and Rickels, 1986; Lader and Olajide, 1987) (30,31). Both carbamazepine (Klein et al., 1986) (32) and phenobarbital (Smith, 1984) (33) have been advocated. Patients often become quite depressed during withdrawal--an observation with intriguing biochemical implications--and may need vigorous treatment with an antidepressant (Olajide and Lader, 1984) (34). The most important elements in helping patients withdraw are psychological reassurance and explanation, relaxation and anxiety management schedules, and perhaps cognitive, individual, or group psychotherapy (Higgitt et al., 1987) (35).

CLINICAL PHARMACOLOGY

Systematic pharmacological studies can be conducted within the framework of clinical studies such as those outlined above. The main problem is the difficulty of mounting long-term prospective studies. One can study the onset of action of a benzodiazepine, and its offset of action after the typical 4-week clinical trial. One can also study long-term users withdrawing from benzodiazepines. Very few studies have linked the two together even in clinical, let alone research, terms. Nevertheless, some fascinating areas have been elucidated, a few of which I shall now outline.

In our laboratory studies, we used a range of subjective, behavioral, physiological, and biochemical measures to monitor the withdrawal process, carried out in patients using rigorous double-blind, placebo substitution, with variable time of withdrawal and compared to drug-free normals (Petursson and Lader, 1984) (15).

Subjectively, patients experienced time-locked increases in anxiety on withdrawal which usually subsided within 2-3 weeks. Symptoms showing significant patterns included anxiety, agitation, shaking, trembling, palpitations, nausea, and muscular tension. Perceptual symptoms usually accompanied the withdrawal, as mentioned earlier. The patients appeared non-specifically "ill" in clinical terms, and body weight dropped transiently. Psychological tests were impaired during withdrawal but this could be attributed to lack of motivation, attention, and concentration because of the anxiety and malaise.

Some physiological measures provided useful correlates of withdrawal. EEG fast-wave activity was increased in the patients prior to withdrawal as compared to normals and decreased during withdrawal to normal levels. Conversely, alpha frequencies increased. The auditory EEG evoked response was no different from normal in the patients, but increased in amplitude during withdrawal before settling back to normal values, thus raising the possibility that this test provides an objective correlate of perceptual hypersensitivity.

Our biochemical measures were somewhat unsophisticated but, despite this, some interesting results were obtained (Petursson et al., 1983) (36). Urinary norepinephrine metabolite concentrations were greatly reduced during long-term benzodiazepine use and slowly returned to normal after withdrawal. At no time was any rebound evident giving no support to the supposition that benzodiazepine withdrawal is accompanied by catecholaminergic overactivity, and incidentally explaining the ineffectiveness of clonidine. By contrast, some data suggested a rebound effect with urinary 5-HIAA, perhaps reflecting transient 5-HT increases.

One aspect of benzodiazepine dependence which interested us was the relationship to tolerance. Why did so few benzodiazepine users show tolerance and escalate their dosage? In our next study, we gave a test dose of diazepam prior to, during, and after withdrawal, and compared psychological, physiological, and neuroendocrine responses with those in normals. Tolerance was demonstrated with respect to most of the variables measured, although the extent to which tolerance had developed to different benzodiazepine effects varied markedly. Thus, growth hormone responses to diazepam showed complete tolerance, while cardiovascular effects were partially tolerant and EEG fast-wave responses showed very little tolerance. The subjective ratings also revealed a significant degree of tolerance, especially to the sedative effects of diazepam, but less so to its euphoriant actions.

We had also become interested in differences among benzodiazepines. Clinically, it was apparent that patients had much more difficulty withdrawing from lorazepam than from diazepam (Tyrer et al., 1981; Rickels et al., 1986) (14a;25). More recently, similar problems are being seen with alprazolam. We were not convinced that this reflected solely pharmacokinetic differences because we had not encountered similar difficulties in patients withdrawing from oxazepam, a low-potency, intermediate-acting compound.

Our next studies involved normal subjects (Higgitt et al., 1988) (16). The development of tolerance over a 15-day period was demonstrated for three different benzodiazepines, the short-acting triazolam, medium-acting lorazepam, and long-acting ketazolam. Tolerance in terms of reduction in various effects of a repeated dose was most noticeable for lorazepam. Tolerance developed to some effects of triazolam but not really to ketazolam, once accumulation had been taken into account. Cross-tolerance to a test dose of diazepam was again most marked with lorazepam. Blunting of the growth hormome response to diazepam was the most sensitive and reliable method of detecting tolerance to the benzodiazepines. Rebound symptoms on discontinuing two weeks' intake of benzodiazepine were marked for all drugs but unrelated either to the tolerance induced or to the elimination half-life.

A further study in patients showed that tolerance persisted in a group of long-term benzodiazepine users for between 4 months and 2 years after abstinence. These ex-long-term users, however, responded to a test dose of diazepam with an immediate symptom reduction followed by exacerbation of these symptoms over the subsequent week. We are currently evaluating the effects of the benzodiazepine antagonist, flumazenil, on such prolonged withdrawal symptoms.

The differences between lorazepam and oxazepam are another current interest. A single-dose comparative study in normal subjects showed that clinically equivalent doses of oxazepam and lorazepam also had equivalent effects on subjective ratings and psychomotor performance. However, lorazepam was much more potent in impairing some aspects of memory (Curran et al., 1987) (37) and in inducing aggressive dyscontrol in a competitive reaction-time task (Bond and Lader, 1988) (38).

BENZODIAZEPINE ABUSE

Sporadic high dose abuse usually occurs within the context of polydrug abuse but is seen increasingly on its own. In the U.K., a particular problem involves temazepam which is available in liquid-filled capsules. These are warmed, the contents extracted with a needle and syringe, and then injected intravenously. Thrombophlebitis is a common complication together with all the other known hazards of I.V. use such as hepatitis, septicemia and AIDS.

Among attenders at a London Drug Dependence Unit, nearly 60% had benzodiazepines detected in their urine on one or more occasions (Beary et al., 1987) (39). Benzodiazepines were easily the second most common drugs used, after methadone. In an alcohol detoxification center in Toronto, benzodiazepines were detected in a third of urine specimens obtained from over one hundred consecutive male admissions (Ogbourne and Kapur, 1987) (40).

The clinical features of benzodiazepine abuse closely resemble those of barbiturate abuse although fatal overdose is much less common. Often, quite heroic and horrific amounts of benzodiazepine are taken orally or intravenously, suggesting very marked tolerance to most of the depressant effects. Abstinence is much more hazardous than stopping an opioid, as fits, confusion, and psychosis are common.

THEORETICAL IMPLICATIONS

I should like now to turn the more general implications of both the clinical and the laboratory studies. The theoretical implications of this and a vast body of human and animal research concern not only benzodiazepines but many other psychotropic drugs as well.

Lader and File (1987) (41) have argued that rebound and withdrawal at both high and low doses are contiguous phenomena and all represent manifestations of the same underlying dependence mechanism. The main difficulty with this hypothesis is that the withdrawal syndrome includes some features that are not seen in rebound, such as the perceptual changes and these features are not obviously in the opposite direction to known benzodiazepine effects. However, little is known of the direct effects of benzodiazepines on perceptual functioning and a depressant action cannot be excluded.

It is more difficult to include tolerance in a unitary hypothesis. Tolerance is itself a complex phenomenon, varying from system to system, as our own research clearly shows. Such differential tolerance might explain the differences across systems with respect to withdrawal phenomena. However, some studies indicate a different time-course for withdrawal and tolerance when the same system is measured, as some of our studies demonstrate for clinical effects. It might be that tolerance is a less sensitive indicator of dependence or develops more slowly than withdrawal.

Finally, dependence and tolerance can be set into the general nexus of drug-organism interactions at the behavioral level and drug-receptor interactions at the biochemical level. They are manifestations of neuro-adaptive processes to drug administration (Haefely, 1987) (42). In turn these processes are a special case of general drug-receptor interactions. Let me remind you that rebound is common on discontinuation from drugs acting on peripheral receptors, such as propranolol on beta-adrenergic receptors and cimetidine on H_2 receptors.

Beyond this, the development of selective agonists, antagonists and inverse agonists on the benzodiazepine receptor promises to provide us with powerful tools to explore the relationships between dependence, tolerance and withdrawal. The convincing identification of the natural ligand acting on this receptor system, assuming such exists, would do much to clarify the biochemical and biophysical processes which underlie these phenomena. The recent elucidation of the structure of the macromolecular receptor complex is an exciting advance which has major implications for the study of dependence mechanisms.

The phenomenon of abuse, on which I have touched, is best examined separately. The behavioral manifestations differ from those of dependence; for example, the benzodiazepines are weak reinforcers (e.g. Ator and Griffiths, 1987; Roache and Griffiths, 1987) (43,44). Tolerance is very marked after sporadic high-dose use and presumably is similar to that following chronic low-dose use, although this remains to be established.

CLINICAL IMPLICATIONS

While few now doubt the reality of benzodiazepine dependence and withdrawal syndromes on normal dosages, controversy continues concerning the clinical importance of these phenomena. In the U.K. with at least twice the prevalence of long-term use of the U.S.A., a major public debate has been in full swing for a decade. Some practitioners avoid the use of benzodiazepines under any circumstances; most reserve them for the short-term management of severe anxiety, in accord with the guidelines of the Royal College of Psychiatrists (1988) (45); others affirm their intention to continue fairly extensive usage (Sussman and Chou, 1988) (46).

One line of argument of those justifying the use of benzodiazepine is that surveys of minor psychiatric morbidity in the community show a prevalence 2-3 times the prescription rate for tranquillizers, suggesting under- rather than over-utilization of benzodiazepines (Nagy, 1987) (47). This, however, assumes that psychological distress should automatically be treated with drugs, a point I shall return to.

The benefit/risk ratio of long-term benzodiazepine therapy was assessed by Rickels and his colleagues (1984) (48). They concluded that a significant percentage (about half) of chronically anxious patients are not in need of continuous diazepam therapy, that intermittent therapy was often more appropriate, and that regular evaluation was essential. A more recent study from this very active group produced some interesting data germane to the natural history of generalized anxiety disorder (Rickels et al., 1988) (49). Patients withdrawing after 6 months treatment with clorazepate had a high incidence of rebound and withdrawal; those discontinuing a non-benzodiazepine tranquillizer showed neither rebound nor withdrawal. This could be interpreted as showing that chronic anxiety disorder is a remitting and relapsing condition rather than one characterized by sustained high levels of anxiety, and that what is often regarded as recurrence of anxiety is usually benzodiazepine-induced rebound.

Another element in the equation is the risks of long-term use. Psychomotor, cognitive and memory impairments are associated with long-term use and these functions may improve on discontinuation of the benzodiazepine (Lader, 1983; Sakol and Power, 1988) (50,51). Benzodiazepine users are significantly more likely than non-users to experience accidents (Oster et al., 1987) (52). Neuroanatomical abnormalities have been reported in association with benzodiazepine usage in three studies (Lader et al., 1984; Schmauss and Krieg, 1987; Uhde and Kellner, 1987) (53,54,55) but not in a fourth (Poser et al., 1983) (56).

Meanwhile, what of the thousands of long-term benzodiazepine users who experience difficulty when they try to discontinue? Research is needed into the optimal schedules for withdrawal and the possible role of pharmacological aids such as carbamazepine and flumazenil. But above all, we need properly organized services to deal with what is essentially an iatrogenic condition. Primary care physicians need training in helping these patients withdraw with proper specialist back-up services for the most intractable cases. Whether the Pharmaceutical Industry should offer to return some of the profits generated from selling benzodiazepines to help these patients is a political not a clinical question, but one that deserves serious debate.

SOCIAL IMPLICATIONS

This brings me back to the wider implications of dependence on prescribed medication. It is important to recognize that the widespread use of tranquillizers is not a new phenomenon. The barbiturates were consumed by the ton. Thus, the total amount of use of sedative and hypnotic medications has increased rather slowly (Rabin and Bush, 1974) (57). Surveys of prescribing patterns show that most prescriptions for benzodiazepines represent continuing therapy for chronic problems. Indeed, in the U.K., the proportion of repeat to total prescriptions for tranquillizers has risen in the past 20 years from less than a quarter to almost 80 percent (Marks, 1983) (58). This implies that few newly-presenting patients are started on benzodiazepines and that a cohort of chronic users has accumulated. Only about a half of those given prescriptions for benzodiazepine tranquillizers have a primary diagnosis of a mental disorder, the rest being for a wide range of somatic disorders (Williams, 1978) (59), especially circulatory, digestive and musculo-skeletal problems, as well as even more ill-defined conditions (Mulvihill et al., 1985) (60). About a third of the patients who received a tranquillizer were judged appropriately treated; 12% of those not given a tranquillizer were judged to need one. In most countries with primary care physicians most of benzodiazepine tranquillizers are prescribed by them (Koch and Campbell, 1983) (61). The remainder of the prescriptions are spread across almost all specialities.

The most direct data come from surveys of use by representative samples of the general population. Two surveys, one in 1971 and the second in 1981, roughly bracket the peak of benzodiazepine use in the U.S.A. and some other western countries. The 1971 study established the 1-year prevalence of tranquillizer use to range between 9.7 and 16.8% of the adult population across the various countries surveyed (Balter et al., 1974) (62). The later study revealed a slightly wider range of prevalence of users (7.4-17.6%), but with some overall fall off in use (Balter et al., 1984) (63b). Across all countries, usage was higher in females than males, in the U.S.A. and the U.K. in a 2:1 ratio. In females, peak usage was in the 45-65 age range, in males it was more uniform across ages. Data were available on duration of use. Chronic use, i.e. for at least the previous 12 months, ranged from 0.5% of the adult population in Sweden to 5.8% in Belgium, the figures for the U.S.A. and the U.K. being 1.8 and 3.1%, respectively. As a percentage of all users, these figures translate into 14.2% and 27.4% in the U.S.A. and U.K. It is hardly surprising that public concern in the U.K. is greater than that in the U.S.A.

The correlates of long-term use in the U.S.A. were evaluated in a survey which showed such users to be mainly older and female, with high levels of emotional distress and chronic somatic health problems (Mellinger et al., 1984) (63a). Most are monitored by a physician. Thus, the usage is within a medical context but nevertheless this begs the question of whether other forms of therapy might not be more effective and more safe. Also, it does not go far to reassure medical opinion in other countries where long-term usage is much higher than in the U.S.A.

The development of long-term use has been studied by Williams and his colleagues (1982) (19). A prospective longitudinal survey showed that 19% of patients given a psychotropic drug continued on that medication beyond 6 months. The factors most predictive of long-term use were age over 45, previous use of psychotropic drugs, severity of psychiatric disorder and chronic social problems (Murray et al., 1982) (64). Many attributed the onset of their symptoms to a life crisis and they tended to lack social support.

Much of the defense of the extensive and long-term use of benzodiazepine tranquillizers revolves around the argument that users are anxious and need the symptomatic relief provided. Anxiety equates to a benzodiazepine prescription. But many other treatments for anxiety disorders are available including a range of psychological therapies (Gelder, 1986) (65). These can be adapted so that any doctor can use them. One study has addressed this issue by evaluating the effects of withholding tranquillizers (Catalan et al., 1984a,b) (66a,b). The general practitioners in two group practices in Oxford identified over 90 patients with minor affective disorders for whom tranquillizers would normally have been prescribed. Half the patients were allocated randomly to tranquillizers chosen by the general practitioner and half to counselling by the G.P. without medication. The counselling was brief, directive and non-specialized, comprising mainly listening, explanation, advice, and reassurance. When standardized assessments were repeated after the start of treatment, the proportions of patients with definable psychiatric disorder fell from 80% before treatment to 40% at one month and 30% at 7 months. The two groups improved at a similar rate and to a similar extent. Thus, two-thirds of the patients did just as well with brief counselling as with tranquillizers, and a third did just as badly. The latter group were characterized by a greater severity of illness. There was no evidence that withholding tranquillizers increased usage of alcohol, tobacco or other drugs. Patients receiving counselling were more satisfied with their treatment than those given tranquillizers. Nor did counselling make increased demands on the general practitioners, compared with prescribing.

CONCLUSIONS

The use of benzodiazepines remains a contentious topic, not helped by exaggerated accounts in the media (Kilwein, 1983) (67). On the other hand, the facile assumption by some doctors and almost all the pharmaceutical industry that psychological distress is an automatic justification for benzodiazepine prescribing (Woods et al., 1988) (68) is not in accord with the facts. Such an acceptance has led to and continues to produce unnecessary long-term use, more so in the U.K. than in the U.S.A.

Long-term use can be criticized on safety considerations but also on efficacy grounds. Rickel's work cited earlier raises doubts after the chronic nature of anxiety disorders. If the condition is largely remitting and relapsing in its natural history, then intermittent but not continuous use might be justified (Rickels et al., 1984) (48). The establishing of long-term efficacy must shift to recognize this; what is needed are studies of the efficacy of intermittent rather than chronic use.

The observation that anxiety tends to recur on discontinuing long-term benzodiazepine usage is not acceptable evidence of long-term efficacy on the grounds, firstly, that outlined above which questions the chronic nature of anxiety disorders and secondly, that the anxiety represents part of a rebound or withdrawal syndrome and not recrudescence of the original anxiety. Obviously, if long-term efficacy cannot be established, then there are no valid indications for such use.

Long-term use can be criticized on two other grounds. The moral one is that tranquillizers are the "opium of the masses" since they suppress emotional symptoms while the underlying social and political causes remain the same (Lader, 1978) (11). Feminist groups have accused the male-dominated medical profession of using tranquillizers to suppress the symptoms induced by sex inequalities in the social structure. The second argument is that resorting to benzodiazepines may sap a person's motivation to try and cope with his symptoms or to try and resolve his problems (Trethowan, 1975) (9). Both of these arguments are difficult to evaluate scientifically.

Can even short-term use be justified when we know that such usage carries a 20% risk of going on to long-term use; i.e., beyond 6 months (Williams et al., 1982) (19)? Catalan et al.'s studies (1984 66a,b) show the limited efficacy of benzodiazepines and counselling in more severe anxiety disorders and useful efficacy in the less ill. There seems no justification for benzodiazepines in the mildly ill and those reacting to life stresses. Counselling is direct, effective and no more expensive in terms of medical time than prescribing a tranquillizer. Indeed, if counsellors could somehow be incorporated into family practices, useful cost savings could probably be achieved. The more severely anxious patients--those with "excessive or unrealistic anxiety" --need a range of therapies, pharmacological and non-pharmacological. Even here, newer anxiolytics are available or in development and some may eventually prove not to be associated with rebound or dependence. Their overall risk/benefit ratio may well be superior to that of the benzodiazepines.

As I have emphasized throughout, the social costs of benzodiazepine prescribing vary from country to country, as does concern about these costs. The controversy rages with claims of "therapeutic Calvinism" and counter-claims of negligent prescribing. A consensus is emerging that these drugs "have an undoubted use in the short-term treatment of anxiety but they are not the first line of management" (Drury, 1985) (69). We need to research further into the various ways of managing anxiety both that responding to life stresses of people and that excessive type which constitutes a medical disorder (Catalan and Gath, 1985) (70).

We are left, therefore, with a sense of dissatisfaction. Have we failed our patients by not realizing that dependence can supervene without evidence of tolerance and escalation of dosage? The best way we can make amends is to take the lesson to heart and to assume the worst about any drug until proven otherwise. Unfounded optimism has no place when people's health and welfare is at stake.

REFERENCES

1. WHO Expert Committee on Drug Dependence (1974). Twentieth Report WHO technical report series, no. 551; Geneva: WHO
2. Lader MH: (1983) Soma and psyche. British Medical Journal, 287, 1906-1908
3. United Nations (1977) Convention on Psychotropic Substances 1971, United Nations, New York
4. Hollister LE, Motzenbecker FP and Degan RO (1961) Withdrawal reactions from chlordiazepoxide ("Librium")
5. Quality Assurance Project (1985) Treatment outlines for the management of anxiety states. Australian and New Zealand Journal of Psychiatry, 19, 138-151
6. Rickels K, Downing RW and Winokur A (1978) Anti-anxiety drugs: Clinical Use in Psychiatry. In: L.L Iversen, S.D. Iversen and S.H. Snyder (Eds), Handbook of Psychopharmacology, Vol. 13, Plenum Press, New York and London, pp. 395-430
7. Marks J (1978) The Benzodiazepines. Use, overuse, misuse and abuse. MTP Press, Lancaster
8. Editorial (1979) Benzodiazepine withdrawal. Lancet, i, 196
9. Trethowan WH (1975) Pills for personal problems. British Medical Journal, 3, 749-51
10. Tyrer P (1978) Drug treatment of psychiatric patients in general practice. British Medical Journal, 2, 1008-10
11. Lader M (1978) Benzodiazepines--The opium of the masses? Neuroscience, 3, 159-65
12. Covi L, Park LC, Lipman RS, et al. (1969) Factors affecting withdrawal response to certain minor tranquillizers. In: Drug Abuse: Social and Psychopharmacological Aspects, ed. by J. Cole and Wittenborn, pp. 93-108, Charles Thomas, Springfield, Ill
13. Covi L, Lipman RS, Pattison JH et al. (1973) Length of treatment with anxiolytic sedatives and response to their sudden withdrawal. Acta Psychiatrica Scandinavica, 49, 51-64
14a. Tyrer P, Rutherford D, Huggett T (1981) Benzodiazepine withdrawal symptoms and propranolol. Lancet, I, 520-522
14b. Maletzky BM and Klotter J (1976) Addiction to diazepam. International Journal of Addiction, 11, 95-115
15. Petursson H and Lader MH (1984) Dependence on Tranquillizers. Maudsley Monograph no. 28, Oxford University Press, Oxford, 1984
16. Higgitt A, Fonagy P and Lader MH (Eds.) (1988) The natural history of tolerance to the benzodiazepines. Psychological Medicine, Mono-

graph Suppl. 13, Cambridge University Press, Cambridge
17. Hallstrom C and Lader M (1981) Benzodiazepine withdrawal phenomena. International Pharmacopsychiatry, 16, 235-44
18. Winokur A and Rickels K (1981) Withdrawal and pseudo-withdrawal from diazepam therapy. Journal of Clinical Psychiatry, 42, 442-444
19. Williams P, Murray J and Clare A (1982) A longitudinal study of psychotropic drug prescription. Psychological Medicine, 12, 201-206
20. Kales A, Soldatos CR, Bixler EO, Kales JD (1983) Rebound insomnia and rebound anxiety: a review. Pharmacology, 26, 121-137
21. Lader MH and Lawson C (1987) Sleep studies and rebound insomnia: methodological problems, laboratory findings, and clinical implications. Clinical Neuropharmacology, 10, 291-312
22. Fontaine R, Chouinard G and Annable L (1984) Rebound anxiety in anxious patients after abrupt withdrawal of benzodiazepine treatment. American Journal of Psychiatry, 141, 848-852
23. Herman JB, Brotman AW and Rosenbaum JF (1987) Rebound anxiety in panic disorder patients treated with shorter-acting benzodiazepines. Journal of Clinical Psychiatry, 48, (10 Suppl), 22-26
24. Ashton H (1984) Benzodiazepine withdrawal: an unfinished story, British Medical Journal, 288, 1135-1140
25. Rickels K, Case WG, Schweizer EE et al. (1986) Low-dose dependence in chronic benzodiazepine users: a preliminary report on 119 patients. Psychopharmacology Bulletin, 22, 407-415
26. Tyrer PJ and Seivewright N (1984) Identification and management of benzodiazepine dependence. Postgraduate Medical Journal, 60, (Suppl.2), 41-46
27. Higgitt AC, Lader MH and Fonagy P (1985) Clinical management of benzodiazepine dependence. British Medical Journal, 291, 688-690
28. Editorial (1987) Treatment of benzodiazepine dependence. Lancet, 1, 78
29. Goodman WK, Charney DS, Price LH, Woods SW and Heninger GR (1986) Ineffectiveness of clonidine in the treatment of the benzodiazepine withdrawal syndrome: report of three cases. American Journal of Psychiatry, 143, 900-903
30. Schweizer E and Rickels K (1986) Failure of buspirone to manage benzodiazepine withdrawal. American Journal of Psychiatry, 143, 1590-1592
31. Lader MH and Olajide D (1987) A comparison of buspirone and placebo in relieving benzodiazepine withdrawal symptoms. Journal of Clinical Psychopharmacology, 7, 11-15
32. Klein E, Uhde TW and Post RM (1986) Preliminary evidence for the utility of carbamazepine in alprazolam withdrawal. American Journal of Psychiatry, 143, 235-236

33. Smith DE (1984) Benzodiazepine dependence potential: current studies and trends. Journal of Substance Abuse Treatment, 1,163-167
34. Olajide D and Lader M (1984) Depression following withdrawal from long-term benzodiazepine use: a report of four cases. Psychological Medicine, 14, 937-940
35. Higgitt A, Golombok S, Fonagy P and Lader M (1987) Group treatment of benzodiazepine dependence, British Journal of Addiction, 82, 517-532
36. Petursson H, Bond PA, Smith B and Lader MH (1983) Monoamine metabolism during chronic benzodiazepine treatment and withdrawal. Biological Psychiatry, 18, 207-213
37. Curran HV, Schiwy W and Lader M (1987) Differential amnesic properties of benzodiazepines: a dose-response comparison of two drugs with similar elimination half-lives. Psychopharmacology, 92, 358-364
38. Bond A and Lader M (1988) Differential effects of oxazepam and lorazepam on aggressive responding. Psychopharmacology, 95, 369-373
39. Beary MD, Christofides J, Fry D, Ghodse AH, Smith E and Smith V (1987) The benzodiazepines as substances of abuse. Practitioner 231, 19-20
40. Ogbourne AC and Kapur BM (1987) Drug use among a sample of males admitted to an alcohol detoxication center. Alcoholism: Clinical and Experimental Research, 11, 183-185
41. Lader MH and File S (1987) The biological basis of benzodiazepine dependence. Psychological Medicine, 17, 539-547
42. Haefely W (1986) Biological basis of drug-induced tolerance, rebound and dependence. Contribution of recent research on benzodiazepines. Pharmacopsychiatrica, 19, 353-361
43. Ator NA and Griffiths RR (1987) Self-administration of barbiturates and benzodiazepines: a review. Pharmacology Biochemistry & Behavior, 27, 391-398
44. Roache JD and Griffiths RR (1987) Lorazepam and meprobamate dose effects in humans: behavioral effects and abuse liability. Journal of Pharmacology and Experimental Therapeutics, 243, 978-988
45. Royal College of Psychiatrists (1988) Benzodiazepines and dependence: a college statement. Bulletin of the Royal College of Psychiatrists, 12, 107-109
46. Sussman N and Chou JCY (1988) Current issues in benzodiazepine use for anxiety disorders. Psychiatric Annals, 18, 139-145
47. Nagy A (1987) Long-term treatment with benzodiazepines: theoretical, ideological and practical aspects. Acta Psychiatrica Scandinavica, 76, 47-55

48. Rickels K, Case WG, Winokur A and Swenson C (1984) Long-term benzodiazepine therapy: benefits and risks. Psychopharmacology Bulletin, 20, 608-615
49. Rickels K, Schweizer E, Csanalsoi MD et al. (1988) Long-term treatment of anxiety and risk of withdrawal. Archives of General Psychiatry, 45, 444-50
50. Lader M (1983) Benzodiazepines, psychological functioning, and dementia, in M.R. Trimble (Ed) Benzodiazepines Divided, pp. 309-325, Chichester, Wiley
51. Sakol MS and Power KG (1988) The effects of long-term benzodiazepine treatment and graded withdrawal on psychometric performance. Psychopharmacology, 95, 135-138
52. Oster G, Russel MW, Huse DM, Adams SF and Imbimbo J (1987) Accident and injury-related health-care utilization among benzodiazepine users and nonusers. Journal of Clinical Psychiatry, 48, 12 (Suppl)., 17-21
53. Lader MH, Ron M and Petursson H (1984) Computed axial brain tomography in long-term benzodiazepine users. Psychological Medicine, 14, 203-206
54. Schmauss C and Krieg JC (1987) Enlargement of cerebrospinal fluid spaces in long-term benzodiazepine abusers. Psychological Medicine, 17, 869-873
55. Uhde TW and Kellner CH (1987) Cerebral ventricular size in panic disorder. Journal of Affective Disorders, 12, 175-178
56. Poser W, Poser S, Roscher D and Argyrakis A (1983) Do benzodiazepines cause cerebral atrophy? Lancet, 715
57. Rabin DL and Bush PJ (1974) The use of medicines: historical trends and international comparisons. International Journal of Health Services, 4, 61-87
58. Marks J (1983) The benzodiazepines--for good or evil. Neuropsychobiology 10, 115-126
59. Williams P (1978) Physical ill-health and psychotropic drug prescription--a review. Psychological Medicine, 8, 683-693
60. Mulvihill MN, Suljaga PK, Falkenstein J and Ehr AP (1985) Patterns of diazepam prescribing in primary care: a case control study. Mount Sinai Journal of Medicine, 52, 276-280
61. Koch H and Campbell WH (1983) Utilization of psychotropic drugs in office-based ambulatory care. National Ambulatory Medical Care Survey, 1980 and 1981. Adv. Data, 90, 1-12
62. Balter MB, Levine J and Manheimer DI (1974) Cross-national study of the extent of anti-anxiety/sedative drug use. New England Journal of Medicine, 290, 769-774
63a. Mellinger GD, Balter MB, Uhlenhuth EH (1984) Prevalence and correlates of the long-term regular use of anxiolytics. Journal of

the American Medical Association, 251, 375-379

63b. Balter MB, Manheimer DI, Mellinger DG and Uhlenhuth EH (1984) A cross-national comparison of anti-anxiety/sedative drug use. Current Medical Research Opinion 8 (suppl. 4), 5-18

64. Murray J, Williams P and Clare A (1982) Health and social characteristics of long-term psychotropic drug takers. Social Science and Medicine, 16, 1595-1598

65. Gelder MG (1986) Psychological treatment for anxiety disorders: a review. Journal of the Royal Society of Medicine, 78, 230-233

66a. Catalan J, Gath D, Edmonds G and Ennis J (1984) The effects of non-prescribing of anxiolytics in general practice. I. Controlled evaluation of psychiatric and social outcome. British Journal of Psychiatry, 144, 603-610

66b. Catalan J, Gath D, Bond A and Martin P (1984) The effects of non-prescribing of anxiolytics in general practice. II. Factors associated with outcome. British Journal of Psychiatry, 144, 603-610

67. Kilwein JH (1983) Valium and Values. American Pharmacy, 12, 5-7

68. Woods JH, Katz JL and Winger G (1988) Use and abuse of benzodiazepines. Journal of the American Medical Association, 260, 3476-3480

69. Drury VWM (1985) Benzodiazepines--a challenge to rational prescribing. Journal of the Royal College of General Practitioners, 35, 86-88

70. Catalan J and Gath DH (1985) Benzodiazepines in general practice: time for a decision. British Medical Journal, 290, 1374-1376

chapter 14

Sexual Medicine 1939 To Today

Domeena C. Renshaw, M.D., F.A.P.A.

While noting the biochemical and genetic advances that have been recently made in psychiatry. I must say that I have no comparable information in the field of human sexuality, but it may be a relief to hear that we have not reached the molecular age of sex! The electrobiology of sex is not what we have today. We have had no explosion of cellular enzymes and transmitters in the field. We have, and pardon the pun, barely reached the physiology. To link with Sir Martin's paper on the elderly, the oldest patient that I have yet been called upon to see as a sexual emergency was a 96-year old man. There was a family crisis because he was visiting in Chicago and had gone into the room of the 15-year old grand-niece and propositioned her. The son-in-law tried to cover all this up: "he was only disoriented and thought it was the bathroom." His daughter was upset lest this be told to school teachers. He reluctantly came in, an M.D./Ph.D. whose cognitive functioning was far better than mine. He informed me that it was all a "tempest in a teacup," because, "Doctor, I never let an opportunity go by, and she was so vivacious at supper" that he thought it was a come-on, but he left when the girl said no. His second wife was 78 and they had intercourse regularly every Saturday night, and had for many years. There was no problem--he had partial erections with fine penetration. I told him that the child protection climate was very different today from that of many years ago and if reported he could spend great effort and expense to prevent going to jail because at 15 she is classified in Illinois as a minor. The law is very drastic for sexual abuse today (6).

I feel privileged to have a "bifocal specialty microscope" in the field of sexuality because I see children at Wednesday Child Clinic and for the past 17 years the adult evening outpatient sexual dysfunction training clinic, so see a wide spectrum of problems.

In the 16th century, Montaigue, the French essayist, remarked,

"There is an A-B-C ignorance that precedes knowledge and a doctoral ignorance that comes after it," and every open-minded scholar finds as study proceeds that the more is known about a subject, the more there is to learn. The Chinese philosopher Lao-Tse wrote in 550 B.C., "To the ignorant man, a tree is a tree, a river is a river; to the learned man, a tree is not a tree, and the river is not a river; to the wise man, a tree is a tree and a river is a river, but they are not the same tree or the same river as an ignorant man sees." When we try and relate these axioms to sexuality, we find that courageous researchers have built, each on the scientific shoulders of earlier scholars: Sir Richard Burton, Havelock Ellis, who had his encyclopedia of sexuality published in Germany at the turn of the century because they did not understand the English and publication was forbidden in England, and Sigmund Freud, who began to explore sexual motivations in the late 19th century.

Robert Dickinson, I was surprised to find, may be the first person who ever considered conjoint therapy, at the Cleveland Clinic in 1928. There was an incredibly high rate of sexual ignorance in the couples he saw as a gynecologist for unconsummated marriages. We still see this in Chicago. In the middle of the so-called sexual revolution, we have now treated 89 unconsummated marriages. Male virgins are not even classified anywhere, but we have treated 47 healthy, bright, athletic, college-educated men who were sexually reserved or inhibited.

Robert Dickinson, in the 1920s, made life-size sectioned female pelvis models, going beyond ancient Chinese dolls. These genitally explicit surgical sections are beautifully displayed in the Cleveland Clinic Museum still today. He brought the husband in, explained where the penis should go, showing the genital anatomy of the woman to both. He began the classical sex education therapy work upon which William Masters (also a gynecologist) built. Masters went a step further; he used the real patient for a conjoint sexological exam which now is a routine part of sex therapy.

In the 1930s, urology and gynecology separated from surgery to become specialties. Endocrinology was not even thought of at the time. It was in the 1970s that the sub-specialty of endocrinology and allergy immunology formed. So, too, sexual medicine is very recently on the scene, with a newly coined word "sexology." We still used rabbits for the pregnancy test when I went to medical school in Capetown in the 1950s. Penicillin had just a 10-year birthday, I think, when I got there. The pill was unknown when I graduated in 1960. So, when you look back, we have come a long way, and our A-B-C ignorance cannot be reversed. In the 1940s came Alfred Kinsey (3), who did the demographic studies that were so important because he literally broke the past sexual secrecy by doing personal interviews of 8,000 men.

In the 1950s Kinsey and Pomeroy studied the sex lives of 12,000 women (4). That data is still a gold mine. In 1955, a fellow South African-American, Joseph Wolpe, at Temple University did a little paper on reversing frigidity (now an outmoded pejorative word) with 2 patients by using self-relaxation. On that Masters built sex therapy for women, and James Semans in 1956 invented the stop-start sex therapy for premature ejaculation. Semans used relaxation (as Wolpe had used with women) to have the man who was so anxious about not holding his erection to just stop lovemaking and let the erection go down. This was later called the "Stop-Start Method." Masters applied a 15 second squeeze at the frenulum of the penis in the way a sneeze could be stopped by pressure at the nasal septum; this became "the squeeze technique."

At Baylor, Texas, Ismet Karacan had been working since the 1960s in a sleep lab and he began to recognize sexual changes in men and boys during sleep (2). Fisher similarly began to work with girls (1). Now at Baylor, another psychiatrist, Connie Moore, is studying females in Karacan's Sleep Lab because female sexuality has been grossly neglected.

To understand what happens to genital physiology, the unconscious, uninhibited state of sleep gives us a "window." We can now measure vaginal transudate and the nocturnal sleep erections. When a man becomes anxious with his partner and cannot have erections, but in sleep has excellent erections, relationship conflict must be explored for the somatopsychic interface of selective impotence.

Then, in 1975, a facetious young urology resident presented a Urology Convention paper on the "postage stamp test" where he had the patient take six 1-penny stamps and encircle the root of the penis at bedtime. In the morning, if he had nocturnal erections, he would have popped the serrations and so show normalcy. The nocturnal erection 8-hour test on the EEG machine was more reliable but very costly. Out of these beginnings grew what is now a "penis industry" in the U.S., an extraordinary explosion of treatments with companies falling over each other to produce the newest testing equipment, aphrodisiac, penile implant injection and gadget to help the estimated 11 million impotent men seeking help.

Gorm Wagner, at Copenhagen Panum Institute (where they do postmortems unless the family says no) began to work in the 1950s on the gross anatomy of the penis and found that this had not been done for more than a hundred years (8). When I started the Loyola Sex Clinic in 1972, I cheerfully accepted from the Chief of Urology who taught penile anatomy that there were little polster valves in the crurae which closed up when the blood peripherally started an erection, and then after an ejaculation they opened up and blood went back into general circulation. Gorm Wagner found no polster valves in the penis, but thousands, millions probably, of striated smooth muscles which are in constant contraction to keep the penis flaccid. For erection they relax to allow the blood flow to go in, which is how papaverine penile injections are thought to work.

So, that's the stage we are in now in this whole new field of sexual medicine. It is lonely since there are very few M.D.s in the field. It is still one that is considered somewhat suspect and the biology is still in the early process of being studied. I was surprised when I began to look at the changes since I wrote a paper in 1983. In only the last six years, there has been an incredible explosion of penile research. There was skepticism already in 1929 when Thurber wrote a wonderful book, *Is Sex Really Necessary?* about "wasting energy on deep and lugubrious books on sex and marriage and other students of misbehavior who while pursuing sex to the last ditch have gotten it down and are breaking its arm." I hope I don't do that! Occasionally, people will accuse me of making sex mechanical and taking away the mystery and the mystique of it. I don't feel powerful enough to do that. What we try to do is to provide sex education which is essential in treatment. So few of us have had a wholesome sex education at home; if I were to ask those present at the seminar: how many of you think you had a good sex education at home from mom or dad, or both, who sat you down and said, "My child, sex is good; let me tell you about it." How many hands? I cannot raise my own hand. My mother who died two years ago, at age 86, wondered for all of her life where she went wrong that her only daughter talked so much about sex, sex, sex, sex, sex! So, where do we learn? We still learn from other children, much of it inaccurate, and many don't correct it.

Many couples who can talk about almost anything, cannot talk about sex. So, part of what we do is to teach them to dialog about sex. There is a wide difference (which I try to teach teens, children, parents) between the 3-letter word "sex" and the 4-letter word "love" with ingredients of caring, sharing, and commitment. Many couples don't get together because of anger, a barrier to intimacy. We spend much more time teaching bowel control to our children than teaching about their own God-given genitals, thus ignorance prevails. Children discover the genitals completely normally as in a very old line drawing of a masturbating baby with a fever cloth, implying that it is only when sick that the child touches the genitals. Babies discover the penis very early in life and also the clitoris, which is less written about. Orgasm in babies has been reported within the first months of life. If the brain is connected to the spinal cord, babies are able to have an orgasm. Kinsey reported it, there is a wonderful journal article from 1888, where a family physician, Sloan, reports a full orgasm in a little girl, eight months of age, that he personally observed after the mother observed the child kicking her legs, rubbing, rocking, all of which may be masturbation equivalents (7). It shocks us as adults to recognize that there is sexuality in children, still a big taboo.

The myth of the enormous penis is still a problem for many men of any age. I have a six foot millionaire who is double Ph.D.'d who says, "I was cheated in the organ business and I have a small organ," which is inaccurate but an ongoing inhibition. We didn't know until Masters began to do his studies in 1960 and opened up the myth to find that penises differ in the flaccid stages much as do fingers and noses, and the smaller penis will add two to four times in length and volume, whereas the longer penis will only add a little, maybe a half an inch, and so in the erect phase there is less than half an inch difference. This is important to know because men worry, "If my penis were bigger, would she have an orgasm during intercourse?" We now know that coital orgasm only occurs in 20-30% of women because of the tremendous timing difference--a woman's sexual cycle takes 13 minutes, a man's less than 3 minutes, on average with an individual range of difference.

The asymmetry of the testes is normal but eight men thought they were deformed. Why? "Because my testes are unequal." "What do you mean unequal?" "Well, they are not straight." The Lord made form and function closely related, one testis is lower so a man can cross his legs in peace, ride a bicycle, jog. If we don't know, we worry. The sexological exam teaches normal sex structure in sex therapy.

The graph (Fig. 1) from Masters and Johnson shows many of the factors that effect sexual functioning. At baseline, we are talking about sexuality, and this is in the higher cerebral centers in thinking, desire and satisfaction.

In the process of arousal, for both men and women there are general changes in the body: increased temperature, increased breathing rate, increased heart rate, increased blood pressure to a peak for the orgasmic response in both sexes (5). There is tension in all of the muscles, every single muscle in the body, from the toes to the head, little muscles, big muscles, including pubococcygeus muscle, and the uterine musculature, tonic first, then small clonic contractions and complete relaxation after a climax occurs. It is not a grandmal seizure as some women worry, "If I let go I'll have a seizure." It is the closest thing without loss of consciousness. We lose control very briefly, but we don't lose consciousness.

Sexual fantasy is now for the first time being studied in a number of people, although it is extraordinarily difficult; it is the lever which allows arousal to happen in an individual. I tell the patient that fantasy is like turning the ignition key to start a car,

MALE	FEMALE
A - Impotence	E - Female coitus
B - Partial erections	F - Arousal, inhibition, pelvic congestion prolonged resolution
C - Premature ejaculation	G - As F with distraction and loss of arousal
D - Average male coitus	H - Prolonged plateau/resolution/ no climax
E - Sustained male coitus	I - As E with multiple orgasms
X - Point of ejaculatory inevitability	

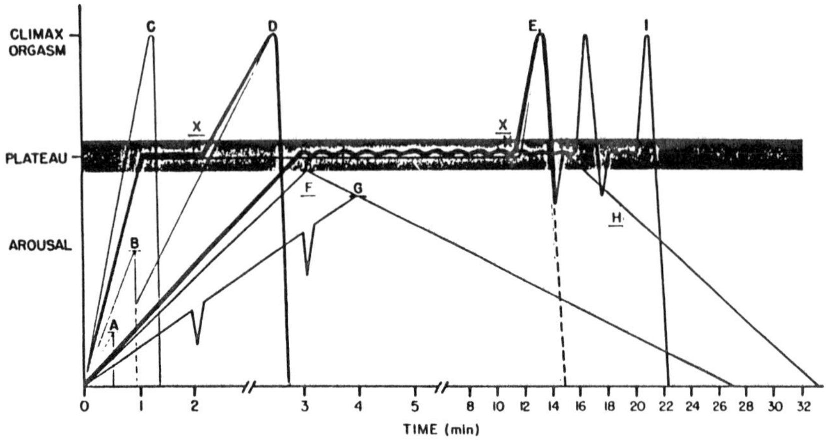

FIGURE 1. COITAL GRAPH

if they have nothing sexual happening in the head, nothing sexual is going to happen in the body. This is very important for individuals who have inhibited sexual desire, now called "DD" in the new DSM-III-R Desire Disorders. We had them when we began the clinic in 1972; they were not listed in Masters and Johnson's book in 1970, I just called them DDs. We treated them with the same technique of relationship therapy and sex education, and it worked.

Our brief sex therapy program at Loyola is once a week for seven weeks. Because we have no space, we are the step-children who use outpatient medicine rooms in the evenings for an intensive 5 hours. We achieve in 35 hours a result that is extraordinary by previous standards of treating impotence and anorgasmia, vaginismus, dyspareunia plus all of the sexual symptoms that bring couples to us in the sexual clinic. Our reversal rate of the symptoms is 80% overall. With unconsummated marriages, full coitus is about 50% at the end of the seven weeks, a further 20% by one year later. We have a 17-year follow-up but we lose touch with many when they move. Couples have lately been open enough to go on national television with me and talk about the sex problems they had, slowly coming out of the darkness. Since the Loyola Sex Clinic began, we have reached a waiting list of 200 couples, without spending one dollar on advertisement, which tells of the number of people who have sexual problems and are waiting for help.

If a man (19-50 years old) has privacy and sexual thoughts, alone or with a sexual partner, he will have these genital changes: first a partial erection and then a full erection, a sustained plateau, then a moment of inevitable reflex ejaculation, detumescence and return to the pre-excitement phase, average timing about 2.8 minutes. This is based on Masters and Johnson studies which were duplicated at Suny in New York, at Maudsley in London, and at Panum in Copenhagen, so Masters' work, criticized as it was at the time in 1966, has stood up to scientific validation. A period of refractoriness follows where no erection is possible. A woman does not have a refractory phase; she can go again and again if she wants to (she may not want to), which is why Masters called women the superior sex as far as sexual expression. A woman, same age group of 19-50, will have first clitoral dilatation which includes throbbing, lubrication of the vagina in the upper two thirds; of which she may not be aware if she is lying supine, she then has a sustained plateau of arousal, she has inevitability of orgasm which occurs at this point even if the phone rings, or the baby cries. She is potentially multi-orgasmic and then returns to the pre-excitement phase. Her average timing by all of these labs is about 13 minutes. So it takes women about four times longer than men. There are women who climax more quickly, and there are men who learn to last longer. It depends on the state of mind and mood. The true physiological payoff is the total body relaxation after the pleasurable climactic high point.

Some men may be so tense and anxious that they ejaculate almost as they begin to erect. At telephone intake we hear: "It is a touch of impotence," which usually means rapid ejaculation because he hardly feels or sees his erection. Therapeutically the squeeze technique then needs to be applied the moment he feels that stirring of an erection, and it works. We have premature ejaculators who don't reach the bed, who don't reach the vagina but ejaculate intracrurally. We treated one such virgin mother who still had her hymen intact because he never penetrated, yet sperm entered. Changes after the age of 50 for the man will be naturally occurring, partial erections, because the connective tissue in the penis is less elastic, and the vascular crural spaces have arteriosclerotic changes. If he knew (which we teach in the presence of the partner) that he needs longer, stronger, direct on the penis foreplay, he could build a better erection--enough for penetration. If he does not know, and sees only the partial erection, he gets upset, loses the erection and she's upset that he is upset. She does the laundry, and they don't get together. Twenty percent of our couples are over the age of 50, and 50% of those are over the age of 60; the oldest we have treated as a couple in the clinic was 86 years old. The older couples usually come because the man is impotent, but the oldest woman who had her first orgasm through Loyola Clinic was 78 years of age. There is hope for everyone and elders do remain interested in sexual functioning.

Our approach is not to do a huge battery of tests. We use sex therapy itself as a diagnostic test. If love play erections are not occurring, we will send the patient for the penile blood flow tests now much improved. They did not exist when we started in 1972. Inaccurately, the then Chief of Urology said that 95% of impotence was psychogenic; now it is said that 50% are organic and 50% are psychogenic. If you include alcohol and chemicals, needed medication and other kinds of drugs that are taken, about 60% are really related to physical causes, and there are those impossible to disentangle who have *both*, somatic with psychogenic overlay. Of all human behaviors, sexual functioning is at the interface of the psyche and the soma. We have healthy young 28 year olds who are impotent. A 31-year old newly married executive on the stock market deals daily in millions of dollars. He is already a millionaire, but he presents with impotence. He jogs (not excessively, which can be a source of fatigue impotence). These young persons are becoming very much a factor in the practice of psychiatry as well as other specialties which tend to dismiss their sexual distress and do not regard it as a legitimate factor in their personal and marital adjustments or maladjustments.

Returning to the physiology of erection, the initial phase of sustained arousal is, we think (confirmed from the sexual side effects of drugs), parasympathetic. The orgasmic phase for both sexes is sympathetic dominance. Study is embryonic in this field of sexual medicine. Certain needed drugs like beta-blockers and antihypertensives are dismissed by some internists as causative of impotence yet they definitely are (5,8). Switch to one of the newer calcium channel blockers and erections return. Certain diuretics such as hydrodiuril may be an immediate cause of potency loss in some men, but not in others. Believe the patient and select another. There are many drug-drug interactions which we do not understand that have negative sexual side-effects. What about for women? A woman on antihypertensives returned her medication to the doctor and said, "these have killed my sex life." He said he was so shocked because he did not realize she had a sex life at 78. A receptionist went on a diet as well as salt reduction and lost 40 pounds to get off her antihypertensives: "It will ruin my marriage if I go on taking this because I am dry, I get no arousal."

Sleep studies, on the scene for the last 20 years, showed REM episode sexual changes, blood pressure changes, heart rate changes, respiratory changes, erections, ejaculation, vaginal lubrication--exactly the same as an orgasmic response with one exception. There was not the tonic-clonic response, but there was the complete muscle relaxation as after a climax. It was found that 80% of REM dreams were sexual in men and women. There were men burned at the stake in the 1600s, for a normal nocturnal ejaculate. If a monk ejaculated in his bed it was believed a harlot of the devil had to have visited him.

Art always precedes science, and this wonderful drawing of baby discovering daddy's sleep erection was done by an anonymous Hungarian artist in Paris about 1832, long before we had invented the EEG machine. Wives discover their "impotent" husband's sleep erection "You lied to me; you are not impotent. I am not going to waste this wonderful erection," she leaps on him; he panics and he loses it--it is not easy to rape a man.

In the penis, there are two lateral crura and the bulbus crura. Papaverine treatment of impotence is by injecting papaverine into the crura. I thought that this would not reach the U.S. because it was invasive and in the U.S., malpractice shapes practice. I was wrong. A full page ad in the Chicago Tribune in January 1987 advertised a papaverine clinic, where men were taught to inject the papaverine (combinations) into the vascular anastomatic tissue of the corpora. Within 20 minutes smooth muscles relax, erection occurs, lasts 20 minutes or more. If it lasts over 4 hours, it becomes an emergency, needing a counter-injection to detumesce the penis and prevent gangrene. It has been in wide use for almost 2 years. Side effects are sexual and physical: one death is reported in the literature from vasovagal shock; one reported delayed erection 8 hours later, 20 miles from his wife. Refrigerated home injections may be abused for papaverine sex parties hoping for "guaranteed" erections. Sclerotic penile tissue may develop and within six months half of the papaverine users are said to need an implanted penile prosthesis (on the market since the 1960s, ranging from $2,000 to $12,000).

In Copenhagen a 19-year old presented: "I'm impotent." The Sex Clinic said: you are young without experience. Go find a prostitute, and it will be fine." He said, "The penis gets wide, but it does not get hard with my girlfriend." He found an experienced prostitute but failed penetration, shot himself, leaving a note: "I can't even get it up with a prostitute." In an autopsy of this young man, researcher Gorm Wagner found a hiatus between the corpora and bulbus crura, a leak. Subsequently, they have with x-ray dye studies found similar penile hiatae, then closed surgically with 50% success rate. This is a whole new research field with vital clinical application where various specialties must collaborate.

New non-invasive Vacuum Erection Devices ($250 to $350) are also now offered as alternative helps. The idea is excellent if the partner is cooperative, if humor is used as they practice. However, conflict may escalate between a couple if now she knows he can attain an assisted erection but he refuses to respond to her overtures.

Post-prostatectomy impotence occurs in a certain percentage regardless of technique or skill. It depends on how the hyperplasia impacts the internal sphincter of the bladder and how it heals whether or not there will be post-prostatectomy retrograde ejaculation into the bladder. Perhaps a synthetic valve now used for incontinence may yet help the post-prostatectomy retrograde ejaculator. One 78-year old who had been impotent 7 years, directly correlated it with the prostatectomy. He had erections and all of subjective and objective signs of an orgasm except the ejaculate went backwards. The couple successfully resumed coitus. He said: "But it feels different now." I replied, "Correct, the warm feeling of an outside ejaculate you will not feel, but you have to get used to feeling the inside one." So the physician can teach patients that the retrograde ejaculate is a real orgasm.

Pituary adenomata can be diagnosed by elevated prolactin levels. Surgical removal or medical treatment (bromocriptin) are possible. If there are no erections after 4 sex therapy visits, then hormone studies are essential.

There are endless men who do not consider morning erections a real erection. "What do you mean?" "It's not a real erection; it is only a urinary erection." "It's very real; the penis is saying "Good morning, head." This question is important for a patient who says, "I'm impotent." "Do you have an erection in the morning?" Some men turn to the wife and say, "Do I?" "You have it at the end of your own body. This week, please look." The penis is visible, therefore, vulnerable. We must teach women how vulnerable men can be when there is not an erection. The penis has three functions: it urinates, procreates, and recreates. For the woman, her analog, the clitoris, is a unique anatomical organ. It is there only for arousal--it has nothing to do with urination or procreation. Because women menstruate, gestate, and lactate, the organs are internal and concealed to protect the growing embryo. So, the woman is taught where her clitoris is during the routine sexological examination. Women are raised to expect a man will "do it to me and give me a climax." No man *gives* a climax. He can facilitate arousal. It's like dying and death. One can help another with dying, but death is a solitary task. Each can be part of arousal but she has to allow the self to attain orgasm. When a woman accepts the responsibility to self-explore for release, it greatly frees a couple to then share and enjoy sexual expression.

Conquering anorgasmia (primary, secondary or situational) has been possible brief sex therapy: sex education, home practice of conjoint loveplay and solo/mutual masturbation. Dyspareunia, vaginismus and desire disorders must have physical causes excluded or treated: such as local infections, intact hymen, atrophic vaginitis requiring hormonal replacement, myxedema etc. Then sex therapy can proceed and reverse the symptoms of many years.

Much progress has been made in the past 50 years to assist patients with the secret pain of the bedroom that too often has had destructive consequences. Sexual health and research must remain the domain of 21st century healers.

REFERENCES

1. Fisher C, Gross J, Zuch J, et al: Cycle of penile erections synchronous with dreaming sleep (REM), Archives of General Psychiatry, Vol 12:29, 1965
2. Karacan I, Williams RL, Thornby JL, et al: Sleep-related penile tumescence as a function of age, American Journal of Psychiatry, 132:932, 1975
3. Kinsey AC, Pomeroy WB, Martin CE: Sexual behavior in the human male, Saunders, Philadelphia, 1948
4. Kinsey AC, et al: Sexual behavior in the human female, Saunders, Philadelphia, 1953
5. Masters W, Johnson V, Kolodny R: Sex and human loving, Little, Brown & Co., Boston, 1986
6. Renshaw DC: Sex talk for a safe child, A.M.A., Box 10946, Chicago, Illinois 60610, 1986 (2nd Edition)
7. Sloan MG: Sexual desire in infancy, JAMA, 10:731-732, 1888
8. Wagner G & Green R: Impotence, Plenum, New York, 1981

chapter 15

Psychiatry And AIDS

Stuart E. Nichols, Jr., M.D.

In AIDS, organic and functional psychiatric symptoms are frequently interwoven and call for a careful differential diagnosis. Since psychiatrists are trained both in medicine and psychology, their expertise is often needed for optimal clinical care. HIV infection, therefore, offers psychiatry the opportunity to gain respect as a medical speciality, but unless it mounts a vigorous response to the epidemic it may lose professional esteem.

Psychiatry's role, however, should not be exclusively biologic in orientation. To treat HIV-infected patients successfully, psychiatrists must understand the science of brain function and also be compassionate psychotherapists. They should be distinguished from other physicians, in part, by their focus on how the HIV virus is locked in battle with the human spirit. Paul Adams, a renowned child psychiatrist, has eloquently stated what makes us unique: instead of collecting a list of symptoms from patients, we ask them to tell us the story of their illness (1). We must remain aware of what having AIDS means to our patients and their loved ones.

AIDS is a national health emergency: the United States Public Health Service has projected that there will be 323,000 cumulative cases in the United States by the end of 1991, and perhaps 10 times that number will be infected with the Human Immunodeficiency Virus (2). The Surgeon General has predicted that we will not have an effective vaccine until the next century. Psychiatrists, especially those working to change addictive behaviors, should assist in devising prevention strategies, yet few addiction specialists are currently involved. Psychiatric expertise is sorely needed in the national prevention effort.

There is, however, a problem in our conceptualization of the epidemic. Few people grasp the reality of HIV infection. The oft-repeated CDC statistics dominate our concepts, yet they represent only

Psychiatry: Past Reflections–Future Visions
B.T. Taylor and I.J. Taylor, Editors

full-blown AIDS cases and not new viral infections. The CDC data cause us to envision the epidemic as it was several years ago, when it was much smaller in size and distribution.

Although the antibody test was licensed in 1985, HIV seropositivity has been assayed only within special groups (drug addicts, prison inmates, and army recruits, for example), clearly not representative of the general population. The CDC only recently has begun determining the incidence of HIV infection in other groups, despite the fact that surveys for the antibody throughout the population are needed if we are to have an up-to-date picture of the epidemic. These surveys should be anonymous so that the persons tested are not self-selected. Repeated surveys could tell us where the new cases of infection are occurring most frequently.

Indeed, the planning of effective prevention services requires data which show where new cases are occurring, permitting us to know where education and counseling are most needed. When epidemiologic surveys indicate that the virus is invading a new area (e.g. high school seniors in a particular city), we could then mount a vigorous prevention campaign of personal and immediate importance to the targeted population.

Of course, large scale testing is expensive. The lack of data on new cases, however, reenforces denial and prevents us from even recognizing the pressing need for anonymous surveys. This pennywise, shortsighted approach allows us to continue underestimating the extent of the epidemic.

The HIV antibody test itself continues to cause confusion. The test can be used in several ways, some of which it performs well, others not so well, and we need to understand the limitations of its usefulness.

HIV testing was originally developed to protect the nation's blood supply, and it does this quite well, although virus-contaminated transfusions do occur, albeit rarely, even today. As mentioned above, the test can also be used anonymously in epidemiologic surveys, and in this regard it is also quite helpful. Clinical use of the procedure, however, is more problematic because of rare false negative and false positive results, and the emotional turmoil testing may produce. Finally, the test may be used as an adjunct in the attempt to change risk behavior. This area of use may be compromised by faulty reasoning, e.g. the concept that merely knowing the results of the test will, by itself, enable an individual to change sexual or drug practices. This last use of antibody testing needs further scientific study.

The most important goal in prevention lies in making sure that uninfected individuals remain uninfected. To meet this goal we must eliminate the widespread belief that physical appearance and social background can identify individuals infected with the virus. We must instead view everyone as a potential transmitter of the virus. We must not think of people as being "safe" because they "look OK." We must not think of "good" and "bad" drugs. To stop thinking of people in stereotypes, however, we must examine the assumptions we harbor about human behavior and confront deeply engrained attitudes. We also need straight talk about sex and drugs. Drug abuse is easier to prevent than cure. We need to learn a lot more about the drug-taking practices and the sexual lifestyles of our society. Sex must be discussed openly long before children become sexually active. Safer sex must become the standard for everybody and condoms readily available to everyone.

As public policies are proposed to contain this viral attack, psychiatrists should also participate in thinking through their ramifications. Many proposals are initiated by a sense of desperation and are likely to be counterproductive if enacted. Alan Brandt in *No Magic Bullet* pointed out how often emotion has interfered with the fight against sexually transmitted diseases (3). With AIDS, calls for quarantine and other measures which attempt to stop seropositive individuals from infecting "innocent victims" pose several problems. Even if one is willing to assume that government is capable of stopping dangerous behavior, what would it cost in terms of civil liberties and loss of the vitally needed cooperation of infected individuals? Such policies also focus attention on people rather than behavior and, in so doing, may promote the dangerous assumption that people can tell who is infected.

In analyzing proposed AIDS policies psychiatrists should maintain a professional stance, distant from the emotion of the times. This is difficult for we too get caught up in the general reaction to AIDS. Nevertheless, the cool analytic assessment of HIV policy is especially needed since this epidemic involves taboo and prejudice in such a major way.

Our present prevention strategy seems to rely on pouring money into the vaccine race while paying lip service to AIDS education and counseling. Why? Could it be that AIDS patients are viewed as being uneducable, or inferior and expendable? Are we gambling that there will be an effective vaccine before large numbers of white, middle-class individuals are infected? This shocking point of view would also explain, in part, why we continue to underestimate the epidemic. Because we conceptualize the disease as infecting persons of low status, we are not eager to spend scarce resources on the expensive effort to change behavior through education.

If, however, we are serious about AIDS prevention, the education needed must extend far beyond mere cognitive learning. It must attempt to change attitudes and teach people practical skills regarding the assessment of safety and the ability to "just say no" to dangerous sexual and drug-related behaviors.

In 1986, nine psychiatric institutions were funded by the National Institute for Mental Health (NIMH) to develop innovative approaches to AIDS education. These programs have been found to be effective, especially in the difficult area of attitude modification. Recently, however, NIMH decided to fund future AIDS prevention programs only in HRSA (Human Resource Services Administration) Centers which have ignored affective learning, minimized psychosocial issues, and emphasized traditional, cognitive-oriented education. AIDS education is being weakened by this new policy, and years of expertise may be lost. Integration of affective learning into the HRSA Centers might be better accomplished by funding psychiatric educators with the stipulation that they affiliate with the medical-model centers. Why has NIMH instituted this policy? Does it believe that psychiatry should play an important role in the epidemic? Does it believe its own assessments which indicate the type of education that is needed?

Another important question to be considered is whether our national response to AIDS is planned, or is it uncoordinated and haphazard? President Reagan clearly tried to avoid getting involved with AIDS; the illness of his friend, Rock Hudson, finally moved him to action. Except for the efforts of Surgeon General Koop and Admiral Watkins we would be much less prepared for the battle against AIDS today.

Perhaps the government is able, even now, to deny the full impact of AIDS. Maybe there is no master plan to attempt to contain this global catastrophe. Does AIDS have the potential to destroy our health care system as we know it, to dominate our economy and threaten our civil liberties? To my mind all this and more is possible, and we should be mobilizing a much greater response to oppose its destructive potential. Are my comments inflammatory and counterproductive? My view of the epidemic may be alarming, but it is reality as I experience it, and if it arouses emotion, I see it as the price paid for dislodging denial. But then, I've suffered the loss of too many friends to AIDS, including twenty-some colleagues, and my point of view is hopelessly biased.

To be sure, society has shown little interest in treating the disease among drug users, although they are spreading the epidemic fastest among heterosexuals. We have not been nearly innovative enough in educating the families of addicts about transmission prevention, and health care for addicts and their families remains as inadequate and fragmented as before AIDS. Where are the treatment programs, or the skilled nursing facilities, or even housing for HIV-infected patients? As the epidemic moves beyond the gay community, we are not likely to have the services of so many unpaid volunteers to assist us, and we have come to count upon them for compassionate care and health cost containment.

Although we may minimize the size of the epidemic, we often exaggerate its deadliness. The statement that AIDS is "uniformly fatal" is frequently heard. AIDS, to be sure, is a terrible illness, but not all of its victims have died, and there are individuals who have lived with full-blown AIDS for more than seven years and are in reasonably good health. Moreover, there are asymptomatic individuals who have been infected with the virus for as long as twelve years. In fact, we now estimate the latency period between infection and illness as averaging between 5 and 10 years, and this figure climbs higher with each added year of observation. Unfortunately, conceptualizing HIV patients as persons who are dying permits us to be less vigorous in our treatment of them, conserving scarce resources for the living.

Psychiatry has several specific roles it should play regarding HIV infection, and I would like to begin with an obvious one: behavior change.

Research is urgently needed to show how we can best facilitate the changes in behavior that will prevent further spread of the virus. Existing AIDS prevention programs usually offer counseling in conjunction with the HIV antibody test. However, the training and experience of the counselor and the type of intervention that will produce the desired behavior change remain unknown. What is the role of psychotherapy as contrasted with counseling? For which patients is it needed? How should peer groups be utilized? How often and for what period of time should an intervention be reenforced to maintain changed behavior?

AIDS also gives us an opportunity to re-evaluate psychotherapy and integrate it into the modern practice of technological psychiatry, combining our concern for the mind with our understanding of the brain. Psychiatrists who are biologically oriented, however, may think little of psychotherapy because it is "unscientific." They may need to be more sensitive to the emotional sequelae of the infection and to understand how fear of the virus may lead to additional distress for persons infected or affected by the virus. Psychotherapists, in turn, need to keep abreast of neuroscience and understand how the virus affects the brain, both directly and indirectly. All psychiatrists need to think about the role that prejudice plays in a society, about why humanity needs scapegoats, and whether our profession has a responsibility to enlighten the world about this persistent, contemptible aspect of human behavior.

Additionally, we all need to know more about the elusive interconnections between the mind, body, and spirit, teasing out practical scientific data from the field of psychoneuroimmunology so that it does not become cultish as have some schools of psychoanalysis. We understand quite a bit about the body, less about the mind, but little concerning the role of the human spirit in health and disease. AIDS presents to us an old fashioned opportunity to see the human spirit responding to attack. If we look we can observe how love, respect, companionship, dignity, hope and other attributes of the human spirit are as necessary for health as food, clothing and shelter. It is in this pursuit that we must allow our patients to tell us their stories, reflecting on what AIDS has done to them, but also what they have done with it. We should listen carefully and sympathetically. In this fashion we may eventually be able to prove that a robust spirit is essential for human health, making it the proper concern of physicians and psychiatrists.

Research must show how valid and important psychologic support is to AIDS patients. Even though it may appear to be no more than kindness and a sympathetic ear, it can lessen substantially the effects of the disease.

Yet manpower remains a serious issue. Why have so few psychiatrists gotten involved with HIV infection? Consultation and liaison psychiatrists may have to deal with hospitalized patients, but other psychiatrists have shown a reluctance to work with the disease.

Most of the psychiatrists who have dealt extensively with AIDS have been drawn to the illness because they are personally involved with it. Many of them are themselves gay or bisexual. There are many gay men and women in psychiatry and the great majority of them still feel the need to hide their sexual orientation. In many institutions it is made clear that not just discretion but dishonesty is the price homosexuals must pay for privileges or advancement. What does this say about a profession that counsels patients to face reality? Our attitude toward gay colleagues shows that we set different standards for ourselves. Can deception and dishonesty ever be seen as ethical, accepted practice?

With AIDS we may be experiencing an important battle in the war for therapeutic turf. There are psychologists, social workers, psychiatric nurses and others who are eager to take over the practice of psychotherapy. Unless we integrate our psychologic and biologic interests we may appear to our colleagues as being undertrained in either neurology or psychology. We must set professional standards and hold ourselves to meet documentable outcomes. We must ourselves be clear of our role as a medical specialist and value and respect it. If we do not accomplish these goals we are very likely to lose ground to the other professions fighting for our turf.

If psychiatry is to meet the many challenges of the HIV pandemic, it must broaden its service to both patients and the community. With patients we must become active members of the clinical care team and offer understanding and compassion to them and their loved ones. At times we must be willing to abandon the practice of maintaining professional distance and advocate for fair treatment for patients discriminated against. We must find psychiatrists who are able to help local and national community leaders to better understand human behavior so that our counterattack to this invasion becomes more rational and effective.

REFERENCES

1. Paul Adams, Professor of Child Psychiatry Emeritus, University of Texas, Galveston, personal communication
2. Centers for Disease Control MMWRS Supplement: AIDS and Human Immunodeficiency Virus Infection in the United States: 1988 Update, 5/12/89
3. Alan Brandt, No Magic Bullet: A social history of venereal disease in the United States since 1880. New York-Oxford University Press, 1987